Cancer
Biology and
Management:
An
Introduction

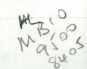

Cancer Biology and Management: An Introduction

C. J. WILLIAMS

CRC Medical Oncology Unit
Southampton General Hospital
Southampton
UK

With contributions by
N. R. DENNIS, D. R. GARROD
R. HILLIER, J. HUGHES
A. D. RAMSAY and **J. SWEETENHAM**

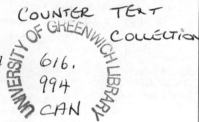
JOHN WILEY & SONS
Chichester · New York · Brisbane · Toronto · Singapore

Other Wiley Editorial Offices

John Wiley & Sons, Inc., 605 Third Avenue,
New York, NY 10158-0012, USA

Jacaranda Wiley Ltd, G.P.O. Box 859, Brisbane,
Queensland 4001, Australia

John Wiley & Sons (Canada) Ltd, 22 Worcester Road,
Rexdale, Ontario M9W 1L1, Canada

John Wiley & Sons (SEA) Pte Ltd, 37 Jalan Pemimpin #05–04,
Block B, Union Industrial Building, Singapore 2057

Library of Congress Cataloging-in-Publication Data:
Cancer biology and management: an introduction/edited by C. J.
Williams.
    p.   cm.
    Includes bibliographical references.
    ISBN 0-471-91781-8 (pbk.)
    1. Oncology. 2. Cancer. I. Williams, C. J. (Christopher John
Hacon)
    [DNLM: 1. Neoplasms.   QZ 200 C2151108]
RC261.I577 1990
616.99′2—dc20
DNLM/DLC   89–16653
for Library of Congress   CIP

British Library Cataloguing in Publication Data:
Cancer biology and management: an introduction
    1. Man. Cancer. Therapy
    I. Williams, C. J.
    616.99′406

    ISBN 0-471-91781-8

Typeset by Photo·Graphics, Honiton, Devon, England
Printed in Great Britain by Courier International Ltd., Tiptree, Colchester.

Contents

Contributors

N. R. DENNIS   Department of Child Health, Southampton General Hospital, Southampton, UK

D. R. GARROD   CRC Medical Oncology Unit, Southampton General Hospital, Southampton, UK

R. HILLER   Countess Mountbatten House, Southampton, UK

J. HUGHES   Department of Psychiatry, University of Southampton, Southampton, UK

A. D. RAMSAY   Department of Histopathology, Southampton General Hospital, Southampton, UK

J. SWEETENHAM   CRC Medical Oncology Unit, Southampton General Hospital, Southampton, UK

C. J. WILLIAMS   CRC Medical Oncology Unit, Southampton General Hospital, Southampton, UK

Preface

Given that cancer is the second leading cause of death in the western world, it is perhaps surprising that very few medical schools have an integrated undergraduate teaching course on the subject. This situation has arisen partly because medicine is often taught in system-based courses. Because cancer can affect any part of body, the result has been fragmentation of teaching so that only rarely is a student presented with an integrated approach which brings together epidemiology and genetics, biology, pathology and a global discussion of all aspects of management.

This failure to integrate teaching is especially disappointing since there have been exciting changes in our understanding of the biology of malignant disease. At the same time there have been steady, but very real, improvements in our ability to control cancer and to cure patients.

This book is intended primarily for medical students, but I hope that it will also prove useful to the newly qualified doctor and those looking for a refresher course. The first part of the book lays the foundations necessary for management. Up-to-date thinking about current concepts in cancer biology and genetics is deliberately emphasised, since the management of malignancy in the next decade or two may be based on modern biological principles. The rest of the first part concentrates on broad principles and details of management referable to different types of cancers. The second part of the book reviews, briefly but systematically, the epidemiology, presentation, investigation and management of the common individual malignant tumours.

Emphasis has been placed on practical management problems and detailed discussion of specific treatments has been avoided. These are matters that are genuinely postgraduate and their discussion is made less useful by the rapid pace of change of current therapies. The importance of quality of life and symptom control is stressed as it is all too easy to concentrate on the illness and forget the patient. In recent years there have been major changes in approaches to patients with malignancy and cancer medicine is leading the way in this; the attitude that we are caring for people and not just treating disease applies equally to all branches of medicine.

The reason for dividing the book into two halves is to encourage the student to read most of the first part, excluding the chapters on paraneoplastic syndromes and cancer emergencies, as a whole and to use part two and the remaining chapters as a reference source when a patient with a particular cancer or problem is seen. In this way, hopefully, the student will have access to integrated information when they are helping care for a patient who has the tumour they are studying. Some information, for example staging systems, is postgraduate in nature but is included in the book for reference in individual cases and because an understanding of the basic framework is useful.

PART
1

Principles of cancer biology and care

INTRODUCTION TO PART 1

The overall aim of this book is to provide an introduction to the practical care of the cancer patient. However, in order to make the best use of clinical information there is a need for a firm understanding of the principles underlying management. The first part of the book, which is wide ranging in its scope, endeavours to provide a rational framework upon which to base the management of individual tumours, which are discussed in Part 2.

The increasing importance of genetics in our understanding of the development of cancer is highlighted by the overlap of information in Chapter 1 (genetics) and Chapter 2 on current thinking about the biology of cancer. Our understanding of these subjects is growing rapidly and *may* lead to new ways of treating cancer. The interaction between genetics, carcinogenesis and epidemiology is evident in Chapter 3, which discusses patterns of cancer around the world and current knowledge of the causes of malignancy.

Remaining chapters in this section are rather more practical in nature, being concerned with the natural history and pathology of cancer as well as the principles underlying the main modalities of treatment (surgery, radiotherapy, chemotherapy). Medical syndromes and emergencies associated with cancer are given considerable space because of the multiple situations which need to be included, even if only briefly. The final chapters in this part of the book cover the very important areas of psychosocial aspects of malignancy and control of symptoms. These have been too long neglected, though they are now starting to receive the attention they deserve since the majority of patients with advanced cancer still die of their disease.

1 | Genetics of Cancer

N. R. DENNIS

What are the essential characteristics of cancer cells and how are they acquired? In particular, are they intrinsic characteristics of the cell or do they represent a response of cells to a change in their environment? If cancer represents an intrinsic property which is transmitted to daughter cells, it must involve the cell's genetic mechanisms. This chapter starts by examining the evidence for genetic involvement, and in particular, for the importance of changes in DNA. Next, familial cancers are looked at. They are rather rare, but their study has led to discoveries of general importance for the more common sporadic cancers. Evidence that mutations cause cancer are summarized below. This chapter considers these data further.

- most carcinogens are mutagens
- susceptibility of some carcinogens is dependent on the ability of enzymes to convert it to a mutagenic form
- defects of DNA repair increase the probability of cancer
- chromosomal instability is seen in many types of cancer
- some cancers are inherited
- malignant tumours are clonal
- some tumours contain mutated oncogenes

There have been major changes in the understanding of the role of genetics in cancer during the past ten years. The identification of cancer-causing genes as normal components of the genotype (until they undergo various changes) is recent. Once these genes (cellular oncogenes) were identified, it became possible to ask two questions, questions that are still being answered. The first is 'by what mechanisms are oncogenes altered in order to contribute to malignant transformation?' The second is 'what are the normal functions of oncogene products, and what is the relationship between these products and the malignant state?' As is often the case in genetics, the identification of an aberrant function has led to important discoveries about normal function, for it is clear that oncogenes have an important role in the control of growth and differentiation. An understanding of cancer genetics can be gained by discussing some basic points.

Are Cancer Cells Clonal?

Most cancers do not show a strong tendency to run in the family. But at the cellular level it has seemed likely for many years that malignant behaviour is passed on from cancer cells to their descendants. Visible chromosome changes arise in cancer cells, and are transmitted to daughter cells, although the number of abnormalities often increases with successive divisions. Much of our thinking about cancer as uncontrolled cell division assumes that a cancer is a clone—a group of cells all descended from a single precursor cell. The morbid anatomy of cancer also suggests this; it often appears to have a unifocal origin.

A good way of demonstrating that a group of cells is a clone is to show genetic identity for a marker for which the tissue of origin was variable. Human tissues do not vary from cell to cell for most of their genes, but for genes on the X chromosome, female cells express either the maternal or the paternal X. For those genes for which she received different alleles from her two parents, a woman is a mosaic. If a genetic difference that can be observed in individual cells is chosen, it becomes easy to type a cancer and find out whether all the malignant cells express a single X-linked allele, where the tissue of origin demonstrably has both (see Figure 1). This has been done for several benign and malignant tumours, most notably by using as a marker *glucose 6-phosphate dehydrogenase*, for which many African and Afro-American women are heterozygous. In almost all cases both benign and malignant tumours show a clonal pattern; neurofibromas in neurofibromatosis being an exception. Similar observations can be made in myelomas and some lymphomas, which arise from a population of B-lymphocytes, each dedicated to the production of a single antibody. The plasma cells and lymphocytes all produce the same antibody.

The Relationship Between DNA and Malignant Behaviour

Before the recent studies of specific chromosomal and gene changes in cancer, two groups of observations strongly suggested the importance of DNA modification.

- First, most recognized carcinogens are also mutagens. Known environmental carcinogens, such as ionizing radiation and various chemicals like vinyl chloride, N-nitroso compounds and polycyclic aromatic hydrocarbons, are known to modify DNA to produce mutations of various types.
- Secondly, DNA repair disorders carry a high risk of cancer. They are a group of rare autosomal recessive disorders. Each has its own pattern of clinical features and cancer susceptibility (see Table 1). In some, the defect in DNA repair can be pinpointed. In others, the defect has not been

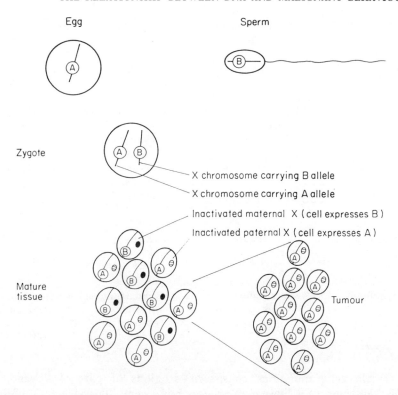

Figure 1. Diagram showing the use of X chromosome inactivation to demonstrate the clonal origin of a tumour. In each cell in the tissue of origin, either the maternal or the paternal X is active, and this remains fixed in the daughter cells when a cell divides. If a polymorphic X chromosome marker which has a cellular phenotype is chosen, heterozygous females can be studied, and their cells can be typed to show whether the maternal or the paternal X is active. (N.B. the difference in appearance between the maternal and paternal X in the diagram is just for illustrative purposes)

localized, but DNA instability is manifest in the form of increased chromosome breakage or sister chromosome exchange (Figure 2). These conditions have focused attention on the normal mechanisms of DNA repair, and suggest that DNA damage is a continual process which is usually corrected. They also provide powerful evidence that mutations are involved in the development of cancer.

The Nature of Mutation

Mutations—changes in the genetic material—are conventionally subdivided into those occurring at the single gene level and those producing visible chromosome alterations. The most localized type is a point mutation—a single base substitution. At the other extreme are alterations in chromosome number.

Table 1. Conditions showing DNA instability and an increased risk of cancer. All are inherited as autosomal recessives

Condition	Main clinical features	DNA repair defect	Main cancer susceptibility
Xeroderma pigmentosum	Light-induced skin damage	Defective excision repair of UV damage	Skin cancers (various types)
Ataxia telangiectasia	Ataxia, telangiectases	Spontaneous chromosome breaks, increased susceptibility to X-ray damage	Lymphomas, leukaemias, carcinomas
Fanconi pancytopenia	Short stature, skeletal anomalies, pancytopenia	Increased chromosome breaks and gaps	Leukaemia
Bloom's syndrome	Short stature, photosensitive skin rash	Increased numbers of sister chromatid exchanges	Lymphomas, leukaemias, carcinomas (very varied)

Many single gene mutations consist of deletions of part of a gene, or, less commonly, insertion of a DNA sequence within a gene. The structural chromosome abnormalities, such as translocations, deletions and inversions, also require DNA breakage, and may result from the same underlying mechanisms as many single gene mutations. The dividing line between gene and chromosomal deletions and insertions is an arbitrary one, as there must be a continuum.

All types of mutation have been found to contribute to the aetiology of cancer, although numerical chromosome abnormalities are less commonly involved than the others. Since 1980, some of the genes involved in these mutations have been identified, and the ways in which they are altered and the effect of these alterations on the behaviour of the cell are beginning to be understood.

Cancer as a Consequence of Cellular Evolution

Mitosis seems designed to equip all body cells with the same genotype. There is, however, a built-in error rate. Changes in the DNA of body cells are known as somatic mutations. Because of the properties of DNA, as long as they do not kill the cell, they are inherited by daughter cells. If a somatic mutation arises in a dividing tissue, a clone of genetically distinct cells will be produced, and there will be mosaicism—the presence in an individual of at least two genetically distinct cell populations, both of which arose from a common ancestral cell.

A mutation which arises in the egg or sperm is known as a germ line mutation, and will normally be present in all the body cells, including the gonads, so that it may be passed on to the next generation. A somatic mutation may or may not involve the gonads.

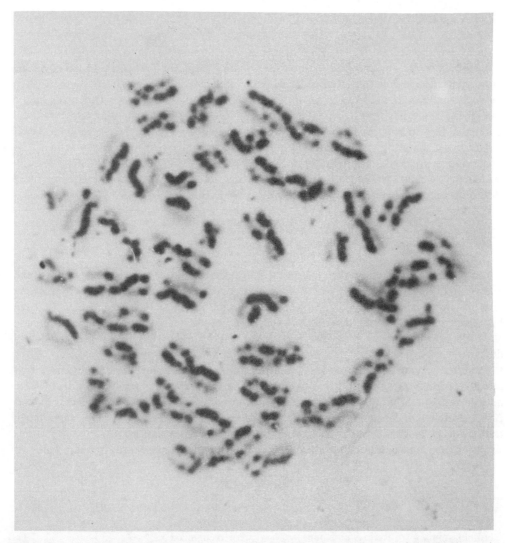

Figure 2. Increased sister chromatid exchange in Bloom's syndrome, one of the DNA repair disorders with an increased risk of cancer. The 'harlequin' appearance is produced by BrDU (bromodeoxyuridine) staining which is initially incorporated in one of the two DNA strands in each chromatid. After a further cell division and DNA replication with the cell not exposed to BrDU, BrDU is present in one of the two chromatids making up each chromosome. Sister chromatid exchanges do occur in normal mitoses, but in far smaller numbers. Reproduced by permission of Wessex Regional Cytogenetics Unit, Salisbury, UK

Most mutations are likely to impair the survival of dividing cells; the resulting new clones will die out. In cancer, we are concerned with those mutations which lead to uncontrolled division. A dividing tissue has the ingredients for Darwinian evolution: genetic variability leading to differential survival. The problem is that it is not in the organism's best interests to generate the 'fittest' cells, but that given time and the dynamics of the situation, cells with an enhanced division rate will inevitably be selected.

Stages in the Development of Cancer

It has been thought for many years that the development of most cancers takes place in several stages. The timing of cancer induction by carcinogens often involves a long latent period. During the latent period, premalignant changes in the tissue can often be recognized, and these also occur in some apparently spontaneous cancers. Once a malignant clone has arisen, it often continues to evolve, acquiring new chromosomal abnormalities and increasingly invasive characteristics.

Now that some of the genetic features of carcinogenesis have been identified, the observations are consistent with a multi-stage process. A single mutation is not generally sufficient to cause a cancer, and in a growing number of examples, two or more different genetic changes in cancers have been identified.

Familial Cancers

Although most cancers do not run strongly in families, there are a few special exceptions. Retinoblastoma, a childhood tumour of the retina, is inherited in some families as an autosomal dominant. In these families, affected people usually have bilateral tumours, although sometimes they can be unilaterally affected or even escape altogether, when the condition may skip a generation. Most retinoblastomas, however, do not occur in such families; they are sporadic and unilateral (see below).

Familial polyposis of the colon is another autosomal dominant condition, in which affected people develop multiple polyps of the large bowel (usually hundreds). By middle age, one or more polyps will almost always have developed a focus of carcinoma. Apart from their numbers, the polyps and carcinomas resemble those seen fairly frequently as isolated, non-familial conditions in older people.

Other inherited conditions with a high risk of specific cancers are listed in Table 2.

Table 2. Some autosomal dominant conditions with a high risk of cancer of specific sites

Condition	Site of cancer	Precancerous condition	Risk of cancer
Retinoblastoma	Retina (and bone)	Not recognized	80–90%
Familial polyposis	Colon and rectum	Polyps	Close to 100% by middle age
Multiple endocrine neoplasia type II	Thyroid (medullary carcinoma), adrenal (phaeochromocytoma)	Thyroid C cell hyperplasia	50% by age 50
Basal cell naevus syndrome	Skin, occasionally CNS	Not recognized (developmental abnormalities of bone also occur)	Around 50% (not usually metastasizing)
von Hippel-Lindau syndrome	Kidney	?Renal cysts (various non-metastasizing haemangiomatous tumours also occur)	Possibly 30% by middle age

Table 3. Nomenclature for describing chromosomal abnormalities

Description	Meaning
−7	Loss of one chromosome 7
+7	Gain of one extra chromosome 7
2q− or del2q	Deletion of part of long arm of chromosome 2
6p+	Addition of material to short arm of chromosome 6
t(9; 22) (q34; q11)	Reciprocal translocation between chromosome 9 and 22 with break points at q34 on chromosome 9 and q11 on chromosome 22
i(8p)	Isochromosome with both arms derived from the short arm of chromosome 8
inv(16) (p13q22)	Part of chromosome between p13 and q22 is inverted

Subsequent sections discuss some of the chromosomal abnormalities associated with cancer. Table 3 summarizes some of the nomenclature used to describe chromosome abnormalities.

The Two Hit Hypothesis

In the 1970s, Knudson put forward a genetic hypothesis to explain these familial cancers with autosomal dominant inheritance of a high and specific risk. In what became known as the two hit hypothesis he suggested that two separate genetic changes were required for tumour development (Figure 3). (The total number of changes

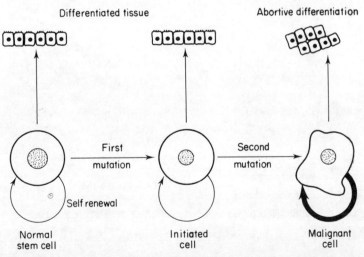

Figure 3. The two hit hypothesis. In this model the normal stem cells and initiated cells have similar properties, both differentiating normally and undergoing normal self renewal. Following a second mutation self renewal becomes greatly increased and differentiation becomes grossly abnormal

necessary could be more than two without materially affecting the hypothesis.) People who inherited the first change, assumed to be a gene mutation, from a parent, would only require the subsequent stage(s) to occur in the target tissue: their tissues would, therefore, be 'primed', and this explains the earlier onset and multiple nature of the familial tumours. In the isolated cases, all the necessary changes would have to occur after the zygote, as somatic mutations; because of this the chances of multiple foci would be far lower. See Figure 4 for a diagrammatic explanation. In genetic terms, one germ line and one or more somatic mutations are contrasted with two or more somatic mutations.

The later mutation(s) need not affect the same gene as the first, but in 1983 this was found to be the case for retinoblastoma and Knudson's hypothesis was confirmed. It was shown that many retinoblastomas carried chromosome rearrangements within the tumour tissue which resulted in only one of the two parental chromosome 13q14 segments being present (see Figure 5). 13q14 was already known to be the site of the retinoblastoma gene (see Figure 6 for a summary of the evidence).

In this case it seems that the first of the two necessary genetic changes is a mutation which can be transmitted as a dominant, but that a second change, to remove the paired normal allele on the other chromosome, is needed before it can be expressed. This second change may involve the whole or a large part of chromosome 13.

The nature of the first mutation varies. In dominant retinoblastoma families it is generally confined to the retinoblastoma gene. In the (usually) sporadic cases of retinoblastoma with other congenital abnormalities and mental retardation, it consists of a chromosomal deletion spanning many genes.

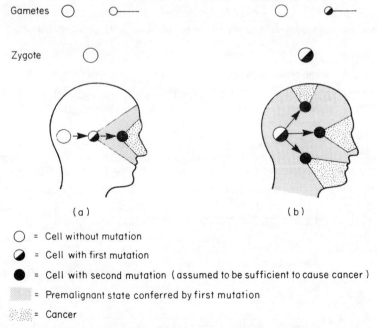

O   = Cell without mutation
◐   = Cell with first mutation
●   = Cell with second mutation (assumed to be sufficient to cause cancer)
▒   = Premalignant state conferred by first mutation
░   = Cancer

Figure 4. The two hit hypothesis. In (a) two somatic mutations produce a cancer. In (b) the first mutation is present in a germ cell and the second mutation has occurred more than once in the already primed tissues

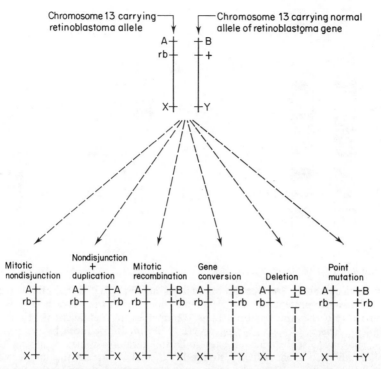

Figure 5. Mechanisms by which a heterozygote for the retinoblastoma gene may lose the paired normal allele to develop a homozygous or hemizygous cell line. rb is the retinoblastoma allele, + is the normal allele. A/B and X/Y are two different genetic marker loci on chromosome 13 for which this person is heterozygous. Adapted from Cavenee *et al.* (1983) Nature, **305**, 779. © 1983 Macmillan Magazines Ltd. Reprinted by permission

The same mechanism seems to operate in Wilms' tumour (nephroblastoma), a childhood kidney cancer, where a gene on the short arm of chromosome 11 must first be altered or deleted and then its normal partner lost. Inherited cases of this tumour, where the first mutation has been transmitted from an affected parent, are rarer than for retinoblastoma, as the prognosis until recently has been poorer.

In carcinoma of the colon, the tumours have been shown to have lost genes on the long arm of chromosome 5, and, in other cases, on the short arm of chromosome 17. It seems likely that the familial polyposis gene represents a mutation of the chromosome 5 gene, since family linkage studies show that it maps to this region.

Although Knudson's hypothesis was built around a rare cancer, it has led to the development of methods which are applicable in common cancers. Several of the 'second hit' mechanisms which remove the paired normal allele affect a whole chromosome or a chromosomal region. Any genes in this region for which the individual is heterozygous will become homozygous or hemizygous in the tumour (Figure 5). Thus, the discovery of loss of heterozygosity for a gene or DNA marker in tumour tissue as compared with normal tissue from the same person suggests that a gene on the same chromosome is involved in tumour genesis. This approach has drawn attention to specific chromosome regions in meningioma and breast, lung and colon cancer.

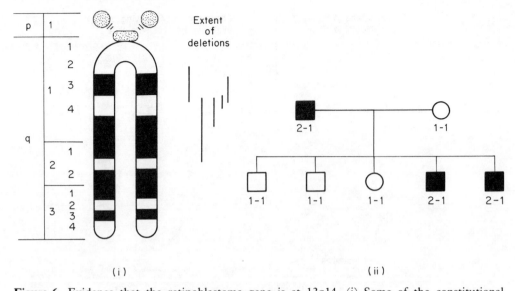

(i)   (ii)

Figure 6. Evidence that the retinoblastoma gene is at 13q14. (i) Some of the constitutional chromosome deletions (present in all the patients' body cells) that have been associated with retinoblastoma. Note that the band 13q14 is common to all the deletions. From Vogel and Motulsky (1986). *Human Genetics*, Springer-Verlag, Berlin. Reproduced by permission.
(ii) Pedigree showing cosegregation of esterase-D and retinoblastoma. Note that the affected offspring have inherited their father's esterase-D '2' allele, whereas the unaffected offspring have inherited his '1' allele. If the two genes were segregating independently, the odds against observing this by chance would be 1 in 16. With the addition of similar pedigrees, the odds of the observed cosegregation arising by chance become less than 1 in 1000. Esterase-D is known to be at 13q14. From Sparks, R.S. *et al.* (1983). *Science*, **219**: 971. © 1983 by the AAAS. Reproduced by permission

Very recently several groups have observed in sporadic cases of heritable tumours that the mutation was carried on the paternal gene rather than as expected on either maternal or paternal genes. It appears from these new findings that in most sporadic cases of both Wilms' tumour and osteosarcoma it is the paternal chromosome that is retained in the tumour, the maternal one being lost (see Figure 7).

Cancer Family Syndromes

In some families, clusters of cancer occur, but predisposition is less specific than in the conditions mentioned above, covering various sites of origin. The usual ones are all relatively common in the general population, such as breast, stomach, large bowel, uterus and ovary, so it is to be expected that familial clustering will occur by chance. But it is generally accepted that these 'cancer family syndromes' (there may be more than one type) occur more often than a chance event. In addition, multiple primary tumours and unusually young onset are often seen in these families. Table 4 summarizes the features of this syndrome and Figure 8 shows a typical pedigree.

Germ line transmission of a susceptibility gene which is directly involved in malignant transformation could be occurring in these families as in inherited retinoblastoma. The

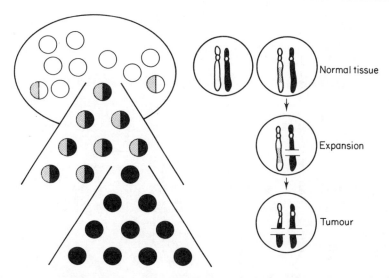

Figure 7. Loss of maternal alleles in tumours. Most cells in the target tissue have maternal (open) and paternal (filled) chromosomes, both of which express either the retinoblastoma gene or the Wilms' gene. On some maternal chromosomes, however, these genes are repressed by methylation imprinting (stippled area). If the first mutation happens to be on a paternal chromosome opposite the relatively inactive maternal allele, this population of cells will expand. This expansion will neither occur with the first hit on a paternal chromosome opposite an active maternal allele nor with the first hit on a maternal chromosome. The expanded population now represents a much increased target for the second event—loss of the maternal allele (by somatic recombination in this case). Note that if the second mutation does not occur, the initial focus of growth may not progress into a tumour. Reproduced by permission from Reik, W. and Surani, M.A. (1989) Genomic imprinting and embryonal tumours. *Nature*, **338**: 112–113

Table 4. Features of the cancer family syndrome

Unusually large numbers of members of the kindred are affected with adenocarcinoma of the colon, uterus and ovary. Adenocarcinoma of the breast and stomach and possibly lymphoma may affect some family members

Colon cancers tend to occur on the right side

Cancers appear at an unusually early age (mean 45 years compared with 65 years in the general population)

Affected family members tend to have multiple primary cancers

The distribution of affected persons in the family is compatible with autosomal dominant inheritance

There are in some cases features of the Muir-Torre Syndrome (sebaceous adenomas, epitheliomas and carcinomas)

Affected persons seem to have an unusually good prognosis

susceptibility would be less tissue specific but this is quite plausible—the retinoblastoma gene is not fully tissue specific, there being evidence of an increased susceptibility to osteosarcoma. So far the genes responsible for the 'cancer family syndromes' have not been identified.

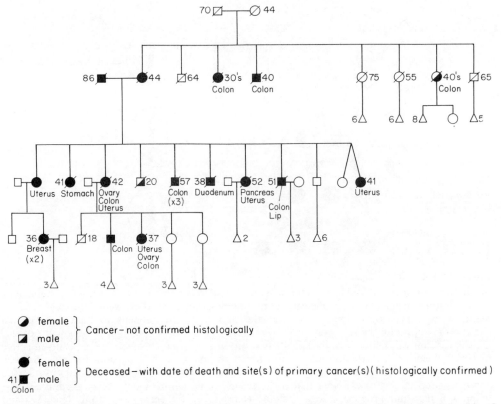

Figure 8. An example of the 'cancer family syndrome'. Part of a family with a high risk of cancer at various sites. From H.T. Lynch *et al.* (1966). *Arch. Int. Med.*, **117**, 206. © 1966 by the AMA. Reproduced by permission

It is worth at this point listing the various mechanisms by which an inherited genetic predisposition to cancer could theoretically occur. Not all of these have been included and not all those included need to be considered in detail.

- Germ line transmission of a mutation with direct effect on cancer promotion in the cells in which it occurs (see above).
- An inherited DNA repair disorder promoting somatic mutation (see above).
- An inherited variation in metabolism of a chemical carcinogen. The lack of examples here probably reflects our ignorance of modes of action and metabolism of chemical carcinogens. Variation in the enzyme aryl hydrocarbon hydroxylase may account for some inherited variation in susceptibility to lung cancer. It is likely that new examples will be discovered in the future as many chemical carcinogens are activated by metabolism and there is certain to be inherited variation in some of the metabolic processes involved.

• Inherited defects in immune surveillance may impair the normal
  removal of malignant cells. Some of the immunodeficiency
  syndromes show an increased risk of cancer, mainly
  leukaemias and lymphomas.

DNA repair disorders and defects of immune surveillance are very rare disorders, most of them autosomal recessive, with a major effect on susceptibility. If the same genes have a small effect in the far more numerous heterozygotes, this could cause more cancers in the population than the effect in homozygotes. Among the DNA repair disorders there is some evidence that heterozygotes for ataxia telangiectasia (identified by their relationship to homozygotes with the full-blown condition as there is no reliable carrier test) have an increased risk of common cancers. One person in 40,000 has ataxia telangiectasia so that about 1 in 100 of the population will carry the gene in single dose.

Identifying Cancer Genes

The recent explosion in knowledge of oncogenes dates from the late 1970s when the genes carried by cancer-inducing retroviruses began to be identified. Retroviruses are RNA viruses which insert a DNA copy of their genome into the host genome. Several of these have been known for many years to cause tumours in various animals. It was found that the retrovirus genes needed to cause cancer were closely related to genes present in normal non-malignant cells from a wide variety of species, including humans. It was also shown, using transfection techniques to transfer DNA between different cells, that some human cancers contained genes which could induce malignant transformation in recipient cells and that these human transforming genes were closely related to some of the retroviral oncogenes.

The conclusions of this work were that there is a class of genes known as cellular oncogenes or proto-oncogenes, widely distributed and preserved in vertebrates, and therefore presumably having important functions, which can in certain circumstances contribute to the development of cancer. This concept, which is briefly discussed in the next few pages, is covered more thoroughly in the next chapter on the biology of cancer.

Studies in cancer cells have shown some of the mechanisms by which these genes may act in carcinogenesis by being expressed:

• inappropriately
• at the wrong time
• at increased levels
• in altered (mutated) forms which are not subject to the normal
  controls

The incorporation of cellular oncogenes into retroviruses, which led to their discovery, is just one of the ways in which oncogenes can be modified to promote cancer. From the retrovirus they are reintroduced into host cells, sometimes with the acquisition of viral promoter sequences or with mutations affecting their expression. This so far has not emerged as an important mechanism in human malignancy.

Protein Products of Cellular Oncogenes

These have obvious importance for the pathogenesis of cancer. Several have been characterized as growth factors or growth factor receptors; thus the normal functions of oncogene proteins seem to be concerned with the control of cell division and differentiation. Many oncogene proteins have tyrosine-specific protein kinase activity and this seems to be an important link in the growth control mechanism. They activate enzymes by phosphorylating tyrosine residues. Growth receptors when triggered by signals from outside the cell send signals into the cell resulting in increased protein kinase activity and activating critical enzyme systems.

Ancestral Oncogene Families?

Different oncogenes may be ancestrally related to each other. Gene families are groups of related but not identical genes which are descended from a common ancestral gene and which share parts of their DNA sequence. Gene duplication has been an important evolutionary mechanism for increasing complexity. The various globin genes on chromosomes 11 and 16 all appear to have been derived from an ancestral globin gene. In the same way, the c-erb B gene on chromosome 7 is similar but not identical to the c-erb B-2 gene on chromosome 17.

Chromosome Abnormalities in Cancer

Many cancers accumulate chromosome abnormalities. For years it was unclear whether these were aetiologically important or whether they were just a consequence of chaotic growth. Certain abnormalities were found to have a high degree of specificity for particular cancers. The best known examples are the Philadelphia chromosome found in chronic myeloid leukaemia, first noted in 1960 and subsequently shown to arise by means of a 9;22 translocation, and an 8;14 translocation characteristic of Burkitt's lymphoma. Both translocations were found to rearrange cellular oncogenes. In chronic myeloid leukaemia the c-abl oncogene on chromosome 9 is translocated to chromosome 22 where it becomes joined to so-called bcr (break-point cluster) sequences. A hybrid protein is produced which has different properties from the normal c-abl protein. The cases of chronic myeloid leukaemia without a visible Philadelphia chromosome have been shown by molecular methods to have a submicroscopic c-abl insertion in the bcr region on chromosome 22.

Burkitt's lymphoma characteristically shows an 8;14 translocation, but sometimes it may be 2;8 or 8;22. In each case the c-myc oncogene from chromosome 8 is being placed near to an immunoglobulin gene. One consequence is that c-myc seems to partake of the high somatic mutation rate of the variable immunoglobulin genes normally used to generate antibody diversity. This may be the mechanism by which a series of c-myc mutations is generated. Those mutations which promote cell division will tend to be preserved; no doubt others resulting in cell death also occur. Alternatively, the translocated oncogene may come under the same controls as the immunoglobulin genes, which are being expressed at a high level.

Gene Amplification

The expression of oncogenes is sometimes altered by multiplication of the number of copies of the gene within each cell—so-called gene amplification. This may lead to visible chromosomal changes in the form of 'double minute' chromosomes and homogeneously staining chromosome regions, which are not always close to the original site of the proto-oncogene. Neuroblastoma, a malignant tumour of childhood arising in the sympathetic ganglia or adrenal medulla, is a well-known example. The *N-myc* oncogene is often amplified to over 100 copies, but only in the more widespread tumours with a poorer prognosis. It is not yet clear whether *N-myc* amplification is a late change occurring in any neuroblastoma (if so it would not be necessary for induction of the tumour), or whether there are two groups of neuroblastomas, permanently with or without *N-myc* amplification, the former behaving more aggressively.

Similar findings in breast cancer concern the *c-erb B-2* proto-oncogene (also known as *HER-2/neu* or *neu*). This gene, which codes for a tyrosine-specific protein kinase, is amplified in some breast cancers, and the number of gene copies correlates well with the prognosis of the tumour as judged by the extent of lymph node involvement and relapse and survival rates. *C-erb B-2* is closely related to but different from the *C-erb B* gene which codes for the epidermal growth factor receptor, another tyrosine-specific protein kinase. This is also over-expressed in breast cancer but the mechanism does not appear to be gene amplification.

Other Types of Cancer-Promoting Changes to Oncogenes

Translocations and gene amplification may well be uncommon ways of achieving aberrant oncogene expression; they are, however, easily recognized because they produce visible chromosome changes. Gene mutations of various types are probably commoner. An example of a point mutation leading to oncogene activation was the discovery in a bladder cancer of a mutated version of the normal c-ras^{H-1} gene. The mutant *ras* gene differed by only a single base from the original.

The effect of this base substitution has been shown to be a loss of normal feedback control in the *ras* protein. The *ras* gene in other tumours can be activated by retroviral transduction (when a modified *ras* gene is acquired from a retrovirus) and by a mutation of the gene's regulatory sequences, when increased amounts of the normal protein are produced.

Much remains to be discovered of the mechanisms by which proto-oncogenes mutate to oncogenes. Mutations which cause inherited disorders usually cause reduced expression of the gene or a defective product. Oncogene mutations are those which confer a *selective advantage* on the cell, and will often result in increased expression, or loss of ability to respond to normal feedback controls, either at the gene or protein level.

The action of mutagens in causing cancer seems to be a non-specific one. There is nothing so far to suggest that certain molecular varieties of mutation are more likely than others to lead to malignant transformation.

Many of the 30 or so human proto-oncogenes so far identified have been found to be over-expressed in particular tumours. There is not much specificity between oncogene and tumour, and a given tumour may have more than one oncogene activated, in accordance with the multiple stage model. For example the *c-myc* gene, whose expression is affected by translocation in Burkitt's lymphoma, is also over-expressed in lung and colon cancers but by mechanisms other than translocation.

The lack of specificity between oncogene and tumour type is not surprising, given the derivations of oncogene names. Most are named after the virally induced animal tumours in which they were discovered. The *ras* genes for example are named after rat sarcoma, *sis* after simian sarcoma, *erb* after avian erythroblastosis and *fms* after feline sarcoma, but homologues of all these genes are involved in the genesis of human tumours.

Inherited Cancers and Antioncogenes

The oncogenes so far identified have not been found to be involved in familial transmission of cancer. The genes responsible for familial retinoblastoma, polyposis and similar conditions are transmitted dominantly but only act when their paired normal allele is removed: they act recessively. Oncogenes on the other hand often act dominantly. It may only need one of the pair of proto-oncogenes present in a cell to be modified in order to transform the cell.

The biochemical action of the familial cancer genes has not yet been clarified but it has been suggested that they may act by suppressing the action of oncogenes. A single dose of the normal gene may well then be enough to retain control. The retinoblastoma gene has recently been cloned and its product characterized, so this hypothesis should soon be tested.

Implications of Cancer Genetics for Prevention and Treatment

It seems clear that the incidence of cancer would be reduced if the somatic mutation rate could be reduced. While much mutation seems to be an in-built property of DNA replication, nobody knows what proportion of cancer-inducing mutations are caused by environmental carcinogens, particularly chemical ones. There may conceivably be a pharmacological or dietary approach to limiting somatic mutation.

The treatment of existing cancer should be greatly advanced when it becomes possible to specify which oncogenes are active in a given tumour. If a mutated oncogene is producing a structurally distinctive cell surface protein, specific immunotherapy may be possible. There are, however, potential problems. Oncogene products are closely similar, and may be identical, to normal gene products expressed, albeit at lower levels, in normal cells. Because of this, they are likely to be difficult therapeutic targets.

Summary and Conclusions

- Various observations suggest that malignant behaviour is a genetic property of cancer cells.

- The genetic differences between cancer cells and normal cells usually arise by *somatic mutation*—changes in the genotype after the zygote stage, which are unlikely to be transmitted to the next generation.
- On rare occasions cancer-inducing mutations are transmitted from generation to generation and account for one important category of familial cancers. Several such mutations act *recessively* in that they require the removal, by a second mutation, of the paired normal allele.
- Another class of cancer-inducing genes, *cellular oncogenes*, are normal genes which have been altered in a way that makes them function inappropriately. Various mutational mechanisms have been identified: chromosome translocations, point mutations, deletions, insertions, gene amplification and (so far mainly in non-human vertebrates) retroviral transduction. These genes act *dominantly*: only one of the pair need to be altered to produce an effect, and their mutations have not so far been found to be passed on from generation to generation, and hence not to contribute to familial cancer susceptibility.
- The normal function of oncogenes seems to be to code for proteins which regulate cell growth and proliferation.
- The existence of genes which control growth, together with the possibility of somatic mutation in dividing tissues, means that cell lines (clones) with an enhanced growth rate will inevitably be selected. In practice, to achieve recognizably malignant behaviour seems usually to require more than one mutation, and perhaps three or four (*multi-step*), often affecting more than one oncogene. The early stage of the process may be recognizable as a precancerous state. Cancers continue to evolve with the accumulation of further growth-enhancing mutations.

These data strongly support the conclusion that cancer is a genetic disease of somatic cells. Development of malignancy probably requires two or more mutations of stem cells in a tissue. Expression of mutations depends on the kinetics of cell proliferation, availability of growth factors, host resistance and other factors.

A few rare tumours are frequently heritable; the precise chromosomal location of genes leading to malignancy have, for instance, been identified in retinoblastoma and Wilms' tumour. Studies in inbred populations suggest that the risk of developing many common cancers is associated with genetic factors, though mutations have not been identified.

Selected Papers and Reviews

Anon (1988) Molecular mechanisms in familial and sporadic cancers. *Lancet*, i: 92–94.
Bishop, J. M. (1982) Oncogenes. *Scientific American*, **246**: 68–78.

Cavenee, W. K., Dryja, T. P., Phillips, R. A. *et al.* (1983) Expression of recessive alleles by chromosomal mechanisms in retinoblastoma. *Nature*, **305**: 779–784.

de Vos, A. M., Tong, L., Milburn, M. V. *et al.* (1988) Three-dimensional structure of an oncogene protein. Catalytic domain of human *c-H-ras p21*. *Science*, **239**: 888–893.

Knudson, A. G. (1985) Hereditary cancer, oncogenes, and antioncogenes. *Cancer Research*, **45**: 1437–1443.

Weber, J. and McClure, M. (1987) Oncogenes and cancer. *British Medical Journal*, **294**: 1246–1248.

2 Biology of Cancer

D. R. GARROD

Introduction

The large group of diseases known as cancer arise because of changes in the growth and behaviour of cells. Unlimited and uncontrollable growth of tumour cells leads to a progressive increase in tumour bulk with consequent impingement on the structure and impairment of function of adjacent normal tissues. In addition to abnormally increased growth, the cells of malignant tumours are able to penetrate into or invade adjacent tissues and to spread from the primary tumour to distant sites in the body, giving rise to secondary tumour masses. It is this ability to spread that characterizes malignant (vs. benign) neoplasms and makes them such a difficult and serious clinical problem (see box).

---

uncontrolled growth → increasing bulk
local invasion
distant spread

The formation of malignant cell populations (i.e. cancers) starts with changes in the genetic material of cells, which then generate, by division and growth, cell populations that retain and express malignant characteristics. There is evidence that human tumours may be clonal in origin, i.e. they may arise from a single defective cell (Figure 1). Such a cell may give rise to a small population of malignant stem cells that have the capacity both for self renewal and for generating large malignant cell populations by clonal expansion. For instance, in haematological malignancies (leukaemias, lymphomas,

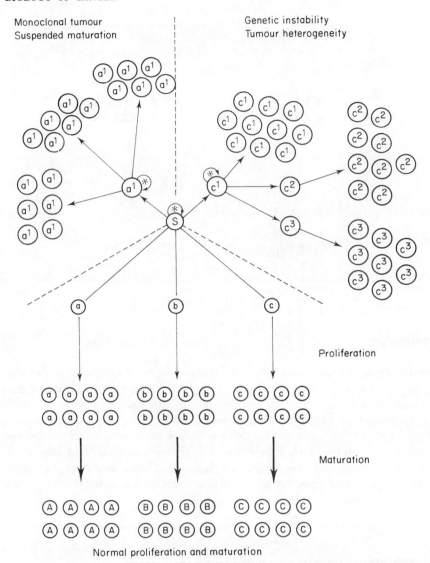

Figure 1. Proliferation and maturation in normal and neoplastic tissues. In normal proliferating tissues, e.g. bone marrow, pleuripotential stem cells (S) divide to undergo self renewal (⋆) and to generate precursors (a, b, c) of various cell types. These precursors proliferate to expand the cell populations and then mature to form differentiated cells (A, B, C). Tumours arise when malignant stem cells (a^1, c^1) arise from normal stem cells. These may proliferate to give rise to clonal populations of immature cells (e.g. leukaemias) or may both proliferate and generate variant clones due to genetic instability (e.g. some solid tumours)

myeloma) enormous populations of malignant cells are produced, all of which possess the same clonal characteristic, such as unique cell surface-associated immunoglobulins (chronic lymphocytic leukaemia, Burkitt's lymphoma) or secreted immunoglobulin molecules (myeloma). The characteristics of leukaemic cells suggest that they are clonally expanded cell populations that have been arrested at some stage on the pathway of differentiation to mature blood cells (Figure 1, top left).

Structurally, the cells of solid tumours may show considerable resemblance to normal cells of the tissue from which they were derived, in which case they are described as well differentiated (page 82). Alternatively, the cells of a tumour may show loss of differentiated characteristics, when they are referred to as poorly differentiated. However, tumours are often heterogeneous, showing a range of cellular differentiation characteristics. A number of human solid tumours have been shown to be monoclonal but in other cases clonal heterogeneity has been demonstrated. Such heterogeneity does not, however, necessarily indicate a polyclonal origin of the tumours since, because of genetic instability, distinct subclones may arise during population expansion from a single initiating cell (Figure 1).

This brief introduction emphasizes two fundamentally important aspects of cancer biology which will form the basis for this chapter. The first is the *genetic changes* that take place in cancer cells and give rise to their malignant properties. What causes these changes? What is their nature? How do they affect cellular physiology and behaviour? The second is the *spread of cancer*—what cellular mechanisms are involved in this devastating process?

Genetic Changes in Cancer Cells

Carcinogenesis

Many factors have been implicated in the causation or promotion of neoplastic transformation on the basis of experiments in tissue culture or on experimental animals, or by epidemiological studies of human populations. These include chemical agents or carcinogens, various types of radiation, and viruses. In general, tumour development is a slow process: there may be a long delay—the latent interval—between contact with a carcinogenic stimulus, such as a dose of ionizing radiation, and the onset of cancer (Chapter 3).

The development of tumours is marked in some cases by well-defined precancerous cellular changes, such as pre-neoplastic dysplasia. With certain exceptions, such as specific childhood tumours, the majority of human cancers are diseases of middle or old age. Indeed, a major reason for the increased incidence of human cancer this century is that, due to better living standards, people are living longer thereby allowing more time for tumour development.

Chemical Carcinogens

The slow development of most tumours probably occurs because carcinogenesis (Chapter 3) is a multi-stage process involving sequential exposure to different agents (Figure 2a). Some examples of chemical carcinogens are shown in Figure 2b. They can cause the formation of tumours in experimental animals when applied in sufficiently high doses. In lower doses they initiate the process of carcinogenesis without causing actual tumour formation. Once carcinogenesis has been initiated, it may be caused to progress either by application of further doses of carcinogens or of another class of

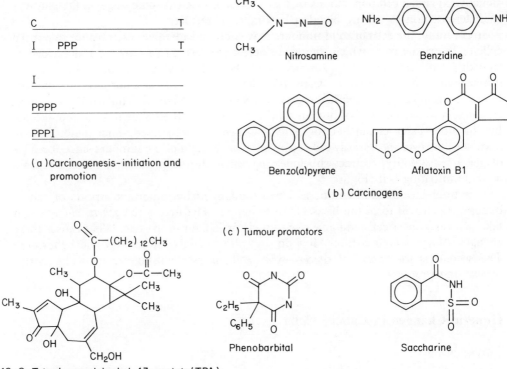

Figure 2. Carcinogenesis, carcinogens and tumour promotors. (a) Carcinogens (C) applied to experimental animals result in formation of tumours (T). Initiators (I) and promotors (P) also cause tumours when applied in the right sequence. However, neither I nor P alone, nor I and P applied in the wrong sequence cause tumours.
(b) Examples of carcinogens. Benzo(a)pyrene, other polycylic hydrocarbons and nitrosamines occur in coal tar and cigarette smoke and may also be derived from other environmental sources. Benzidine and other aromatic amines have been encountered in the dye industry. Aflatoxin B1 is produced by the mould *Aspergillus flavus* and was discovered in mouldy peanuts.
(c) Examples of tumour promotors. TPA is the tumour-promoting agent in croton oil which has been found to promote tumour formation in mouse skin. Phenobarbital may promote liver cancer and saccharine bladder cancer

compounds called tumour *promotors* (Figure 2c). Tumour promotors are not carcinogenic in their own right and are only effective in causing tumour formation if their action follows that of an initiating carcinogen.

Chemical carcinogens either are, or are metabolized to, highly reactive (electrophilic) compounds that can react directly with a variety of cellular constituents. The crucial part of their activity is that they are *mutagens* which react with DNA, causing direct alteration or damage to the genetic material. They may react with the purine and pyrimidine bases of DNA, combining with them to form adducts, alkylating them (adding small alkyl groups, e.g., CH_3-, C_2H_5-) or causing base removal, or they may react with the phosphate residues of the phosphate-sugar backbone. Such modifications to DNA may lead to miscoding, inaccurate replication or chain breakage.

Tumour promotors are generally not mutagens and affect cellular properties in a manner complementary to the genetic damage caused by initiating carcinogens. For example, it has been shown that the phorbolester, 12-0-tetradecanoylphorbol-13-acetate (TPA), is an activator of an important phosphorylating enzyme, protein kinase C, involved in transmembrane signalling in cells (see below).

Carcinogenesis—Initiation, Promotion.
Genetic damage → mutagenesis

Radiation

Various types of ionizing radiation are also mutagenic and cause damage to DNA. Radiation causes damage because it imparts energy to a tissue as it penetrates it. High-energy radiations such as α-particles (e.g. emitted from radon gas which is present in some metal ores and may be inhaled by ore miners) are more likely to cause tissue damage than low-energy radiations such as X-rays and γ-rays because they lose more energy per unit length of path to the surrounding tissue as they penetrate (Figure 3). They are said to have a higher linear energy transfer (LET). Thus there is a greater probability that an α-particle will cause a double-stranded break in DNA than will an

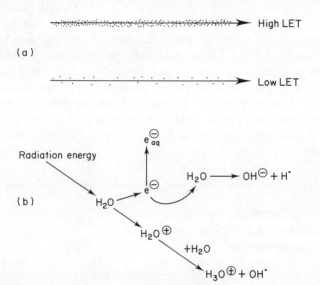

Figure 3. Radiation carcinogenesis. (a) Particles of high linear energy transfer (LET) lose more energy per unit length of path through tissue than particles of low LET. High LET particles are therefore more likely to cause damage.
(b) Ionizing radiation may damage biomolecules directly, or, by causing release of electrons from water molecules and stimulating the production of highly reactive free radicals of hydrogen, hydroxyl groups or hydrated electrons. These free radicals then cause damage by reacting with biomolecules

X-ray. Radiation can damage target molecules either by direct disruption of chemical bonds within them or by generating highly reactive free radicals by fragmentation of water. The free radicals then may diffuse and react with the target molecule.

Radiation may cause loss or alteration of bases from DNA, DNA strand breakage or breakage of chromosomes. Radiation acts synergistically with chemical carcinogens and promotors so that, for example, cigarette smoking exacerbates the effect of radon inhalation in ore miners and TPA increases experimental radiation-induced cell transformation.

Radiation → tissue damage
      → free radicals
      → mutagenesis
      → synergism with carcinogens

DNA Repair

Genetic damage of the type caused by carcinogens and radiation is not necessarily permanent because cells have the capacity to repair damaged DNA. A combination of enzymes enables damaged bases to be excised, and new DNA to be synthesized in the gap and joined to the ends of the undamaged strand. Strand breaks can also be repaired. If a change in the DNA is to become permanent the damaged DNA must undergo replication before repair so that one cycle of cell division is necessary to incorporate a lesion into DNA. Therefore, cells in proliferating tissues (e.g. bone marrow, intestinal epithelium) are more susceptible to tumour initiation because they are dividing. A practical illustration of the importance of repair mechanisms is provided by individuals who lack them. Thus people with the autosomal-recessive disorder, xeroderma pigmentosum, are predisposed to developing multiple skin cancers brought on by sunlight because their cells are unable to repair DNA that has been damaged by ultraviolet light.

DNA repair enzymes
Tumour initiation in dividing cells
Xeroderma pigmentosum

Viruses

Certain viruses are able to cause transformation of cells in tissue culture, e.g. Rous sarcoma virus (RSV) and polyomavirus (Py), and there is direct evidence for the involvement of viruses in cancers of animals, e.g. avian erythroblastosis virus (AEV), mouse mammary tumour virus (MMTV) and feline leukaemia virus (FLV). There are a number of well-established associations between viruses and human cancer, but in no case has the role played by the virus been clearly established and in no case is infection with the virus sufficient in itself to cause cancer. Additional factors, such as exposure to carcinogens or tumour promotors, or immunodeficiency, appear to be required. Examples of viruses associated with human cancer include:

- The human T-cell leukaemia viruses (HTLV-1 and -2) are associated with adult T-cell leukaemia common in individuals born in West Africa, the Caribbean and southern Japan.
- Chronic infection with the hepatitis B virus is a risk factor in primary liver cancer.
- Papillomaviruses are associated with a number of benign and malignant tumours, especially carcinoma of the cervix.
- A type of herpesvirus called Epstein-Barr virus (EBV) is associated with Burkitt's lymphoma, a B-cell malignancy common in children in West Africa and New Guinea, and nasopharyngeal cancer in Asia.

Viral transformation depends upon integration of viral DNA into the genome of the host cell with consequent alteration in structure and activity of genes. Some of the viruses mentioned above have genomes that consist of DNA (e.g. EBV, hepatitis B virus and the papillomaviruses), while others, the *retroviruses*, have genomes consisting of RNA (e.g. AEV, MMTV, FLV, HTLV). The genomes of the latter group must be copied into double-stranded DNA by enzymes called *reverse transcriptases* before insertion into the host genome can take place (Figure 4).

Genetic analysis of viral transformation has revealed that the *transforming genes* of many retroviruses (e.g. RSV and AEV), rather than being true viral genes, are derived from nomal genes of the cells that are infected by the viruses. The viral genes are called *viral oncogenes (v-onc)* while the corresponding cellular genes are called *cellular oncogenes (c-onc)* or *proto-oncogenes*. The viral oncogenes appear to have been acquired and modified from the cellular genes themselves during the course of viral evolution. They have become inserted into the viral genome where they perform no apparent function (see below).

Other retroviruses, including HTLV, and DNA viruses, such as papillomaviruses, possess transforming genes that are not the counterparts of cellular genes but are truly part of the viruses' own genomes. These genes appear to function by modifying cellular function in much the same way as oncogenes.

Viruses associated with human cancer, e.g. HTLV, EBV, papillomavirus, DNA and RNA viruses
Viral oncogenes and cellular oncogenes

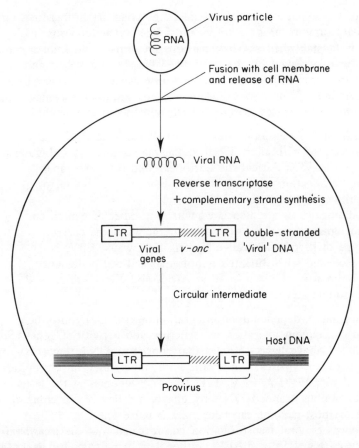

Figure 4. Insertion of viral genome into that of the host cell. The example shown is that of an RNA virus or retrovirus. The viral genome consists of a single strand of RNA that somewhat resembles normal cellular messenger RNA. Once inside the cell the RNA is converted to DNA by the enzyme reverse transcriptsae, then into double-stranded DNA like that of the host. The 'viral' DNA consists of long terminal repeats (LTRs), normal viral genes and a viral oncogene which can cause cell transformation. The viral DNA becomes incorporated into the DNA of the host, at which stage it is known as a 'provirus'. LTRs are strong promotors and enhancers of gene transcription and can cause transformation of cells if they are inserted into the host genome near a cellular oncogene (see below). The HTLV retroviruses insert into the human genome in a manner similar to that shown in the diagram. The genomes of DNA viruses can insert directly into the host genome

Chromosomal Abnormalities in Cancer

Damage to the genetic material of cancer cells caused by the various carcinogenic agents described in the previous section is reflected in the finding that most tumours have structural and/or numerical abnormalities of their chromosomes, some of which are associated with particular types of tumours. These abnormalities have been found by cytogenetic analysis. The dividing tumour cells are arrested in metaphase, the stage of mitosis when the chromosomes are most condensed, by treatment with colchicine, and then spread on microscope slides so that their chromosomes may be examined (Figure 5). The analysis is greatly enhanced by chromosome banding in which the spread chromosomes are treated with trypsin (G-banding) or a quinacrine derivative (Q-banding). In addition complementation studies by whole cell fusion and *in situ* hybridization with radiolabelled nucleic acid probes onto metaphase chromosomes enable the mapping of genes on chromosomes (see below).

Chromosomal abnormalities in tumours may involve *gain or loss* of chromosomes or parts of chromosomes, *translocation* of part of one chromosome to another, *inversion* of part of a chromosome or *duplication* of one arm of a chromosome with loss of the other. Some well-established examples are considered below.

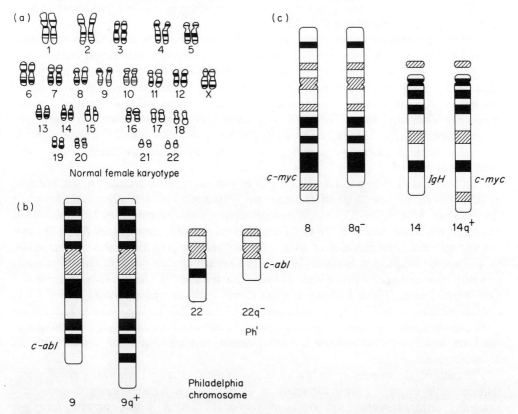

Figure 5. (a) Diagram representing normal female karyotype as seen by G-banding. The male karyotype is identical except for the presence of a small Y chromosome in place of one of the X chromosomes.
(b) 9:22 translocation (as found in chronic granulocytic leukaemia) resulting in formation of a Philadelphia (Ph') chromosome. The normal chromosomes are labelled 9 and 22. The abnormal chromosomes are labelled 9q+ and 22q− to denote lengthening and shortening of their long arms, respectively, as a result of the reciprocal translocation. The translocation involves the *c-abl* oncogene, whose expression is altered in consequence.
(c) 8:14 translocation as found in the majority of patients with Burkitt's lymphoma. The usual chromosomes are labelled 8 and 14, and the abnormal chromosomes 8q− and 14q+ to denote shortening and lengthening, respectively, of their long arms. The translocation involves transfer of the *c-myc* oncogene from the long arm of chromosome 8 to a position adjacent to the immunoglobulin heavy chain locus (IgH) in chromosome 14

The majority of patients with chronic granulocytic leukaemia (CGL) have bone marrow cells containing the Philadelphia (Ph') chromosome, so called because it was first discovered in Philadelphia in 1960. The Ph' chromosome is an abnormally small chromosome 22 that arises through a reciprocal translocation involving the tip of the long arm of chromosome 9 and a large part of the long arm of chromosome 22 (Figure 4).

This translocation involves the interchange of two oncogenes, c-abl and c-sis, between the chromosomes. The c-abl gene has been found to produce an abnormally long transcript when a Ph' chromosome is present and this may be significant in the causation of CGL; the activity of c-sis appears to be unaffected by the translocation. The Ph' chromosome is also present in some cases of acute myeloid leukaemia (AML) and acute lymphocytic leukaemia (ALL).

Burkitt's lymphoma shows a translocation between the long arms of chromosomes 8 and 14 (Figure 5) in about 90% of patients. This involves translocation of the c-myc oncogene from chromosome 8 to a position adjacent to the immunoglobulin heavy chain (IgH) genes on chromosome 14. This results in enhanced transcription of the c-myc gene, probably because the translocation results in separation of the gene from its regulatory elements. Other Burkitt's lymphoma patients show translocation of the immunoglobulin light chains, λ and κ, from chromosomes 2 and 22, respectively, to a position adjacent to the c-myc region of chromosome 8. Similar translocations have been found in ALL.

Gain and loss of chromosomes also occur in various types of leukaemia; for example in AML there may be three of chromosome 8 (trisomy) or only one (monosomy) of chromsomes 5 or 7. In ALL an abnormal number of chromosomes (aneuploidy) is common: chromosomes 6, 8, 18 or 21 may be gained and chromsomes 7 and 20 lost.

Chromosomal abnormalities of solid tumours are less well documented than those of leukaemias because it is more difficult to obtain populations of dividing cells and to make chromosome preparations. However, a number of chromosomal aberrations have been found. These include: translocations between chromosomes 6 and 14 in ovarian carcinoma and between chromosomes 11 and 22 in Ewing's sarcoma; deletions from chromosome 1 in neuroblastoma, from chromosome 3 in small cell carcinoma of the lung and from chromosome 6 in melanoma; and monosomy of chromosome 22 in meningioma.

The childhood tumours retinoblastoma and Wilms' tumour both have heritable and non-heritable forms. Cytogenetic analyses of individuals with heritable disease have located a retinoblastoma locus on chromosome 13 and a Wilms' tumour locus on chromosome 11. Both loci can carry recessive mutations. In individuals with tumours, the normal body cells are heterozygous at these loci, bearing one normal and one mutant allele. However, the cells of the tumour have become either *homozygous* or *hemizygous* for these recessive mutations: i.e. they either possess two mutant alleles (homozygous) or they possess a single mutant allele only (hemizygous) (Figure 6). Hemizygosity or homozygosity may arise by a variety of mechanisms, including chromosome loss or deletion, or mitotic recombination (i.e. crossing-over between homologous chromosomes during mitosis in somatic cells). It is likely that similar effects may arise from chromosomal changes in other tumours.

Other chromosomal abnormalities are associated with *gene amplification*. Thus the formation of *isochromosomes* by duplication of the arms of individual chromosomes (e.g.

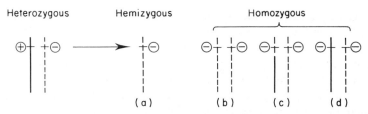

Figure 6. Mechanisms that can result in genetic hemizygosity or homozygosity as found in Wilms' tumour and retinoblastoma. Cells in the normal tissues of the body are heterozygous, i.e. one chromosome of a pair carries a normal gene or allele and the other chromosome carries a mutant allele. Hemizygosity can result from loss of the chromosome bearing the normal allele (a) or by deletion of the allele bearing part of the chromosome (not shown). Homozygosity can result from chromosome loss and reduplication (b) giving two copies of the mutant-bearing chromosome; by mitotic recombination (c); or point mutation of the normal allele to the mutant form (d)

the short arm of chromosome 6 in retinoblastoma) produces extra copies of all the genes on this part of the chromosome. Gene amplification is also denoted by the presence of either *homogeneously staining regions* (HSRs) on chromosomes, or very small acentric chromosomes (without centromeres) called *double minutes* (DMs).

Such changes have been found in association with drug resistance in cultured cells (e.g. amplification of the gene for the enzyme dihydrofolate reductase in methotrexate resistance), and with amplification of oncogenes in cell lines (e.g. *c-myc* in an acute promyelocytic leukaemia line and *N-myc* in a neuroblastoma line).

Translocation—e.g. Ph' chromosome in CGL and 8:14 in Burkitt's lymphoma
Deletion and chromosome loss
Homozygosity and hemizygosity—Wilms' tumour, retinoblastoma
Gene amplification—HSRs and DMs

Chromosomes, Cancer and Cell Fusion

It has now been well established that the ability of a wide range of different malignant cells to form tumours in host animals can be suppressed by fusing the cells with normal fibroblasts. However, some hybrids retain or re-acquire the capacity to form tumours. Hybrid cells formed by fusion have a tendency to eliminate chromosomes, and careful analysis of the karyotypes of cell hybrids has revealed that suppression of malignancy in hybrids is associated with the retention of specific chromosomes. If these chromosomes are lost the hybrids are malignant.

Suppression of malignancy in cell hybrids appears to be associated with the presence of a normal chromosome 4 for mouse tumours and chromosome 1 for human tumours. In addition, evidence for the role of chromosome 11 in suppression of human malignancy has been obtained by introducing a single normal chromosome 11 into cells from uterine carcinoma and Wilms' tumour by *microcell transfer*. This involves fusing a small membrane-bounded vesicle containing a single chromosome to the malignant cell.

The nature and function of the genes involved in suppression of malignancy is unknown. However, since specific chromosomes are able to suppress a range of different malignancies, the genes are likely to be involved in the control of some general cellular property, perhaps control of differentiation.

The data from cell fusion and genetic analysis of Wilms' tumour and retinoblastoma (see above) suggest that malignancy is associated with genetic characteristics of a recessive nature. Thus in Wilms' tumour and retinoblastoma, homozygous or hemizygous cells are malignant, but heterozygous cells possessing a normal allele are not. In cell hybrids the presence of a normal chromosome 4 (mouse) or chromosome 11 (human) overrides the presence of the same chromosome from the malignant cell. Much interest has been occasioned in recent years by the discovery of a considerable number of genes—oncogenes—whose expression is associated with malignancy, and this may be interpreted to suggest that oncogenes exert a dominant genetic role in malignancy. It is not yet clear how this apparent conflict between the data from cell fusion studies and oncogene studies may be resolved. However, before embarking on a discussion of oncogenes it should be stressed that the idea that they play a genetically dominant role in malignant transformation is almost certainly oversimplified.

Cell fusion—suppression of malignancy—chromosome loss
Cell differentiation
Dominance and recessiveness

Oncogenes

Oncogenes are normal genes whose altered expression is associated with neoplastic transformation. As noted above many viral genes that cause cell transformation, so-called viral oncogenes (*v-onc*), are derived from normal cellular genes called cellular oncogenes (*c-onc*) or proto-oncogenes. In order to illustrate the idea of normal and altered gene expression the *c-abl* gene is a useful example as its altered expression has already been mentioned in association with the 9:22 chromosome translocation in chronic granulocytic leukaemia (CGL).

The normal expression of the *c-abl* gene occurs during mid-development of the embryo. Expression of *c-abl* in CGL is therefore inappropriate, being in the wrong place at the wrong time, and expression of the same gene may be amplified 5–10 times. Most other oncogenes have been shown to be expressed during normal development. Some, like *c-abl*, are expressed at a particular time and in a tissue-specific manner. Others, like the *ras* genes, are expressed ubiquitously and throughout development. Some oncogenes, e.g. *ras*, have been conserved during evolution; homologues can be found not only in humans, mammals and birds, but also in fruit flies, nematode worms, yeasts and slime moulds. Such conservation indicates that these genes have an important function in normal cellular physiology. c-abl is the normal cellular counterpart of the retroviral oncogene v-abl, which is present in the Ableson mouse leukaemia virus and also in a feline sarcoma virus. v-abl is one of about 20 viral oncogenes that have been shown by molecular biological techniques (nucleic acid hybridization and sequencing) to have normal cellular counterparts or proto-oncogenes. Some of these, and some human malignancies with which their cellular counterparts have been associated, are listed in Table 1.

Other oncogenes do not have known viral counterparts. Many of these have been identified by the technique of DNA transfection, by which DNA isolated from tumour cells is introduced into 'normal' recipient cells in tissue culture, usually by mixing the DNA with precipitated calcium phosphate in order to facilitate uptake (Figure 8d). Later, the cultures are examined for the appearance of foci of transformed cells, which can be recognized because the cells pile up on top of each other while the normal cells remain as a single, flat layer. Transformation denotes the introduction of an oncogene into the cells. Of course, transfection also detects oncogenes that are related to retroviral genes, and by this means it has been found that ras genes appear to be associated with transformation in about 20% of human tumours. This result is difficult to interpret because the transfection technique may be highly selective for particular genes, and may therefore give a biased impression of the relative contribution of particular genes to human cancer.

Table 1. Some oncogenes associated with cancers

Oncogenes	Associated cancer(s)
abl	Chronic granulocytic leukaemia
erbB	Squamous cell carcinoma, glioblastoma
fes	Myeloid and lymphoid leukaemias
fms	Mammary and renal carcinomas
fos	Choriocarcinoma
mos	Plasmacytoma
myb	Myeloid and lymphoid leukaemias, colon carcinoma
myc	B-cell lymphoma, promyelocytic leukaemia, colon carcinoma, small cell lung carcinoma
N-myc	Neuroblastoma, retinoblastoma, small cell lung carcinoma
Ha-ras	Bladder carcinoma, lung carcinoma, mammary carcinoma
Ki-ras	Lung carcinoma, colon carcinoma, bladder carcinoma, neuroblastoma
N-ras	Neuroblastoma, teratocarcinoma, fibrosarcoma, melanoma, lung carcinoma, rhabdomyosarcoma, mammary carcinoma
sis	Osteosarcoma, glioma
src	Brain tumours

How Does The Inappropriate Expression or Activation of Oncogenes Take Place?

There is evidence that several alternative mechanisms are involved.

(a) Alteration in the control of gene transcription is one possibility. An example of this is insertional mutation, found with some retroviruses that lack oncogenes but nevertheless cause tumours in animals. The genomes of avian leukaemia viruses (ALV) that become inserted into the genome of host cells are flanked by long terminal repeat (LTR) structures (Figure 4)—regions of the DNA that do not code for proteins but possess 'promotors', regulatory elements that initiate gene transcription. B-cell lymphomas in chickens are associated with integration of LTR regions of ALV upstream of the cellular *myc* oncogene, leading to increased transcription of the *myc* gene and greatly increased production of *myc* RNA.

AVL insertion is not confined to this region of the host genome, but only insertion adjacent to *myc* results in leukaemia, demonstrating an association between the disease and the activation of the oncogene. Similar mechanisms of oncogene activation have been found with AEV and MMTV. This process is called *insertional mutagenesis*.

(b) Alteration in *transcriptional control* appears to be important in some human tumours where chromosomal translocations result in a change of the location of an oncogene. Thus, in Burkitt's lymphoma (see above) translocation of part of the long arm of chromosome 8 to chromosomes 14, 2 or 22 results in the association of the *myc* gene with immunoglobulin genes which are actively transcribed in mature B-lymphocytes (Figure 5c). Furthermore, translocation often involves loss of the upstream regulatory sequences of *myc*, enabling it to be influenced by other regulatory elements in its new location and leading to enhanced transcription. (Upstream regulatory sequences are regions of DNA that precede the protein coding regions of genes and control gene expression.) The 9:22 translocation found in the Ph' chromosome of CGL (see above) results in fusion of the *c-abl* gene from chromosome 9 with part of chromosome 22 (Figure 5b). This results in production of a much larger transcript from *c-abl*—9 kilobases instead of 512 bp (1 kilobase = 1000 bp; bp = base pair)—and the synthesis of a longer *abl* protein (molecular weight 210,000 instead of 120,000) with greater protein phosphorylation activity (see below).

(c) Another mechanism of oncogene activation is *gene amplification*. When this is marked it may be associated with chromosomal abnormalities known as HSRs and DMs (see above). Gene amplification in tumours may also be detected by Southern blotting, in which a radiolabelled oncogenic nucleic acid probe is hybridized to tumour DNA on a filter.

First the DNA must be cut into fragments with restriction enzymes, separated according to size by electrophoresis on agarose gel and then blotted from the gel onto a nylon filter. The labelled probe then binds to the specific complementary sequence (the gene) on the filter. The amount of binding when compared with the amount of binding to DNA from normal cells indicates whether the gene is amplified (Figure 7). Examples of gene amplifications found in human tumours are: *c-myc* in promyelocytic leukaemia; *N-myc* in neuroblastoma, retinoblastoma and small cell carcinoma of lung; *c-myb* in AML; and *c-Ki-ras-2* in carcinoma of lung, colorectum and bladder.

(d) Oncogene activation may also occur by *point mutation* in the gene, at least in the *ras* gene family. It has been shown by gene sequencing and site-directed mutagenesis

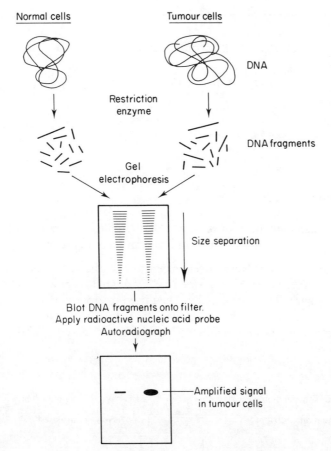

Figure 7. Detection of gene amplification in tumour cells by Southern blotting

(constructing genes with specific sequence alterations by genetic engineering and transfecting them into cells) that mutations resulting in substitution of the amino acid glycine at position 12 or of the glutamine at position 61 in the *p21ras* protein (see below) are associated with oncogenesis in a variety of human tumours.

Much evidence shows that *co-operativity of oncogenes*, i.e. activation of two or more oncogenes, is required for malignant transformation, reflecting the evidence from carcinogenesis studies that malignant transformation is a multi-step process (see page 21). When primary cells from normal tissues are grown in tissue culture they do not establish permanent cell lines. It has been shown that primary embryonic fibroblasts can be immortalized in culture by transfection with activated *c-myc* gene and that transformation requires additional transfection with *c-ras* (activated *ras* alone produces transformation but not immortalization). Thus complementation between oncogenes appears to be required for transformation.

Moreover, it appears that complementation in general may be required between oncogenes that produce cytoplasmic and nuclear protein products (see over).

Oncogenes—normal and abnormal expression
Transfection
Insertional mutagenesis, transcriptional control, gene amplification,
point mutation
Co-operativity

Growth of Cancer Cells

The growth of malignant or transformed cells in culture shows characteristics that distinguish it from that of normal or untransformed cells (Figure 8).

(i) *Anchorage independence*. Normal cells need to be adherent to a surface in order to grow in culture, whereas transformed cells are able to grow in semi-solid media such as 0.3% agar. This property has been used to grow stem cells directly isolated from human tumours. It correlates well with tumorigenicity, i.e. the ability of cells to form tumours in experimental animals, and may be used as an assay for transformation.

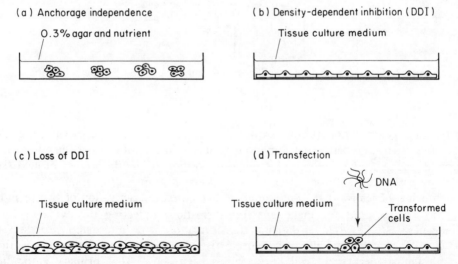

Figure 8. Growth characteristics of tumour cells in tissue culture. (a) Anchorage independence. Transformed cells will grow in suspension in soft agar while normal cells require anchorage to a substratum. (b) Density-dependent inhibition (DDI). Normal cells growing on a substratum continue growing only until the cell density becomes high. This usually results in formation of a confluent monolayer on the culture substratum. (c) Transformed cells growing on a substratum are not subject to DDI but grow to form multilayers. (d) Transfection of normal cells with DNA from transformed cells results in appearance of foci of transformation where an oncogene has entered a cell. This is recognized by local overgrowth of cells in a monolayer

(ii) *Density-dependent inhibition*. When normal cells grow attached to a surface, they continue growing only until the local density becomes high. This usually results in the formation of a continuous single layer of cells (a confluent monolayer) on the culture surface. Transformed cells, by contrast, readily pile up and grow to form multilayers on the culture surface. This characteristic may be used to identify foci of transformed cells, as in the DNA transfection assay (see above).

(iii) *Decreased serum requirement*. Transformed cells usually require serum concentrations of only 1–2% in their culture medium in order to grow, whereas normal cells require 5–10-fold higher concentrations.

Each of these effects is in some way associated with the availability in the culture of polypeptide hormones and growth factors. Thus normal cells may show anchorage-independent growth if appropriate growth factors are added to the medium. Density-dependent inhibition is most likely due to local depletion of growth-promoting substances in the medium adjacent to the cells, and the serum requirements of normal cells can be provided by synthetic media with an appropriate balance of growth factors and hormones.

Growth Factors

The fact that normal and transformed cells have different growth requirements has given rise to the suggestion that 'autocrine secretion' of growth factors may be involved in the uncontrolled growth of tumour cells (Figure 9). Thus, rather than receiving growth factors from a distant site in the body by an 'endocrine' mechanism, or from adjacent cells by a 'paracrine' mechanism, it is suggested that malignant cells stimulate themselves to grow by producing and responding to their own growth factors.

In culture, transformed cells would secrete and respond to their own growth factors rather than being dependent on growth factors in serum. In order to be able to respond to growth factors, cells must possess specific cell surface receptors for those factors.

The growth of normal cells is regulated by the interaction of several polypeptide growth factors and hormones that are present in blood and tissue fluids. Examples of these are epidermal growth factor (EGF), insulin and the insulin-like growth factors (IGFs) or somatomedins, fibroblast growth factor (FGF), nerve growth factor (NGF), and a number of lymphokines, which are substances that regulate growth and differentiation in the immune system. The latter include colony-stimulating factors (CSFs), interleukins (ILs), tumour necrosis factors (TNFs) and interferons (IFs) (Table 2).

Two types of tumour-associated growth factors have been described—*transforming growth factors* α and β (TGFα and β). TGFα, a polypeptide consisting of 48 amino acids, was first detected in association with virally transformed cells, and has since been shown to be produced by human cancer cells that also have receptors for it. This peptide is structurally related to EGF and binds to EGF receptors. It is able to induce anchorage-independent growth of normal fibroblasts. The relationship between TGF and transformation was demonstrated by transforming cells with temperature-sensitive viruses. It was found that TGFα was produced only when the cells were grown at the temperature necessary for transformation. It now appears, however, that TGFα has a role in normal foetal development.

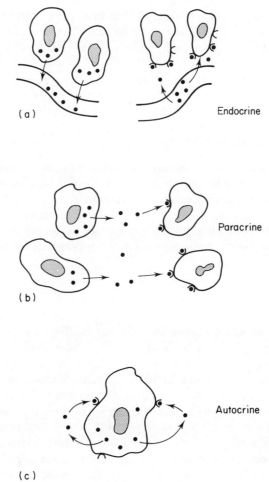

Figure 9. Stimulation of cell growth by hormones and growth factors. (a) Endocrine stimulation. A hormone is secreted into the bloodstream at one site in the body and transported to other sites where it interacts with cells that have specific surface receptors for it. (b) Paracrine stimulation. Cells release a growth factor which interacts with nearby receptor-bearing cells. (c) Autocrine. A cell releases a growth factor that binds to specific sites on its own membrane

TGFβ was also discovered in medium conditioned by transformed cells, but it is quite distinct from TGFα. It is a homodimer (two identical peptide chains) of 109 amino acids. It has been demonstrated in tumour and in normal tissues, and is expressed at specific times in normal development, when it appears to stimulate elaboration of extracellular matrix. Cells that respond to it have specific TGFβ receptors. TGFβ is not mitogenic for cultured cells unless EGF is present in the medium, so that the action of these two growth factors is synergistic. Under some conditions TGFβ can act as an autocrine growth inhibitor rather than a mitogen, and thus has a variety of effects in growth control and differentiation.

A good illustration of the autocrine hypothesis in cell transformation is provided by the PDGF-related product of the oncogene of simian sarcoma virus (SSV) known as

Table 2. Some polypeptide growth factors of interest in transformation

Growth factor	Characteristics
Epidermal growth factor (EGF)	Mitogenic in many cell types, including non-epithelial cells. Abnormal expression of receptor in some tumours
Transforming growth factor I (TFG)	From transformed cells and tumours. Promotes anchorage-independent growth. Homology with EGF. Binds to EGF receptor
Transforming growth factor II (TGF β)	From transformed cells and normal tissues. Mitogenic only in presence of EGF or TGF. Distinct receptor. Inhibits growth of some cells
Platelet-derived growth factor (PDGF)	From platelets. Present in serum. Mitogenic in wound repair
Bombesin	Small cell carcinoma of lung. Autocrine mechanism
Lymphokines	
Colony-stimulating factors (CSFs)	Growth and differentiation of leucocytes. Promote differentiation and inhibit proliferation of leukaemic cells
Interleukin 2 (IL2)	Mitogen of T-cells. Abnormal expression of IL2 in some T-cell tumours
Tumour necrosis factors (TNFs)	From macrophages. Induces tumour necrosis. Growth factor in fibroblasts
Interferon β (INF β)	Growth inhibitory in some cells. Production induced by other growth factors

$p28^{sis}$ (p = protein; 28 = relative molecular mass of protein $\times 10^{-3}$; sis = designation of oncogene). This protein is almost identical to the 109 N-terminal amino acid residues of the β-chain of PDGF. (PDGF can be a heterodimer consisting of an A and B chain, or a homodimer consisting either of two A or two B chains.) PDGF-like molecules are produced by human osteosarcomas and gliomas, probably the products of *c-sis* genes, and many of the cells that produce them have functional PDGF receptors.

Bombesin is a small peptide (14 amino acids) that is produced by human small cell lung cancers (oat cell carcinoma), the cells of which also possess specific receptors for the peptide. The growth of small cell lung cancer cells in tissue culture is stimulated by bombesin, and this effect can be inhibited by a monoclonal antibody which recognizes the C-terminal of the peptide and blocks binding of the peptide to its receptor. Growth of the tumour cells in nude mice can also be inhibited by injection of the antibody.

This example provides both a clear demonstration of the autocrine hypothesis and an illustration of the potential of antibodies or other growth factor antagonists for therapy.

Among the lymphokines, therapeutic possibilities may be envisaged for the CSFs (which inhibit growth and promote differentiation of leukaemic cells), the TNFs (which cause tumour necrosis but are also mitogens for fibroblasts) and interferons (which appear to have autocrine growth inhibitory effects in addition to anti-viral action).

The autocrine hypothesis
Normal and transforming growth factors

Action of Growth Factors

The first step in the action of polypeptide hormones and growth factors is binding to specific glycoprotein receptors on the cell surface. One way in which growth may be promoted in certain tumour cells is by overexpression of growth factor receptors, e.g. EGF receptors on squamous carcinoma cells from head and neck cancers and on A431 vulval carcinoma cells, and IL2 receptors in leukaemia. Binding of a peptide to its receptor initiates a process of transmembrane signalling by a number of different pathways. In this way the effect of the polypeptide, be it growth stimulation or inhibition of growth or some other response, is transmitted to the inside of the cell. It is not known precisely how growth factors influence cell division, but something is known about the mechanisms of membrane transduction of extracellular signals, which are important in relation to the possible actions of oncogenes.

The binding of many hormones to their receptors results in activation of an enzyme called adenylate cyclase, which is associated with the inner aspect of the plasma membrane (Figure 10a). This enzyme mediates the production of cyclic AMP (cAMP), an important intracellular signalling compound, from ATP. Interaction between the hormone receptor and the enzyme is mediated by a so-called G-protein that has GTPase activity (i.e. converts GTP to GDP). The cAMP produced as a result of occupancy of the receptor by the hormone diffuses into the cytoplasm, where it activates enzymes known as cAMP-dependent protein kinases. These are enzymes that bring about the phosphorylation of proteins by adding phosphate groups to specific serine and threonine residues, and thereby modify the action of the protein that is phosphorylated. The phosphorylated proteins, often enzymes, are the mediators of the intracellular effects of the hormones.

Some growth factors—PDGF, EGF and bombesin—use a different transmembrane signalling system, the inositol-lipid pathway (Figure 10b). Here, binding of the peptide to the receptor results in activation, via a G-protein, of a phospholipase enzyme that cleaves a lipid, called phosphatidylinositol (PI), to diacylglycerol (DAG) and inositol

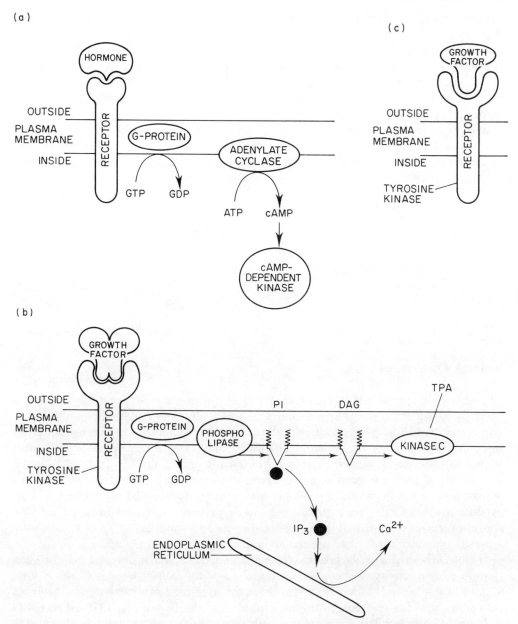

Figure 10. Mechanisms of transmembrane signalling via hormone and growth factor receptors. (a) A hormone binds to a surface receptor triggering the activation of adenylate cyclase, via a G-protein, to produce cAMP. The cAMP diffuses into the cytoplasm to regulate the activity of a cAMP-dependent protein kinase. (b) Growth factor binding to a receptor stimulates, via a G-protein and a phospholipase, the cleavage of phosphatidylinositol (PI) to diacylgylcerol (DAG) and inositol triphosphate (IP_3). DAG activates protein kinase C while IP_3 induces Ca^{2+} release from endoplasmic reticulum. Kinase C is also activated by the tumour promotor TPA. Note that the growth factor receptor bears intrinsic tyrosine kinase activity in its cytoplasmic domain. (c) Binding of a growth factor to the external domain of a receptor activates intrinsic receptor tyrosine kinase activity on the cytoplasmic side of the membrane

triphosphate (IP_3). Both DAG and IP_3 have important signalling roles. DAG remains associated with the membrane where it activates another phosphorylating enzyme, protein kinase C. IP_3 diffuses into the cytoplasm where it causes release of bound intracellular Ca^{2+} from the endoplasmic reticulum and a consequent rise in intracellular Ca^{2+} concentration. Ca^{2+} has important intracellular regulatory functions, mediating the activity of Ca^{2+} binding proteins such as calmodulin, which itself is a modulator of protein and enzyme activity.

EGF does not appear to use the PI pathway. However, the EGF receptor, which like many other membrane receptors is a transmembrane protein, has intrinsic protein kinase activity in its cytoplasmic portion (Figure 10c). In this case the phosphorylating activity is specific for the amino acid tyrosine. Occupancy of the EGF receptor results in enhanced tyrosine phosphorylation within the cell. Intrinsic tyrosine kinase activity is also present in the PDGF and insulin-like growth factor receptors.

Transmembrane signalling
Cell surface receptors
Cyclic AMP, phosphatidylinositol, protein kinases

Role of Oncogenes

The above account of cell surface receptors and transmembrane signalling provides a basis for considering the possible modes of action of some oncogenes that seem to affect the signalling processes involved in growth promotion. Beginning with the receptor component of the signalling pathway, one oncogene in particular has been shown to code for an altered receptor. The v-erbB gene codes for an EGF receptor that does not bind the growth factor because it lacks both part of its extracellular domain and a small part of its cytoplasmic domain. Because of this defect it may produce a continuous growth promoting signal. In some types of human cancer (see above) overexpression of EGF receptors may contribute towards malignancy: however, a v-erbB type mechanism has not so far been detected in human cancer.

Significantly, the v-erbB protein retains the domain responsible for its intrinsic tyrosine kinase activity. Many other oncogenes code for membrane-associated tyrosine kinases (Table 3) and, as has been already noted, tyrosine kinase activity is associated with other proteins that give mitogenic stimuli, i.e. the PDGF and FGF receptors.

Tyrosine phosphorylation normally accounts for only about 0.01% of the phosphoamino acids in cells and yet there are a number of tyrosine kinase genes that are related to cell transformation, suggesting that tyrosine kinase activity is an important cell regulating mechanism.

The oncogenes in the group that includes fos, myb and myc encode nuclear proteins. Transcription of fos and myc mRNA follows rapidly upon stimulation of cells with PDGF—fos within 30 minutes and myc within 4 hours. Treatment of cells with tumour promotors (e.g. TPA) also induces transcription of these genes; this suggests a pathway by which activation occurs, because TPA is an activator of protein kinase C, the

Table 3. Cellular location and function of protein products of oncogenes

Gene	Location of protein product	Function of product
sis	Extracellular	Truncated PDGF
abl	Plasma membrane	Tyrosine kinase
erbB	Plasma membrane	Tyrosine kinase
fes/fps	Plasma membrane	Tyrosine kinase
fgr	Plasma membrane	Tyrosine kinase
fms	Plasma membrane	Tyrosine kinase
met	Plasma membrane	Tyrosine kinase
neu	Plasma membrane	Tyrosine kinase
src	Plasma membrane	Tyrosine kinase
yes	Plasma membrane	Tyrosine kinase
Ha-ras	Plasma membrane	GTP-ase
Ki-ras	Plasma membrane	GTP-ase
N-ras	Plasma membrane	GTP-ase
mil	Cytoplasm	Serine kinase
raf	Cytoplasm	Serine kinase
fos	Nucleus	DNA binding
myb	Nucleus	
myc	Nucleus	
p53	Nucleus	

phosphorylating enzyme that is normally activated by DAG after PI cleavage following ligand binding to the PDGF receptor (see Figure 10b). The *fos* and *myc* proteins are DNA-binding proteins. A correlation between growth, differentiation and *myc* expression has been found in the HL60 promyelocytic cell line, namely high expression during growth and low expression in the differentiated state. These observations suggest that loss of growth control may result from abnormal expression of these genes.

The remaining group of oncogenes is the *ras* family. These encode proteins ($p21^{ras}$) that are membrane associated, possess GTP binding and GTPase activity, and show sequence homology with G-proteins. It seems probable therefore that $p21^{ras}$ is part of the G-protein family and that point mutations (see above) may bring about constitutive stimulation of transmembrane signalling systems—the cyclic AMP system, the PI system or some other growth-related mechanism.

In summary, the abnormal growth of cancer cells may result from one or any combination of a number of factors:

- autocrine secretion of a growth factor
- overexpression of growth factor receptors
- loss of growth inhibition
- malfunction of some transmembrane-intracellular signalling process

The study of growth factors and oncogenes is beginning to provide an understanding of these processes and should lead to a variety of possibilities for inhibiting uncontrolled growth *in vivo*.

The Spread of Cancer: Invasion and Metastasis

Malignant cells are characterized by their capacity to invade the tissue which surrounds them and to spread to distant parts of the body to generate secondary growths. It is this latter property, known as metastasis, that makes cancer so difficult to treat by surgical and radiotherapeutic means, and which makes early detection so vital. Invasion and metastasis are complex and ill-understood processes that probably depend on a number of contributory mechanisms which differ between tumour types.

The development of an *epithelial tumour* (about 90% of human cancers are epithelium-derived tumours or carcinomas) usually proceeds according to the following generalized schemes (Figure 11). A normal epithelium consists of one to several organized layers of cells. At the basal surface of the epithelium the cells are attached to a basement membrane, which overlies a connective tissue stroma penetrated by small blood vessels and lymphatics. The stroma is attached to other tissues, frequently a layer of muscle.

Premalignant and early malignant changes occur within the epithelium itself leading to formation of a localized tumour, a carcinoma *in situ*. Invasion begins when tumour cells penetrate through the basement membrane and into the underlying stroma. This invasion eventually becomes very extensive. For example, in advanced colorectal carcinoma a tumour may penetrate completely through the wall of the bowel.

Once invasion has begun, the possibility exists for tumour cells to penetrate into lymphatics or blood vessels. Here, if they lose contact with the primary tumour, they will be transported to other sites. Thus metastasis is initiated. Metastasis consists of a series of steps, sometimes referred to as the metastatic cascade:

- release of cells from the primary tumour
- dissemination of cells via lymphatics, blood vessels or body cavities
- arrest of cells, usually in small blood vessels
- extravasation or penetration of cells through vessel walls and into the surrounding tissues
- survival and growth of cells at the secondary site

Invasion

The initial step in carcinomatous invasion is penetration of the basement membrane, a lamellar structure consisting principally of type IV collagen, the glycoprotein laminin, and heparan sulphate proteoglycan. It may also contain another glycoprotein, fibronectin, which together with other collagen types and proteoglycans, is always a major constituent of the stromal extracellular matrix beneath the basement membrane. Epithelial cells possess specific membrane receptors that mediate adhesion to these various matrix components. Below normal epithelia the basement membrane is continuous, but adjacent to invading carcinoma cells it is commonly found to be reduced or absent.

This may be due to decreased synthesis or abnormal assembly of components, or degradation of basement membrane. Tumour cells generally release a variety of *lytic enzymes*, including a number of proteases. Among these are:

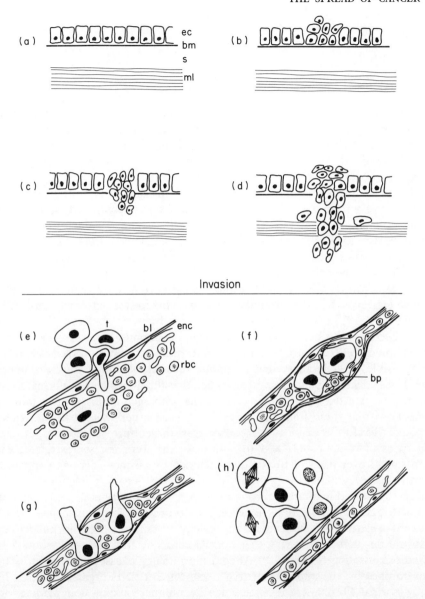

Invasion

Metastasis

Figure 11. Invasion and metastasis. (a) Normal epithelial cells (ec) form an organized layer attached to a basement membrane (bm) above a stroma (s) of extracellular matrix and a muscle layer (ml). (b) Some of the cells have undergone malignant change, forming a carcinoma *in situ*. (c) Carcinoma cells have penetrated the bm and invaded the s. (d) Extensive invasion has taken place so that the cells have penetrated the ml. (e) Invading tumour cells (t) penetrate the bl of the blood vessel endothelial cells (enc) and enter the blood to be transported to other sites. (f) Some tumour cells, associated with aggregated blood platelets (bp) have become arrested in a small blood vessel in a tissue distant from the original tumour. (g) The tumour cells penetrate the endothelial lining of the small blood vessel and extravasate. (h) Tumour cells multiply in a 'fertile soil' to initiate a secondary tumour

- plasminogen activator, which cleaves plasminogen in plasma to
  its active form
- plasmin
- cathepsins
- a specific type IV collagenase

It is likely that these enzymes are of great importance at several stages during invasion and metastasis, including degradation of the basement membrane at the onset of invasion, subsequent penetration of the extracellular matrix, detachment of cells and cell clumps from the primary tumour to initiate metastasis and degradation of the basement membrane of small vessels at extravasation.

Another mechanism that may contribute to the invasive activity of some tumours is *mechanical pressure* resulting from increase in bulk due to uncontrolled growth. However, there are several pieces of evidence to suggest that this is rarely the sole cause of invasion: benign tumours often grow faster than malignant tumours; some types of tumours metastasize when they are still small; and inhibition of DNA synthesis in tumour cells has been shown not to prevent invasion in culture.

A third factor in malignant invasion may be *increased motility* of tumour cells, which may move actively into the surrounding matrix. This idea is extremely difficult to test *in vivo*, but arises from a number of observations. In sections of tumours, single cells that have become detached from the tumour are commonly found in the surrounding matrix. Tumour cells in culture can be seen to move actively into tissues and, though it is impossible to generalize, many tumour cells show altered motile properties in culture. It was demonstrated over 30 years ago that the movement of normal fibroblasts in culture was arrested when they made contact with each other (contact inhibition of movement) so that their ability to spread over each other was greatly restricted and they would therefore remain as a monolayer on the culture substratum. In contrast, certain types of tumour cells and transformed cells were not so restricted, enabling them to spread over parts of the culture occupied by normal cells or to spread on top of them.

The reasons for this altered behaviour shown by some tumour cells are not fully understood, but some indications are emerging from studies of transformed fibroblasts. These cells usually show abnormal morphology in culture; they do not flatten onto the substratum in the same way that normal cells do, and they may show a lack of polarized organization (Figure 12). Altered morphology is associated with: loss of cell surface fibronectin, the adhesive matrix glycoprotein that is organized into a fibrillar array by normal fibroblasts; reduction in the number of adhesion plaques or focal contacts which the cells form with the substratum; and disorganization of the actin cytoskeletal stress fibres which insert into the cytoplasmic faces of the adhesion plaques (Figure 13). These observations suggest that the transformed cells are less adhesive than their normal counterparts, and this may enable them to move more readily and to climb on top of each other. In cells transformed with the Rous sarcoma virus (RSV) it has been found that the *pp60*[src] tyrosine kinase protein localizes to the adhesion plaques, suggesting that phosphorylation of some component of the adhesion plaques by this oncogene product may bring about the disorganization.

Tyrosine phosphorylation of three components of the adhesion plaques has been demonstrated. These are the transmembrane glycoprotein, integrin, which is the cell surface

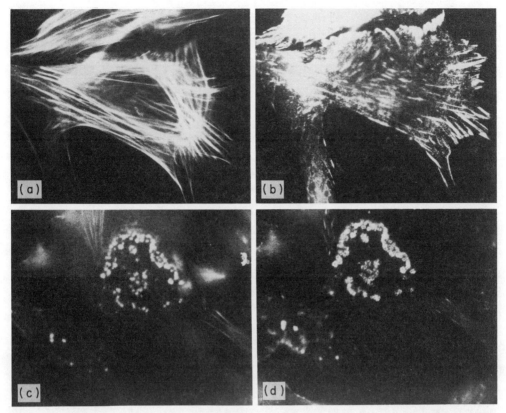

Figure 12. Morphology of normal and transformed cells in culture. (a) Normal fibroblasts adopt a flattened, well-spread shape on a substratum. Their cytoplasm is characterized by a well-ordered cytoskeleton, part of which consists of stress fibres, mainly comprised of actin. (b) At their distal ends many of their stress fibres insert into adhesion plaques or focal contacts. These are regions where the underside of the cell is very close (<10 nm) to the substratum. Fluorescent antibody staining shows that the proteins vinculin and talin, and the glycoprotein/integrin, the fibronectin receptor, are localized in focal contacts—points at which the cell adheres to the extracellular matrix. (c) Transformed fibroblasts generally show less flattened morphology than normal fibroblasts, have a less well-organized cytoskeleton and fewer adhesion plaques. (d) In fibroblasts transformed by RSV, the *pp60*^{src} protein can be localized to the adhesion plaques by fluorescent antibody staining. (Photographs provided by Dr S. Kellie, Department of Biochemistry, Royal College of Surgeons and reproduced by permission)

receptor involved in adhesion to fibronectin, and two cytoplasmic proteins, talin and vinculin, which are involved in attachment between the membrane receptors and the actin stress fibres. It has also recently been shown that increased activity of the *c-src* gene can reduce intercellular adhesiveness of epithelial cells. Tyrosine kinase activity therefore affects cell shape, adhesion and motility, as well as cell growth control (see above).

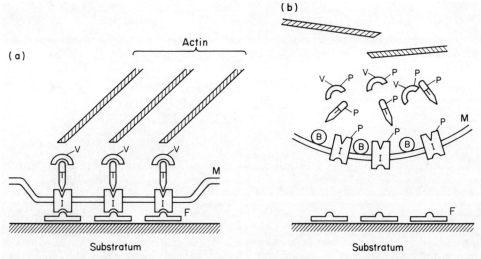

Figure 13. Diagram to show possible structure of adhesion plaque in normal and RSV-transformed fibroblasts. (a) In the normal cell the well-ordered actin stress fibre inserts into the inner face of the plaque where vinculin (V), talin (T) and integrin (I) interact. Integrin, a transmembrane glycoprotein, binds to fibronectin (F), which is adsorbed to the tissue culture substratum, thus mediating adhesion. (b) In the cell transformed by RSV, the *pp60*[src] protein (B) is localized to the inner leaflet of the plasma membrane (M) in the region of the plaque. The other plaque components have been phosphorylated (P) by the tyrosine kinase activity of *pp60*[src] resulting in disorganization of the plaque, reduced adhesion and disruption of the stress fibres. Reproduced by permission of Dr S. Kellie and Cambridge University Press

---

Invasion

Cell adhesion—extracellular matrix
Lytic enzymes
Mechanical pressure
Cell motility

Metastasis

Reduced cell adhesion may be responsible for release of cells from the primary tumour into lymphatics, blood vessels or other body cavities at the onset of metastasis, but experimental proof of this is not yet available. An important factor in cell release from solid tumours appears to be *tumour necrosis*. There are clinical data to suggest association between tumour necrosis, invasion and presence of tumour cells in the blood, and some experimental results suggest that cells are more readily released from necrotic tumours than from non-necrotic tissue. Necrosis may arise from: release of lytic enzymes by the tumour cells themselves or from invading lymphoid cells; from tumour necrosis factors; from vascular insufficiency in the centre of a rapidly growing tumour; or even from tumour cell death as a response to radiotherapy or chemotherapy. Release of tumour cells may also be promoted by mechanical factors such as blood flow in veins, muscular activity, and clinical examination and treatment.

Although it is a crucial step in the metastatic cascade, release of cells from primary tumours does not determine how many metastatic tumours will form. On the contrary, *metastasis is an extremely inefficient process*. It has been estimated that enormous numbers (many millions) of cells may be released into the circulation from primary tumours each day and yet relatively few metastatic deposits will form. It has also been shown in experimental studies that when cancer cells are introduced into the venous circulation of mice, the majority of them are very rapidly trapped in the capillary bed of the lungs but less than 1% of them remain after 24 hours. The reason for this is not understood, but death of trapped cells may occur through a variety of causes, such as mechanical stress imposed by the circulation, poor nutrition, toxicity due to high oxygen levels (which will be considerably above those in the tissues where the cells originated), or immunological effects such as provided by T-lymphocytes, polymorphs, macrophages and natural-killer cells. Thus *the circulation is a very hostile environment for tumour cells*.

Metastasis—cell adhesion, necrosis
Inefficiency

What Determines Where Metastases Will Develop?

The most common sites of occurrence of secondary tumours in human cancer are the lungs, liver, lymph nodes and brain. However, some tumours apparently show preferential metastasis to certain sites, e.g. prostatic carcinoma to bone, and melanoma of the eye to liver.

One view of metastasis suggests that the site of secondary tumour formation is determined principally by *haemodynamic factors* because the vast majority of tumour cells, both single cells and cell clumps, are most likely to be trapped in the small capillaries of the organs that they encounter first. This organ will be the lungs for tumour cells that enter blood draining into the vena cava, and the liver for tumour cells entering the hepatic portal system. (Lymph nodes appear to be the predominant site of entrapment of cells that enter the lymphatic system.)

An alternative view is the so-called 'seed and soil' hypothesis in which differential survival of tumour cells is supposed to occur, so that tumour cells of a given type, though distributed to many organs, will survive and grow only where local conditions (nutrition, growth factors, oxygen tension) are suitable.

In all probability both of these considerations are important for most tumours, while the 'seed and soil' hypothesis may account for cases of apparently highly specific metastasis. It has been suggested that specific adhesion of tumour cells to the capillary endothelium may account for organ specificity of metastasis. However, this seems unlikely, except in the case of some lymphomas whose cells may have organ-specific adhesion receptors.

Arrested tumour cells are frequently found to be associated with fibrin and aggregates of blood platelets. This may occur either because the tumour cells become arrested by emboli already formed in association with damaged endothelium or because the tumour cells themselves promote platelet aggregation and embolus formation. Platelet aggregation is controlled by the antagonistic action of two prostaglandins, prostacyclin (which is produced by endothelial cells and is inhibitory) and thromboxane (which is produced by platelets and stimulates aggregation. Damage to endothelium would promote aggregation by reducing prostacyclin, while some circulating tumour cells have been shown to promote platelet aggregation.

Drugs that promote prostacyclin synthesis or inhibit thromboxane synthesis have anti-metastatic effects in experimental systems, but results with 'anticoagulants' such as aspirin are contradictory. The possible importance of embolus formation in metastasis has been suggested by experiments in which fibrinolytic agents have been shown to reduce the incidence of metastasis, whereas anti-fibrinolytic agents may promote metastasis. Adhesion of tumour cells to the endothelial basement membrane may be a determinative step in the extravasation process. Some experimental work has centred around the role of the laminin receptor in this adhesion. Monoclonal antibodies against the laminin receptor have been shown to inhibit attachment of human melanoma and colon carcinoma cells to basement membranes *in vitro*, and in experimental animals the metastasis of tumour cells specially selected for adhesion to laminin (as opposed to other extracellular matrix components) can be inhibited by blocking the laminin receptor. More recently, short peptides derived from the regions of fibronectin and laminin that bind to the cell receptors for these matrix components have been shown to inhibit metastasis in experimental systems. The peptides are composed of the amino acids Arg-Gly-Asp in the case of fibronectin, and Tyr-Ile-Gly-Ser-Arg in the case of laminin.

Development of metastases
Haemodynamics
Cell adhesion
'Seed and soil'
Fibrin—platelets—prostaglandins

Extravasation of tumour cells requires penetration through the endothelial cell layer, the endothelial basement membrane, and into the surrounding tissue. The lytic enzymes produced by tumour cells may be crucially important in this process too, as they may be in the initiation of invasion and metastasis.

Once tumour cells have penetrated into the tissue beneath the basement membrane, local conditions presumably determine whether or not they will proliferate to form large secondary tumours. Little information is available concerning factors that determine this. However, if secondary tumours are to grow beyond a certain size they will require a blood supply. It has been shown that some tumours produce angiogenesis factors that promote the growth of blood vessels into them.

Extravasation
Lytic enzymes
Angiogenesis factors

Much work on the experimental analysis of metastasis in animals has depended upon selection of cell lines with high metastatic potential. While such work has produced much interesting data, highly selected cell lines may bear little resemblance to the original tumours and even less to metastatic cells in human cancer. On the other hand, genetic instability in human solid tumours may generate metastatic cell populations that differ in properties from those of the cells of the original tumour. There has also been a report that transfecting non-metastatic cells with DNA from a human metastatic tumour confers metastatic potential, but metastasis cannot yet be ascribed to any particular biochemical property. There are essentially three models for tumour metastasis. These are not mutually exclusive and may apply to different tumours:

- Metastasis is a random event depending only on random survival of tumour cells.
- Tumours contain a population (probably very small) of metastatic cells.
- A small population of metastatic cells might be in dynamic equilibrium with a non-metastatic cell population so that cells would express metastatic properties during the process of metastasis but non-metastatic properties would be re-established as the secondary tumour grows.

If the third model were correct, it would greatly increase the difficulty of determining what cellular properties are crucial for metastasis.

Acknowledgements

I thank Dr Terry Kenny and Professor Peter Alexander for thorough and constructive criticism of the manuscript.

Selected Papers and Reviews

Berridge, N.J. (1986) Cell signalling through phospholipid metabolism. In A.V. Grimstone, H. Harris and R.T. Johnson (eds), 'Prospects in cell biology'. *J. Cell Sci.* (Suppl.), **4:** 137–153.

British Medical Journal (1988) *Basic Molecular and Cell Biology*. BMJ Publications, London.

Franks, L. M., and Teich, N. (eds.) (1986) *Introduction to the Cellular and Molecular Biology of Cancer*. Oxford Scientific Publications, Oxford, New York, Tokyo.

Harris, H. (1988) The analysis of malignancy by cell fusion: the position in 1988. *Cancer Research*, **48**: 3302–3306.

Kellie, S. (1988) Cellular transformation, tyrosine kinase oncogenes, and the cellular adhesion plaque. *BioEssays* **8**: 25–30.

Marshall, C. J. (1986) Oncogenes. *J. Cell. Sci.* (Suppl.), **4**: 417–430.

Sporn, M. B. and Roberts, A. B. (1985) Autocrine growth factors and cancer. *Nature*, **313**: 745–747.

Tannock, I. F. and Hill, R. P. (eds.) (1987) *The Basic Science of Oncology*. Pergamon Press, New York.

3 Environmental Causes of Cancer

C. J. WILLIAMS

Epidemiology is the study of the frequency of a disease in populations living in different conditions and in different parts of the world. It has given many clues to the causes of cancer and in some cases has suggested strategies for avoiding environmentally caused cancers. Thus the real importance of the search for 'environmentally related' cancers is that some may turn out to be avoidable. This possibility has been assessed by Doll and Peto (1981) in their monograph on the causes of cancer in the United States of America. Their assessment of the importance of environmental causes of cancer was based on several different types of information, which are considered below.

Variations in Incidence of Cancer Around the World

The cancer incidence[*] and mortality[†] of different communities in different parts of the world have been studied for most of this century. In Britain cancer causes a very significant proportion of deaths at all ages (Figure 1). Although efficiency in diagnosis and reporting may vary considerably, useful data may be accumulated. This will still be severely affected by the age distribution of the population under study. However, this can be overcome by studying specific age groups or by using standardized populations adjusted for age. International agencies have collated this type of data and have shown an extraordinarily large variation in the incidence of certain tumours in different parts of the world (Table 1).

As can be seen, this ratio of variation from highest to lowest is never less than 6 and in some cases is more than 100. Whilst some of the variation may be artifactual, as discussed above, the true range of variation may be even greater as many parts of the world have not been studied: the least developed areas are not amenable to study

---

[*] The *incidence* (rate) is the total number of new cases of a cancer reported per year.
[†] The *mortality* or *death* (rate) ignores the non-fatal cases (per year).

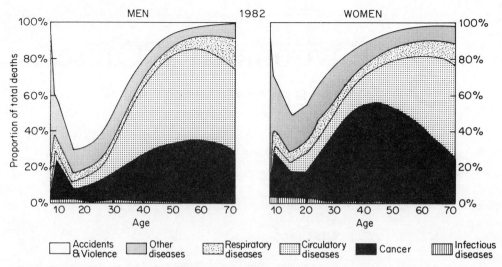

Figure 1. The importance of various causes of death (1982). The proportion of deaths from varying causes are plotted according to age. From *Living with Risk* (1987) B.M.A. Guide. Wiley, Chichester; reproduced by permission

but are likely to give the largest contrasts with developed countries. Although there is a very wide range of variation for individual tumours, the overall incidence of cancer in different communities varies much less. Examination of Table 1 shows that a country may have the highest incidence of one tumour and the lowest of another; for example, England is highest for lung and lowest for liver and nasopharynx. Because of this, the variation in overall cancer rate around the world is only about three-fold.

Apart from skin cancer, where the risk is much greater in people with little skin pigmentation, it does not seem that the large variation in cancer incidence from community to community is caused by genetic factors. One way of examining for this is to study the incidence of cancer in people migrating from one community to another.

Changes in Incidence of Cancer on Migration

Changes in the incidence of cancer in people migrating from one part of the world to another would be good evidence of a non-genetic factor in the causation of that tumour. However, good data are hard to come by because:

- The migrants may intermarry with the host population.
- Prolonged data collection is needed since the migrants require time to adopt the 'habits' of the local population.
- The migrating population needs to come from a clearly defined community.

Study of cancer incidence in the Black population in the United States might seem a promising exercise, since good data on cancer incidence are available, but this has not proven to be the case. Unfortunately, the ancestors of Blacks taken to North

Table 1. Incidence rates of the common cancers in men and at certain sites restricted to women. Reproduced by permission from R. Doll and R. Peto (1981). *The Causes of Cancer.* Oxford University Press, Oxford

Primary site	Cumulative incidence* (%) in highest incidence area	Highest incidence area	Ratio of highest rate to lowest rate†	Lowest area
Skin	>20	Australia, Queensland	>200	India, Bombay
Oesophagus	20	Iran, northeast	300	Nigeria
Lung, bronchus	11	England	35	Nigeria
Stomach	11	Japan	25	Uganda
Uterine cervix	10	Colombia	15	Israel, Jewish
Prostrate	9	USA, Blacks	40	Japan
Liver	8	Mozambique	100	England
Breast	7	Canada, British Columbia	7	Israel, non-Jewish
Colon	3	USA, Connecticut	10	Nigeria
Uterine corpus	3	USA, California	30	Japan
Buccal cavity	2	India, Bombay	25	Denmark
Rectum	2	Denmark	20	Nigeria
Bladder	2	USA, Connecticut	6	Japan
Ovary	2	Denmark	6	Japan
Nasopharynx	2	Singapore, Chinese	40	England

*By age 75 yr, in absence of death from other cause.
†By ages 35–64 yr, standardized for age as in International Agency for Research on Cancer (1976).

America as slaves came from parts of Africa with different patterns of cancer. In addition, intermarriage has taken place with the local inhabitants.

The best available data come from comparison of cancer rates in Japanese living in Hawaii and in Japan. A large population of Japanese moved to Hawaii at the turn of the century. They have not intermarried, but have adopted many Western habits. This allows a comparison between the incidence of cancer among the Japanese in Japan and that among Hawaiian Japanese, as well as with that among Caucasians in Hawaii (Table 2).

Table 2 shows that for every type of cancer, apart from lung, the incidence in Hawaiian Japanese was more like that in the local Caucasians than in Japanese in Japan. Such data strongly suggest that environmental factors play a major part in cancer causation.

Table 2. Comparison of cancer incidence in native Japanese and in Japanese and Caucasians in Hawaii. Reproduced by permission from R. Doll and R. Peto (1981) *The Causes of Cancer*. Oxford University Press, Oxford

Site of cancer	Sex	Annual incidence per million people		
		Japan	Hawaii	
			Japanese	Caucasians
Breast	F	335	1221	1869
Uterine cervix	F	329	149	243
Colon	M	78	371	368
Uterine corpus	F	32	407	714
Lung	M	237	379	962
Oesophagus	M	150	46	75
Ovary	F	51	160	274
Prostate	M	14	154	343
Rectum	M	95	297	204
Stomach	M	150	46	75

Changes in Cancer Incidence Over Time

Since the genetic make-up of a population cannot change substantially over a short time-span, major changes in the incidence of cancer in a population over time are good evidence of an environmental cause. Such data are not easy to collect as the accuracy of diagnosis and efficiency of data collection may have also changed with time. However,there are good international data on major changes of incidence for several common tumours. Two tumours that have changed dramatically in incidence in the last 3–4 decades are stomach and lung cancer (Table 3).

In the time period studied stomach cancer decreased in incidence universally whilst lung cancer became more common. These data conclusively implicate environmental factors, though these may of course operate together with genetic factors.

More recently, there is evidence of a worldwide increase in malignant germ cell tumours in industrialized countries. This is well shown by data from Denmark, where accurate data have been collected (Figure 2).

Identification of the Causes of Cancer

It often seems that everything causes cancer, but in general this feeling is based on circumstantial evidence since the appropriate scientific experiments are not possible. In many of the cases where there is information, this has come from industrial exposure (e.g. asbestos), though occupational cancers are relatively uncommon (Table 4). Examination of the role of potential carcinogens (e.g. tobacco smoke) in the general population has helped elucidate the cause of several human cancers, though the cause of many malignant tumours remains unknown.

Table 3. Changes in the incidence of lung and stomach cancer around the world (1950–1975)

Country	Percent change in mortality*	
	Stomach cancer	Lung cancer
Australia	−53	+146
Chile	−56	+38
Denmark	−62	+87
England and Wales	−49	+33
Ireland	−54	+177
Japan	−37	+408
Netherlands	−60	+89
Norway	−59	+118
Switzerland	−64	+72
United States	−61	+148

*Since nearly all patients with these tumours die these figures approximate to incidence.

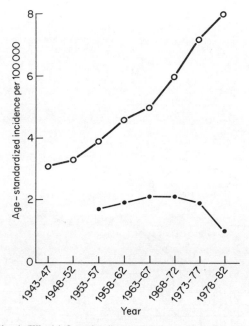

Figure 2. Age-standardized (World Standard) average annual incidence rates (○) and mortality rates (●) of testicular cancer in Denmark, 1943–1982. Reproduced by permission from A. Osterlind (1986) *British Journal of Cancer*, **53**: 501–505

Much has been made of the risks of radiation, food additives and other aspects of life in an industrialized society. So far, these risks appear small. For example, the National Radiological Protection Board estimate that 87% of the radiation exposure experienced by an average person is from natural sources (Figure 3). Only 1.5% was

Table 4. Cancers that can definitely be produced by occupational hazards. Reproduced by permission from R. Doll and R. Peto (1981) *The Causes of Cancer*. Oxford University Press, Oxford

Site of cancer	No. of deaths	No. of deaths ascribed to occupational hazard (%)†
Mesentery and peritoneum	1349	133 (9.9%)
Liver and bile ducts	2796	82 (2.9%)
Larynx	3459	64 (1.9%)
Lung	95,086	11,855 (12.5%)
Pleura and other airways	1353	239 (17.7%)
Bone	1737	47 (2.7%)
Skin (not melanoma)	1814	139 (6.7%)
Prostate	21,674	217 (1.0%)
Bladder	9849	831 (8.4%)
Leukaemia	15,391	1203 (7.8%)
Miscellaneous tumours	30,266	1230 (4.1%)
Total	184,774	16,022 (8.7%)

*The estimates of total occupational hazard (including those tumours with suspected or no proved risk) is 14,777 of 218,337 males (6.8%) and 2292 of 183,618 females (1.7%).

†Occupational hazards are more common in men than women: of 131,867 male deaths, 14,046 (10.7%) were ascribed to occupational hazard; the respective figures for women were 52,907 deaths with 1976 (3.7%) related to occupation.

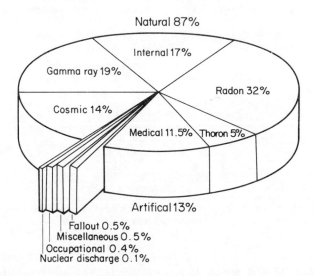

Natural 87%
Internal 17%
Gamma ray 19%
Radon 32%
Cosmic 14%
Medical 11.5%   Thoron 5%
Artifical 13%
Fallout 0.5%
Miscellaneous 0.5%
Occupational 0.4%
Nuclear discharge 0.1%

Figure 3. The overall effective dose from radiation of natural and artificial origin is about 2 mSv (200 millirems) on average. The percentage contribution of each source to the overall value is shown here. Natural radiation contributes almost 90%, with about half of that coming from radon. From *Living with Risk* (1987) B.M.A Guide. Wiley, Chichester; reproduced by permission

felt to be associated with the peaceful use of nuclear power or fall-out from atomic weapons. Similarly, the potential carcinogenic risks of food additives are likely to be far outweighed by the carcinogenicity of the 'natural' food itself or by traditional methods of preservation.

Environmental Risks

Doll and Peto have evaluated the current data and have made estimates of the importance of likely factors implicated with cancer causation in the United States (Table 5). Of these environmental factors the first three are most easily manipulated.

Smoking and Alcohol

Cigarette smoking is an extremely important cause of cancer in all parts of the respiratory and upper digestive tract as well as other diseases (see Table 6 for an assessment of the importance of the risk). Its effect on cancers of the larynx and oesophagus is also largely dependent on alcohol consumption. It seems that the effects of smoking and alcohol on these two sites are synergistic (i.e. they are more than additive). If the risk for a non-smoker, non-drinker is 1.0:

- the risk of a non-drinking smoker of 20/day is 1.7
- the risk of a non-smoking drinker of 100 g of alcohol/day is 7.2
- the risk of a smoker of 20/day who drinks 100 g of alcohol/day is 12.1

Other synergistic effects of tobacco are important, especially that between asbestos exposure and smoking. Smoking is also implicated in the causation of bladder, pancreatic and probably other carcinomas.

Table 5. Best estimates of the importance of different factors in the causation of cancer in the United States. Reproduced by permission from R. Doll and R. Peto (1981) *The Causes of Cancer.* Oxford University Press, Oxford

Factor	Proportion of all cancer deaths (%)	
	Best estimate	Range of estimates
Tobacco	30	25–40
Alcohol	3	2–4
Diet	35	10–70
Food additives	< 1	−5*−+2
Sexual and reproductive behaviour	7	1–13
Occupation	4	2–8
Pollution	2	< 1–5
Industrial products	< 1	< 1–2
Medicines and medical procedures	1	0.5–3
Geophysical factors	3	2–4
Infection	10 ?	1–?
Unknown	?	?

*Allowing for a protective effect of antioxidants and preservatives.

Table 6. Risk of an individual dying in any one year from various causes

Cause	Risk
Smoking 10 cigarettes a day	1 in 200
All natural causes, age 40	1 in 850
Any kind of violence or poisoning	1 in 3300
Influenza	1 in 5000
Accident on the road	1 in 8000
Leukaemia	1 in 12,500
Playing soccer	1 in 25,000
Accident at home	1 in 26,000
Accident at work	1 in 43,500
Radiation while working in radiation industry	1 in 57,000
Homicide	1 in 100,000
Accident on railway	1 in 500,000
Hit by lightning	1 in 10,000,000
Release of radiation from nearby nuclear power station	1 in 10,000,000

Smoking is now declining in Britain, though there is a worrying increase in young women. Lung cancer deaths in men have peaked but in women there is still a rapid rise in the number of deaths and this has become the commonest malignant tumour killing Scottish women. Further public health education on the hazards of cigarette smoking are needed, though changes in smoking habits are most likely to follow changes in 'fashion' and developing awareness of the unsocial nature of the habit. The government has much to contribute by increasing taxation and introducing legislation on smoking in public places.

Passive smoking appears to cause a definite but small increase in the risk of non-smokers developing lung cancer. Though the risk is not large it is important since the majority of the population are exposed.

Diet

Data on the effects of diet on cancer causation vary from definite evidence to inferred evidence of a link. For instance aflatoxin, a fungal contaminant of peanuts, is clearly implicated in the development of liver cancer in certain tropical countries. Similarly, the consumption, in Japan, of bracken has been linked to oesophageal cancer. On the other hand data linking increased dietary intake of fat with breast cancer (Figure 4) has not been fully substantiated by prospective case-control studies. If such a link exists it may well be related to changes in the metabolism of sex-steroid hormones in obesity. Malignant tumours which are more common in overweight individuals include:

- breast
- endometrium
- gall bladder and bile duct
- ovary

Diet low in roughage has been associated with an increased risk of large bowel cancer; the link remains attractive but so far unproved. Consumption of large amounts

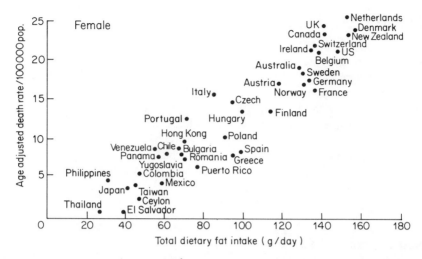

Figure 4. Correlation between breast cancer mortality and fat consumption in various countries. Reproduced by permission from Carroll, K.K. (1975) *Cancer Research*, **35**: 3374–3383

of nitrate and nitrite appear to increase the risk of upper gastrointestinal cancer. This risk may be reduced by consuming vitamin C, which may be able to reduce the formation of nitrosamines, powerful carcinogens, in the stomach.

- Although manipulation of diet as a way of preventing cancer holds promise, we do not have the knowledge to recommend an appropriate diet. Much information is on the crude level of simply correlating risk with dietary intake.
- An increase in vegetable and fibre consumption together with a reduction in animal fat intake may be beneficial and is unlikely to be harmful.
- Simple correlation of a cancer rate with a possible causative factor is not proof of an effect. For instance, the rising importation of bananas at the same time as an increase in lung cancer is unlikely to represent a causal link!

Oral Contraceptives

There has been much debate about the possible carcinogenic effects of oral contraceptives. The argument is not resolved and current data, based on patients receiving oral contraceptives in the past, may be irrelevant to current practice since new lower dose contraceptive pills are now used. Although some studies have suggested an increased risk of breast cancer, others have failed to substantiate this. There does, however, appear to be a *protective* effect with regard to endometrial cancer. Early age at first sexual intercourse and multiple partners are risk factors for carcinoma of the cervix uteri.

Conclusions

- Study of the patterns of cancer around the world, changes in incidence in migrants and in incidence with time all strongly suggest that many cancers have an environmental cause.
- Estimates of the importance of various environmental factors in westernized countries can be made.
- The most important factors are tobacco, diet, alcohol and sexual habits. These factors can all be easily modified to reduce risk, though there is currently insufficient information on diet.

Selected Papers and Reviews

Armstrong, B. and Doll, R. (1975) Environmental factors and cancer incidence and mortality in different countries with special reference to dietary practices. *International Journal of Cancer*, **15**: 617–631.

Doll, R. (1980) The epidemiology of cancer. *Cancer*, **45**: 2475–2495.

Doll, R. and Peto, R. (1981) *The Causes of Cancer: Quantitative Estimates of Avoidable Risks of Cancer in the United States Today.* Oxford University Press, Oxford.

Haenszel, W. and Kurihera, M. (1968) Studies of Japanese immigrants: 1. Mortality from cancer and other diseases among Japanese in the United States. *Journal of the National Cancer Institute*, **40**: 43–68.

Mould, R. F. (1983) *Cancer Statistics.* Adam Hilger, Bristol.

4 Cancer Screening

C. J. WILLIAMS

The early detection of cancer, before it has caused any symptoms, is an intrinsically attractive approach to treating cancer. The potential advantages are obvious:

- The patient is fit and well at the time of treatment.
- A precursor lesion can be treated to prevent the development of cancer.
- The cancer may be picked up when it is small, so there is the best chance that it has not spread.
- Because it has been found at an early stage, less extensive surgery is needed.
- If adjuvant chemotherapy is indicated this is more likely to be effective since the tumour burden will be small.

To the general public this all adds up to a fail-safe way of detecting cancer at a stage when '*treatment has the very best chance of producing a cure*'. However, this result will only be achieved if several criteria can be met:

- A highly sensitive test that can reproducibly detect the cancer at an early stage.
- A treatment capable of curing patients found to have a small cancer.
- A test acceptable enough to those being screened so that they are willing to attend on a regular basis.
- A test specific enough so that not too many people are treated unnecessarily.

In addition, cancer screening is only likely to become generally available if it can be shown to be sufficiently cost effective for the community to afford it. This stricture makes it likely that screening will only be a practical proposition for common types of cancer.

Although the ideas behind screening seem so sensible and obvious, it is important that the effectiveness of any screening programme is rigorously tested before being widely introduced. Among the disadvantages associated with screening is anxiety produced both in the general population and in individuals. Ineffective screening may highlight the problem of an untreatable cancer, only heightening the fears of those already apprehensive about developing such a tumour. Amongst those screened a proportion will be found to have an abnormality which on further investigation turns out to be benign; these people will have suffered severe anxiety and depression, imagining that they probably have cancer. Because of these effects and the financial cost, it is essential to show that screening really does achieve its goal of curing more people of cancer.

The process of testing new methods of cancer screening is laborious and expensive. The prerequisities are:

- A thorough evaluation of the 'screening test' in terms of its sensitivity, specificity and predictive value in the target population. Only tests which can reliably detect small tumours are suitable for the next stage.
- An assessment of the impact of screening on the outcome of the disease (size of the primary tumour and its stage at diagnosis; time to recurrence in those who relapse; and, most importantly, the survival pattern of the population).

When suitable tests have been developed which can identify small tumours with appropriate sensitivity and specificity they should ideally be tested for their potential as a screening tool in prospective controlled trials. In these a large population is randomized into two groups—those offered screening and a control group who are offered no specific screening programme. An alternative to this approach is to offer screening to everyone in a defined population and to compare the outcome in them with an apparently similar group of people not offered screening (a case control study). Although such studies can be easier to set up they may be subject to major criticisms about the make-up of the control group. Although there are a number of end-points for such studies—size and stage of tumour at diagnosis for instance—the most important measure of success is overall survival.

Selecting Tumours for Screening

Because the sole aim of screening is the early detection of small tumours, it is essential that treatments capable of curing such small tumours are available before screening can be contemplated. The natural history of individual tumours is, therefore, of major importance. Some tumours appear to pass through a premalignant and/or *in situ* tumour stage before development of a frankly malignant tumour. These cancers, best exemplified by cervical cancer, are clearly likely to be ideal candidates for screening programmes. Other tumours appear to be poor candidates since they are rarely cured by current treatments even if detected when small. Tumours such as non-small cell lung cancer and pancreatic cancers fall into this group.

Screening for Cancer at Specific Sites

Cancer of the Cervix

Because there is a detectable premalignant phase (cervical intra-epithelial neoplasia—CIN grade I–III) before the development of invasive tumour in many cases of cervical cancer, this tumour should theoretically benefit from screening. Fortunately, this has proven to be the case, and there has been a dramatic decline in deaths from this tumour in some countries. However, there are still areas where our understanding is incomplete.

- The decline in incidence from invasive cervical cancer started in 1935 in the USA (Figure 1), whilst screening programmes were not introduced until the 1950s.
- Although severe dysplasia and *in situ* cancer is regarded as a precursor of invasive malignancy this is not always the case. In a Danish study, for instance, only one-third of 127 *untreated* women with dysplasia and *in situ* cancer developed invasive cancer within 9 years.

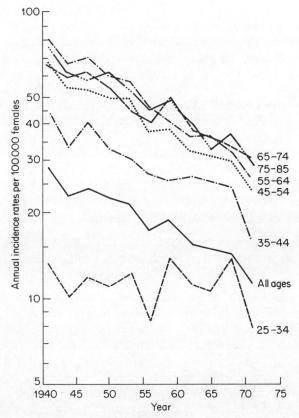

Figure 1. Cervix cancer incidence rates in New York state (except New York City) 1940–72. Reproduced by permission from Silverberg (1975) American Cancer Society

- Debate still surrounds the age at which screening should start and its subsequent frequency.

Much of this uncertainty over the exact role of cervical cancer screening stems from a failure to conduct large-scale controlled studies at the beginning. Though comparison with historical data or matched controls is always fraught with difficulty, the consensus view is that screening does appear to have reduced mortality for cervical cancer.

- In Iceland, where 85% of women were screened and where good records are available, the death rate from invasive cervical cancer fell from 32.1 per 100,000 women to 14.6 per 100,000 women in the 6 years after the opening of a screening clinic in Reykjavik. The frequency of late stage tumours at diagnosis was also reduced.

There is no international consensus opinion about how to run a screening programme, but the following points can be made:

- Dysplasia usually precedes carcinoma *in situ* by 5 to 10 years.
- The mean duration of carcinoma *in situ* is 8 years.
- Regression of abnormal smears, if it occurs, usually does so within 1 year, so that two smears 1 year apart are a good indicator of spontaneous regression.
- Most screening programmes which appear to have reduced mortality have used a screening interval of more than 1 year.
- The International Agency for Research on Cancer has, based on ten European and North American studies, estimated that a screening programme commencing at 25 years with three-yearly screening to age 60, will result in a 91% reduction in expected mortality.
- The American Cancer Society estimates that yearly re-screening will only detect one cancer for every 50,000 women examined. They recommend that cervical smears are only repeated once every 3 years after an initial negative test. A similar policy is practised in Great Britain.

Although this cost-effective policy of less intensive screening would seem to be able to prevent nearly all deaths from cervical cancer, there are still several potential difficulties:

- Those at greatest risk of cervical cancer (women in poor socio-economic groups, those starting sexual intercourse at an early age and with multiple partners) are the groups least likely to participate in a screening programme.
- Some tumours which are unduly aggressive may arise in the interval between screening visits.
- National screening call and recall programmes are complicated and expensive. In Britain, they have, so far, not been run efficiently and an effective programme has yet to be introduced. A computer-based call and recall system is

currently being developed to try to improve the present muddle.

- The concept that the full histological spectrum of CIN I–III is a precursor lesion which should be treated has effectively reduced the specificity of the test. About 4% of women will show evidence of some degree of CIN, although only 0.04% develop cervical cancer.

Breast Cancer

There is no easily recognizable premalignant stage in the development of breast cancer, so that screening can only be successful if treatment of early stage invasive carcinoma is potentially curative. Luckily, this is the case in breast cancer (Table 1).

The introduction and refinement of xeromammography of the breast in the last three decades has given us a potential tool for screening. This may be coupled with physical examination of the breast, either by a trained person or as self-examination. Current recommendations about screening are based on mammography; self-examination and routine examination are as yet of uncertain significance.

Mammographic Screening. The catalyst for current thinking was a study in New York, organized by the Health Insurance Plan (HIP) in 1963. In this, 62,000 women aged 40–64 years were randomly assigned to either four annual screening mammograms or to no screening at all. The results of this controlled trial consistently showed a reduced mortality in the group offered screening (Table 2), despite the short period of screening. However, this advantage for screened women was only statistically significant in women over 50 years of age.

Other controlled trials and case control studies, in Europe and North America, of mammographic breast screening have in general yielded similar results. In Britain, the Forrest committee has assessed the available data on breast screening up until 1986 and have drawn the following conclusions:

- Trials showing significant survival benefit have all used mammography: the value of breast self-examination and clinical examination remains to be proven.

Table 1. Prognostic significance of clinical stage at presentation in breast cancer. Reproduced by permission from A. H. Paterson *et al.* (1984) *Reviews on Endocrine Related Cancer*, Suppl. 14 pp. 35–39

UICC Stage	No. of patients	No. of developing metastases (%)	Survival of those with metastases	
			3-year (%)	5-year (%)
I	630	75 (12)	66	38
II	982	240 (24)	59	38
III	463	218 (47)	46	30
IV	186	186 (100)	25	10

Table 2. Breast cancer deaths by age, at 5 and 14 years (HIP study)

Age at entry	No. of deaths at			
	5 years		14 years	
	Mammography	Control	Mammography	Control
40–49	19	20	46	61
50–59	15	33	53	68
60–64	5	10	19	24
Total	39	63	118	153

- There is, currently, no role for screening in women under 50 years of age. This conclusion may change as current studies are recruiting more younger women and the use of adjuvant therapy may change the outlook in these women.
- Mammographic screening should be offered to all women over the age of 50 years, until 65 years of age.
- Routine mammography should be repeated every 3 years.
- Mammographic screening should be performed by specialist centres since expertise is required in mammography, ultrasound, fine needle aspiration, cytology and the management of benign and early malignant breast disease.
- The National Health Service should set up a breast screening service based in specialist units in each Regional Health Authority. This is currently being implemented and will include facilities for call and recall.

Since much anxiety is engendered by breast cancer screening it is imperative that the system runs efficiently, with no women waiting for prolonged periods before investigation if they turn out to have a positive mammogram. The majority of those with abnormal mammograms are found to have benign disease on further tests and would suffer unnecessary anxiety if this diagnosis was delayed. Similarly, for patients found to have breast cancer the quicker the diagnosis is made the better.

Other Cancers

There is no established role for screening for other malignant tumours. Pelvic ultrasound is being evaluated as a screening test for ovarian carcinoma. So far it appears capable of detecting small tumours. However, randomized prospective trials are needed to see if the test will result in improved survival in screened patients compared with an unscreened control.

Simple demonstration that tumours are picked up early does not guarantee that survival will be improved. For instance, a randomized American study has screened men for lung cancer using 6-monthly chest X-rays and sputum cytology. Although screened patients had smaller tumours than their unscreened counterparts, survival was identical.

In Japan, where gastric carcinoma is much more common than Britain, screening for stomach cancer appears to be beneficial. However, routine gastroscopy is included in the screening and it is not felt to be appropriate in countries which have a lower incidence and possibly tumours with a different natural history.

In the United States, screening programmes for colorectal cancer have mainly used occult blood testing, with further invasive tests reserved for those with blood in their stool. Currently there is no consensus that such an approach would reduce mortality for these tumours.

Bladder cancer is more common in those exposed to certain chemicals in industry, and urinary cytology is recommended for such people as a screening technique, though its utility is uncertain.

Skin cancer is more common in Caucasians exposed to excessive sunlight, and in Australia public health campaigns appear to have resulted in earlier diagnosis of malignant melanoma. Their utility is now being tested in Europe.

Conclusions

- Although an attractive way to approach the problem of cancer, screening is expensive and may engender unnecessary anxiety.
- The decision as to whether to offer screening should be based on scientifically valid trials which show that screening can reduce mortality from that tumour. Ideally these trials should be randomized, comparing a screened group with an unscreened control group.
- Currently screening is only offered for two tumours in Britain: cervical cancer and breast cancer.
- Screening programmes are only likely to be beneficial if they are taken up by the population at risk and are managed in such a way that 'customers' attend regularly. This probably means that screening should be concentrated in specialist centres—this is certainly the intention in the case of breast cancer.

Selected Papers and Reviews

Draper, G. J. (1982) Screening for cervical cancer: revised policy. The recommendations of the DHSS Committee on Gynaecological Cytology. *Health Trends* **14**: 37–40.

Forrest, P. (1986) *Breast Cancer Screening: Report to the Health Ministers of England, Wales, Scotland and Northern Ireland.* HM Stationery Office, London.

McPherson, A. (1986) *Cervical Screening. A Practical Guide.* Oxford University Press, Oxford.

Miller, A. B. (ed.) (1985) *Screening for Cancer.* Academic Press, New York.

Prorok, P. C. and Miller, A. B. (eds.) (1984) *Screening for Cancer. UICC Technical Report Vol. 78.* International Union Against Cancer, Geneva.

Shapiro, S. (1982) Ten to fourteen year effects of breast cancer screening on mortality. *Journal of the National Cancer Institute,* **69**: 349–355.

5 The Histopathological Diagnosis of Cancer

A. D. RAMSAY

Almost since the time of Virchow (1821–1902) the treatment of cancer has been based on a 'tissue diagnosis', meaning that a precise identification of the type of malignancy present in each patient is required for the correct treatment. To obtain such a diagnosis a sample of the cancer is sent for histological or cytological examination, allowing the cells present to be identified and the type of malignant neoplasm to be defined. Histology deals with specimens of tissue, or biopsies, whereas cytology looks at individual cells, which can often be obtained more readily. Histopathological examination frequently includes the study of both hisotological and cytological material, and incorporates light microscopy, electron microscopy, and enzymatic and immunological methods of identifying cellular characteristics.

In oncology, the pathologist detects the presence of malignant disease and identifies the specific type of cancer present. In addition, the pathologist will grade the neoplasm, assessing the degree of malignancy, and frequently helps to stage cancer, assessing how far the tumour has spread. Only when a specific diagnosis has been made, and the cancer has been staged and graded, can the correct therapeutic measures be taken.

The Role of the Histopathologist

The histopathologist plays a major role in the diagnosis of almost every form of malignant neoplasm. Histopathology involves the study of disease (pathology) at the level of the tissues and their constituent cells. The present-day classification of neoplasms is based upon the cell of origin of the tumour, regardless of the site at which the tumour is found. So squamous cell carcinoma can arise in the lung, mouth, oesophagus or on skin, and yet the cells, although malignant, are usually still identifiable as squamous cells. Table 1 gives a brief summary of modern cancer classification, listing the commoner malignancies and the normal tissue from which they arise.

Table 1. Classification of cancer

Tissue or cell of origin	Malignant neoplasm
Epithelium	Carcinoma
Squamous epithelium	Squamous cell carcinoma
Glandular epithelium	Adenocarcinoma
Urothelium (transitional epithelium)	Transitional cell carcinoma
Basal cells of skin	Basal cell carcinoma
Mesenchyme	Sarcoma
Fibrous tissue	Fibrosarcoma
Cartilage	Chondrosarcoma
Bone	Osteosarcoma
Smooth muscle	Leiomyosarcoma
Striated muscle	Rhabdomyosarcoma
Lymphocytes	Lymphoma
Haemopoietic cells	Leukaemia
Germ cells	Teratoma
Melanocytes	Melanoma
Glial cells of central nervous system	Glioma
Primitive neural cells	Neuroblastoma

Since cancers are classified by the cell of origin, it is clear that histopathology is essential to modern oncology. Both treatment regimens and epidemiological data rely on the correct identification of the various types of cancer, either from cytological or histological specimens. Histopathologists also perform post mortems, which provide valuable information regarding the efficacy of cancer therapy and enable precise death certification, contributing to the epidemiology of cancer.

The aim of histopathology is to produce a 'tissue diagnosis' in each cancer patient. This is clearly required in the distinction of benign from malignant neoplasms, ensuring that, for example, a benign skin naevus (mole) and malignant melanoma, which may look very similar to both patient and doctor, are not treated in the same manner. Similarly, until a breast lump is examined histologically or cytologically, it may be impossible to tell if it is benign or malignant.

The value of the tissue diagnosis is also apparent when dealing with different forms of malignant disease. For example, histopathological examination may be the only way in which primary and secondary neoplasms in the brain can be distinguished. The finding, at frozen section, of the former will direct the surgeon to consider the possibility of surgical excision whereas surgical removal is usually contraindicated if it is a metastasis. The histopathologist can also suggest the most likely primary site of the cancer, enabling investigations and treatment to be directed to the region of the body concerned.

Histopathological Techniques

Routine histopathology consists of macroscopic and microscopic assessment of tissue specimens. With large specimens like colon, lung, breast or uterus it is obviously inappropriate to examine the whole organ under the microscope, so the macroscopic assessment is critical. All specimens are described, indicating what normal tissue is present and what pathological abnormalities can be seen with the naked eye. Selected blocks of tissue are then cut from the specimen and processed for microscopic examination. The blocks are chosen to be representative of the tumour and of the apparently normal tissue, and frequently include margins of surgical resection and lymph nodes contained within the specimen. Any unusual areas or unexpected findings will also be sampled. Small biopsies are processed in their entirety.

The blocks selected for microscopic examination are fully fixed, dehydrated and embedded in wax. Thin sections are cut from the wax-embedded tissue, stained, and mounted on glass slides. The standard histopathological stain is haematoxylin and eosin, which tends to stain nuclei blue and cytoplasm red-pink. However, a wide variety of other stains can be applied to the tissue sections, and these allow the pathologist to visualize material that helps in defining the cells present. For example, stains indicating the presence of mucin in lung carcinoma cells will identify it as a glandular (mucin-secreting) adenocarcinoma rather than a squamous cell carcinoma. A short list of commonly used special stains is given in Table 2.

Traditionally specimens are sent to the histopathology laboratory in a fixative (usually formalin), which preserves histological detail by preventing autolytic changes. In a modern laboratory, however, specimens will often be sent fresh, in an unfixed condition. This allows the pathologist greater scope for investigating the specimen. Fresh tissue can be stored in liquid nitrogen, and subsequently used for immunological staining methods. Living cells can be extracted from fresh specimens of tumours, and these may then be grown in tissue culture and analysed cytogenetically to identify abnormalities in the cancer genome. Prior to fixing the main specimen in formalin, the pathologist is able to place samples of tissue in other fixatives, some of which enable better preservation of ultrastructural detail and so are used for electron microscopy. Figure 1 summarizes the way in which specimens are dealt with, and indicates the options available when tissue is received fresh.

When required, a rapid histological section can be produced from fresh tissue. By freezing, sectioning and staining the specimen in around 5–10 minutes, an 'instant' tissue diagnosis can be achieved. This 'frozen section' is often used whilst a patient is under anaesthetic, enabling the surgeon to proceed with the correct operation for the pathology concerned. Similar frozen sections can be cut from tissue stored in liquid

Table 2. Special stains

Stain	Demonstrates
PAS* and diastase-PAS	Carbohydrates (glycogen) and mucins
Alcian blue	Acid mucins
Grimelius	Biogenic amines (carcinoid tumours)
Van Gieson	Collagen fibres
Masson-Fontana	Melanin pigment
Perl's prussian blue	Iron pigment

*PAS = periodic acid-Schiff

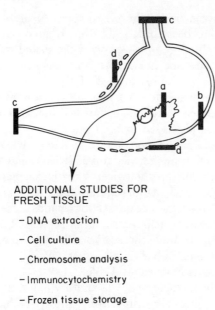

1. Macroscopic description

2. Select blocks

    a = Tumour
    b = Normal tissue
    c = Resection margins
    d = Lymph nodes

3. Fix and process

4. Cut sections

5. Stain

6. Mount on slides

7. Light microscopy

ADDITIONAL STUDIES FOR
FRESH TISSUE

– DNA extraction

– Cell culture

– Chromosome analysis

– Immunocytochemistry

– Frozen tissue storage

– Process for electron microsopy

Figure 1. Diagram showing the histopathological method of examining specimens, and the additional studies that can be carried out on fresh tissue

nitrogen, and because such sections retain many of the cellular antigens present in life, they are ideal for the immunological methods of staining discussed below.

Cytopathology

Cytological methods of diagnosis, used extensively in screening for and detecting carcinoma and premalignant disease of the uterine cervix, are often used in conjunction with histological methods. It is often easier to obtain a cytological specimen than a histological biopsy, and many malignancies can be diagnosed on cytology alone.

Cytology deals with cells rather than tissues, and the specimens are collected in many different ways. Masses close to the surface (breast lumps, lymph nodes, salivary tumours) can be examined by fine needle aspiration, where a sample of the cells is sucked into a syringe needle. Brushings or washings can be taken at bronchoscopy or endoscopy, and pleural and other fluids can be drained and spun down to concentrate the contained cells. Urine and sputum can be collected and examined, and smears can be taken from regions like the cervix. In general the decreased cell-to-cell adhesion of malignant cells means that if a tumour is malignant, cancer cells will usually be present in the specimen.

The staining of cytological preparations differs slightly from the methods used in routine histology, with the Papanicolaou and Giemsa stains being most commonly used. Although cytological specimens lack the architectural features of a histological biopsy, the cellular features of malignancy (see below) are present, and enable the examining pathologist to make a diagnosis in many cases. As the specimens do not require a lengthy fixation and processing stage, cytology often gives a more rapid diagnosis than histology. There are limitations to cytological diagnoses, however, and it may be necessary to proceed to a biopsy for more precise tumour typing or for tumour grading (see below).

Histochemistry and Immunohistochemistry

Histochemistry is a means whereby substances within histological and cytological material can be demonstrated by specific chemical reactions. The technique can be used to demonstrate cellular enzymes and other proteins, nucleic acids, lipids and some metals. It is often carried out on frozen sections as many enzymes and lipids are destroyed or inactivated in fixed or processed tissue. The demonstration of a cellular or tissue component relies upon a chemical reaction whereby the component is made visible by the subsequent production of a coloured indicator substance.

For example, nuclear DNA can be stained by the Feulgen technique. The tissue is first treated with hydrochloric acid, which hydrolyses the deoxyribose chain forming aldehyde (-CHO) groups. Schiff's reagent is then added: this reacts with aldehyde groups, converting a colourless dye (basic fuchsin) in the reagent to a deep magenta-coloured dye. Aldehyde groups on the hydrolysed DNA are thus visualized, and in the material examined DNA is stained magenta.

Immunohistochemistry is a recently developed technique which has had a major impact on diagnostic histopathology. The development of antibodies, both polyclonal and monoclonal, to cellular antigens means that pathologists can now identify specific cell types by their immunological phenotype as well as their morphological appearance. The technique is termed 'immunohistochemistry' or 'immunocytochemistry', and relies on the applied antibody binding to the antigen in a tissue section or cytological preparation. An indicator system is then used to stain the areas where the antibody has bound so that the examining pathologist can visualize specific antigenic components of cells and tissues. The indicator often consists of a second antibody that is complexed with an enzyme (commonly horseradish peroxidase).

After application of the first (primary) antibody, the material under study is washed so that the only antibody remaining is that bound to the complementary antigen. The second (indicator) antibody is then applied, followed by a similar washing process. A complex of antibodies (both primary and secondary) and enzyme is bound to the original antigen. A colourless substrate for the enzyme is added, and enzymatic activity results in a strongly-coloured reaction product wherever the complex is bound. The end result is that the antigen is specifically stained and can be clearly identified by the examining pathologist.

There are many variations on this theme, with avidin-biotin complexes replacing the antibody-antibody binding, and various enzymes being used as indicators, but the overall principle remains the same. The process of immunocytochemical staining is shown diagrammatically in Figure 2.

The specificity of immunological staining depends upon the specificity of the primary antibody used. Monoclonal antibodies are highly specific, identifying a single antigenic epitope, and form the basis for most immunocytochemistry. Although many cellular

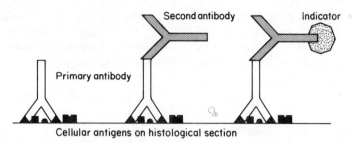

Figure 2. Diagrammatic representation of immunocytochemical staining

antigens can only be demonstrated in unfixed or frozen tissue, some antigens survive the fixation and subsequent processing, and so the technique can be used alongside routine staining methods. Monoclonal antibodies that are active in routinely-processed formalin-fixed and wax-embedded tissues are available for many antigens, and the search continues for other such antibodies. In addition to their greater convenience, these antibodies allow the retrospective study of tissue blocks, enabling previous diagnoses to be confirmed (or refuted) by immunological means.

Although the list of monoclonal antibodies against tissue or cellular antigens is almost endless, a selection of useful antigens that can be recognized in paraffin section is given in Table 3. Of particular value are antigens found in specific cell types. The leucocyte common antigen (LCA) is restricted to white cells, and so staining with an anti-LCA usually indicates that the tumour is a lymphoma. The intermediate filament desmin is characteristic of muscle cells, and so positive staining will be found in

Table 3. Useful immunocytochemical antigens

Antigen	Class of substance	Associated malignancy
Leucocyte common antigen (LCA)	Cell surface macromolecule	Lymphomas, leukaemias
Immunoglobulin heavy and light chains	Surface and cytoplasmic immunoglobulins	B-cell lymphomas
Cytokeratins	Intermediate filament	Epithelial neoplasms
Desmin	Intermediate filament	Muscle-derived neoplasms
Vimentin	Intermediate filament	Mesenchymal neoplasms
GFAP*	Intermediate filament	Glial (CNS) neoplasms
CEA†	Onco-foetal antigen	Carcinomas (lung, bowel)
AFP‡	Onco-foetal antigen	Germ cell neoplasms Hepatocellular carcinoma
S100 protein	Cellular transport protein	Neural tumours, melanoma
Leu M1	Cell surface polysaccharide	Hodgkin's disease (Reed-Sternberg cells)

*GFAP = glial fibrillary acidic protein
†CEA = carcinoma-embryonic antigen
‡AFP = alpha-fetoprotein

leiomyosarcomas and rhabdomyosarcomas. Cytokeratins are the intermediate filaments of epithelial cells, so positive staining is a feature of carcinomas. There are exceptions to these general rules, and it is histopathological dogma that panels of antibodies should be used, and a diagnosis should not be based on the result of a single antibody alone. It must also be said that immunocytochemistry will only help identify the cells present; it will not enable a diagnosis of malignancy to be made on its own. The diagnosis of a malignant neoplasm is based on the macroscopic and microscopic morphological features; immunocytochemistry indicates the cell of origin of the neoplasm.

Ultrastructural Examination

A further option open to the pathologist is the examination of the neoplastic cells by electron microscopy. Prior to immunocytochemistry, ultrastructural examination was used to distinguish morphologically similar tumours, specific cellular organelles or structures identifying the neoplasm. For example, the presence of desmosomes usually indicated epithelial cells, thick and thin myofilaments were seen in striated muscle tumours, and melanomas contained melanosomes. Although much of this role has been subsumed to immunological methods of staining, electron microscopy provides a useful back-up in tumour diagnosis, particularly in the face of unusual or conflicting immunocytochemical results.

Molecular Biological and Genetic Analysis of Cancer

With increasing use of modern molecular biological techniques, pathologists often find themselves in close collaboration with molecular biologists and geneticists when faced with interesting or problematic malignancies. Techniques such as gene probing, Southern blotting, chromosome banding and karyotypic analysis can be carried out in these cases, increasing both the amount of information obtained from the pathological specimen and our knowledge of cancer as a whole.

Pathological Characteristics of Malignant Neoplasms

Macroscopic Features of Cancer (Figure 3)

The most important macroscopic features of cancer are *invasion* and *metastasis*. Whilst benign neoplasms grow as well-circumscribed, smooth, rounded masses, cancer grows in an irregular fashion, infiltrating into surrounding tissues in a manner analogous to the claws of a crab. Thus benign tumours are usually enclosed within a fibrous capsule, whereas malignant tumours often have no clearly defined edge, and lack such a capsule. Invasion of a squamous cell carcinoma is illustrated in Figure 4.

Naked eye examination of a malignant tumour often shows the effects of this invasion, so that an adenocarcinoma of the intestine, which arises at the mucosal surface, can frequently be seen to have eroded through the full thickness of the bowel

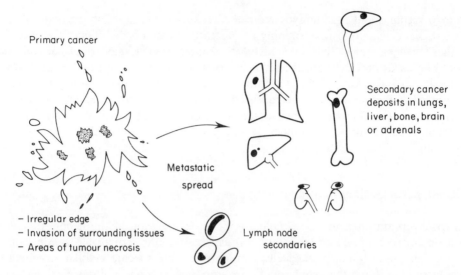

Figure 3. The macroscopic features of malignant neoplasms

wall, with tumour present at the serosal surface. Similarly, a carcinoma of the breast may invade the overlying skin, producing an exophytic ('fungating') mass, or infiltrate the underlying chest wall muscle leading to a fixed, immobile mass needing extensive surgical removal.

The rapid growth of many cancers means that they outgrow their blood supply, and regions of the tumour undergo spontaneous necrosis. For this reason yellow-white

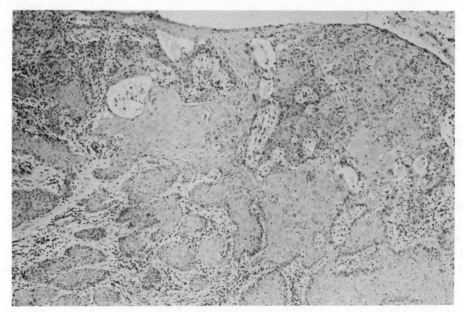

Figure 4. Low-power photomicrograph showing a squamous cell carcinoma arising from laryngeal epithelium (top of picture) and invading into underlying connective tissue

areas of necrosis, sometimes with accompanying haemorrhage, are frequently seen on the cut surface of malignant neoplasms.

Metastasis is the most reliable diagnostic feature of malignant neoplasms. Invasion involves the extension into and destruction of local tissue by cancer, whereas the metastatic process allows cancers to spread widely throughout the body, reaching sites distant to and separate from the original (primary) location. It is clearly preferable to diagnose (and treat) most malignancies before metastasis takes place, and it is the problem of metastasis that prevents the successful treatment of many forms of cancer.

Although all malignant neoplasms have the ability to metastasize (the property being one of the definitions of cancer), not all cancers do so. Different cancers metastasize with differing frequencies, to different sites, by different routes. The basal cell carcinoma of the skin, a fully malignant tumour that can show extensive local destruction, never metastasizes. Primary cancer arising within the central nervous system will metastasize to sites in the CNS, but rarely spreads outside the neuro-axis. In general the more rapidly growing, more *anaplastic* (see below) cancers are those that spread early, producing multiple metastases at various sites. Metastasis commonly results in secondary deposits of cancer in lymph nodes, lungs, liver, central nervous system, adrenals and bone. The histological appearance of the tumour at these sites is identical to that seen at the primary site.

Metastatic spread may occur by several routes. Malignancies may spread through the lymphatic system, with deposits of cancer in lymph nodes; through the bloodstream (haematogenous spread), with tumour emboli producing distant secondaries in sites like lungs or liver; through the body cavities, the tumour spreading via the peritoneal or pleural cavity; or by direct physical transplantation, which is a rare complication of operative and investigative procedures. In addition malignant tumours in the central nervous system may metastasize via the cerebrospinal fluid circulation. The primary mode of spread of carcinomas is lymphatic, with local and then regional lymph node secondaries. In contrast, most sarcomas metastasize primarily through the bloodstream. It should be stressed however, that both varieties of cancer can metastasize by either route, and that lymphatic and haematogenous spread are often inseparable.

The pathologist will encounter metastasis in a variety of situations. When examining a specimen the lymph nodes may be sampled to detect secondaries—with carcinoma of the colon the nodes in the pericolic fat are studied, whereas with breast carcinoma the axillary lymph nodes must be examined. In some cases blood vessels may be sampled. Renal carcinoma, for example, shows a marked tendency to infiltrate the renal vein, and a pathological assessment of an involved kidney would include the resection margin of this vessel. A sample from a presumed secondary, at the site of a pathological fracture, for example, may be sent for analysis, the pathologist's task being to identify the type of cancer and the probable primary site. In fact, when examining any tumour, the possibility of metastatic disease must always be considered, and the distinction of primary and secondary malignancies is a major part of the histopathological diagnosis of cancer.

Microscopic Features of Cancer (Figures 5, 6 and 7)

Although different cancers show different features under the microscope, there are some characteristics common to all malignancies. Cancer cells show an increase in

Normal epithelium   Malignant epithelium

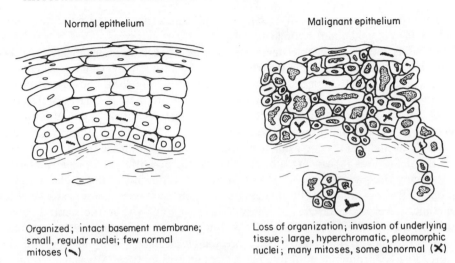

Organized; intact basement membrane;   Loss of organization; invasion of underlying
small, regular nuclei; few normal   tissue; large, hyperchromatic, pleomorphic
mitoses (↘)   nuclei; many mitoses, some abnormal (✘)

Figure 5. The microscopic features of malignant neoplasms

nuclear size over their normal counterparts, so that the ratio of nucleus to cytoplasm is increased. Normally this nuclear:cytoplasmic ratio is around 1:5, but in malignant neoplasms it can approach 1:1. The nuclei are usually darker staining (hyperchromatic), reflecting this increase in nuclear material. Karyotypic analysis of neoplastic cells confirms a greater amount of nuclear DNA in malignant cells, with polyploidy and aneuploidy being common. There is also an increased variability in nuclear size and shape when compared to normal cells, this feature being termed nuclear pleomorphism.

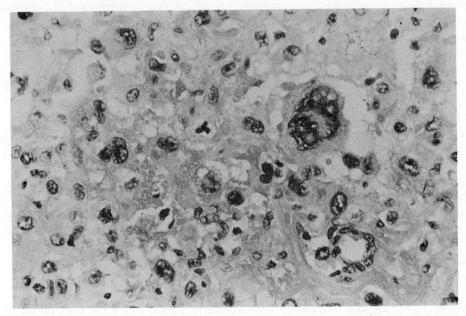

Figure 6. Nuclear atypia in a low-power photomicrograph from a malignant glial tumour

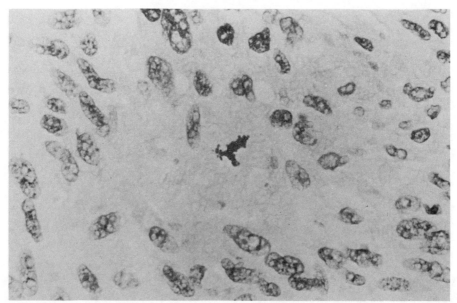

Figure 7. Tripolar mitosis (centre) in a malignant tumour of smooth muscle (leiomyosarcoma)

The growth rate of malignant neoplasms is higher than that of the normal tissue from which they arise, and this is reflected in an increased number of mitoses in cancer cells. It should be noted that a high mitotic rate does not always imply malignancy, as normal processes of hyperplasia and repair can show a similar increase in cell divisions. However, the mitotic figures seen in cancer are frequently abnormal, with bizarre tripolar or quadripolar mitotic spindles, or fragments of condensed chromatin disseminated at random throughout the dividing cell. Such abnormal mitoses can result in the formation of tumour giant cells, with two or more nuclei, or bizarre tumour 'monster' cells with huge misshapen nuclei. Collectively these nuclear changes seen in cancer cells are termed 'nuclear atypia'.

Cancer cell cytoplasm shows some degree of loss of specialized features, the cells being less well differentiated than the normal population from which they arose. Thus malignancies of striated muscle may not contain cross-striations, and squamous cell carcinomas may or may not produce keratin.

The overall organization of the cells with respect to one another and to the surrounding tissues is lost. Normal tissues show a clear pattern of growth, typified by squamous epithelia in which the basal layers divide and the superficial layers keratinize and desquamate. In a squamous cell carcinoma this pattern is lost, and mitoses, keratinization and cell death can be seen anywhere within the tumour.

Invasion is seen at the microscopic level as well as the macroscopic level, with cancer cells penetrating through basement membranes and other structures, and malignant cells infiltrating the surrounding tissues. This infiltration may occur along tissue planes, may involve microscopic invasion of blood vessels or lymphatics, and can be seen in such areas as the perineural sheaths of nerves (Figure 8).

Other histological features of cancer include changes in the stromal tissues in and around malignant tumours, and evidence of a host response to the malignant cells.

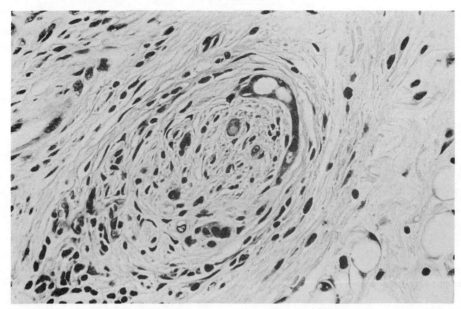

Figure 8. Photomicrograph showing perineural invasion by an adenocarcinoma. Neoplastic glands are seen in the perineural sheath

Some carcinomas excite a fibrous stromal reaction (typically breast carcinomas), producing a firm, hard 'scirrhous' tumour. In others the fibrous tissue can become soft and mucoid. Host lymphocytes are seen around the malignant cells in a proportion of malignancies, malignant melanoma in particular showing this feature.

Pathological Grading of Cancer

As discussed above, cancer cells lose the specialized functions of their normal counterparts, and show a spectrum of nuclear abnormalities. The degree of these changes is variable, and provides the basis for the pathological grading of cancer. Cancers which resemble the normal tissue of origin fairly closely, both in terms of morphological appearance and function, are well-differentiated. Such tumours show many of the architectural and cytological features of the normal tissue, often with little nuclear atypia, and are usually readily categorized by the pathologist. For example, a well-differentiated adenocarcinoma will form glands and produce mucin; a well-differentiated squamous cell carcinoma will show keratin formation (keratin 'nests' or 'pearls'); and a well-differentiated rhabdomyosarcoma will show cross-striations.

At the other end of the spectrum, poorly-differentiated tumours show little resemblance to their tissue of origin and an increased degree of nuclear atypia. Categorizing such tumours may be very difficult, as all poorly differentiated neoplasms tend towards the same histological appearance. Thus a poorly-differentiated adenocarcinoma lacks gland and mucin formation and may resemble a poorly differentiated squamous cell carcinoma, which will similarly lack keratin formation. A poorly differentiated rhabdomyosarcoma will lack cross-striations and other evidence of its striated muscle origin.

Between well- and poorly differentiated categories there is an intermediate category of moderately differentiated. Much of the assessment of the degree of differentiation is subjective, and yet it is generally true that the less differentiated a cancer, the more aggressive is its clinical course. In this way the tumours are grouped into low-grade (well-differentiated) and high grade (poorly differentiated) categories. Such categories are often important in the treatment of the cancer, the high-grade neoplasm receiving more aggressive therapy.

The microscopic features described above as being characteristic of malignant neoplasms are grouped together under the umbrella term of *anaplasia*. The more anaplastic a cancer, the greater the nuclear atypia, and the more undifferentiated the tumour. The lack of identifiable histological features may make the more anaplastic tumours difficult to define, such lesions often being fitted into general descriptive categories, for example anaplastic carcinoma or anaplastic sarcoma. Anaplastic malignancies tend to show marked nuclear abnormalities, a hgh mitotic rate, and rapid growth and metastasis; they are clearly high-grade tumours. Distinction of such tumours using routine histology may be difficult, with anaplastic carcinoma resembling anaplastic lymphoma or melanoma. Increasing use of immunohistochemistry has enabled the correct identification of many previously uncategorized anaplastic neoplasms.

Specific Diagnostic Features of Selected Malignancies

The diagnosis of specific types of cancer is frequently made by the identification of certain diagnostic pathological features. Some of these have already been mentioned, like keratin formation in squamous cell carcinoma. Others are obvious—for example, the presence of melanin pigment in malignant melanoma. This section gives a brief overview of the key histopathological features of the more common malignancies encountered in oncological practice.

- *Squamous cell carcinomas* (lung, larynx, skin, oesophagus) are identified by the presence of keratin pearls in well-differentiated examples and individual cell keratinization in more undifferentiated lesions. Between the squamous cells there should be a row of 'prickles' or intercellular bridges, which represent the desmosomes connecting adjacent cells (Figure 9).
- *Adenocarcinomas* (arising in stomach, bowel, lungs and breast, to name but a few possible sites of origin) will show gland formation if well differentiated. In addition special stains are used to look for mucin secretion. Intracellular droplets of mucin are seen in the less well-differentiated tumours. In a particular form of adenocarcinoma, often seen in stomach but not restricted to that site, the tumour cells are distended by a large cytoplasmic globule of mucin that pushes the nucleus to one side. Such cells are said to resemble a signet ring, and the tumour is described as 'signet ring carcinoma'.

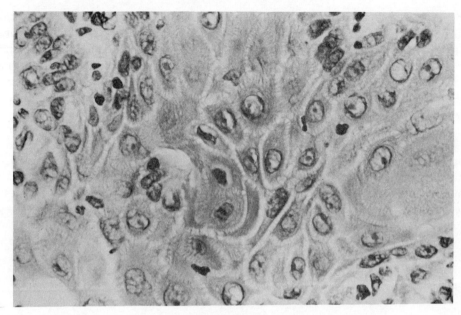

Figure 9. High-power photomicrograph of a well-differentiated squamous cell carcinoma showing the intercellular bridges or 'prickles'

- *Sarcomas* are usually composed of long, spindle-shaped cells. In the rhabdomyosarcoma evidence of striated muscle differentiation is indicated by the presence of large amounts of pink cytoplasm, often containing cross-striations. Glycogen is abundant in rhabdomyosarcomas, and the tumour cells may adopt long 'strap-like' forms that resemble the syncytial arrangement of normal striated muscle.
- *Malignant lymphomas* are divided into Hodgkin's disease and non-Hodgkin's lymphomas. The diagnosis of Hodgkin's disease rests mainly on the detection of a specific cell type, the Reed-Sternberg cell. Classical Reed-Sternberg cells have a bilobed nucleus, each lobe having a prominent pink nucleolus, and abundant pale-blue cytoplasm when examined in routine histological sections. Non-Hodgkin's lymphomas are a diverse group, but those derived from B-lymphocytes are unique in that immunocytochemistry can be used to distinguish reactive from neoplastic populations (and hence to identify malignant lymphomas, as there are no benign lymphoid neoplasms). Heavy and light chain production in B-cells can be detected by immunological staining. A reactive (non-neoplastic) population of B-cells will show a mixture of heavy and light chain types, whereas neoplastic B-cells, all being derived from a single transformed precursor, will all show the same heavy and light chain type.

If immunohistochemistry indicates a light chain restriction to one subtype (either κ or λ) in a collection of B-cells, then the population is identified as neoplastic. The neoplastic B-cells may also show heavy chain restriction. So immunological techniques form a powerful tool for the analysis of lymphoid malignancies. More recently molecular biological methods have been added to this field, with genetic analysis being used to detect clonal populations of both B- and T-lymphocytes.

Summary and Conclusions

Key points in the histological assessment of cancer are:

- Assessment and treatment of cancer patients depends upon the correct identification of the type of malignancy present.
- Malignant neoplasms are classified according to their histogenesis.
- Identification of types of cancer depends upon a tissue (pathological) diagnois.
- Pathologists diagnose cancer in histological and cytological specimens.
- Macroscopic features of cancer include invasion and metastasis. Metastasis occurs through lymphatics, blood vessels, cerebrospinal fluid, body cavities and by physical spread at surgery.
- Microscopic features of cancer cells include nuclear pleomorphism, nuclear hyperchromatism, high mitotic rate, raised nuclear:cytoplasmic ratio and abnormal mitoses. The cytoplasm shows loss of differentiated features.
- In addition to light microscopy pathologists use electron microscopy, special stains and immunocytochemistry. Genetic and molecular biological methods are just becoming available.
- Immunocytochemistry allows the histological identification of specific tissue antigens using polyclonal and monoclonal antibodies.
- Histologically cancers can be divided into three grades: well-differentiated; moderately differentiated; and poorly differentiated. The less differentiated or more anaplastic a cancer, the more rapid its growth and spread in the patient.
- Specific types of cancer show specific histological and immunological features that enable their precise identification.
- Malignant lymphomas can be identified using immunological analysis to reveal light chain restriction. Molecular biology can detect clonal gene rearrangements in lymphocytes.

Selected Papers and Reviews

Filipe, M. I. and Lake, B. D. (1983) *Histochemistry in Pathology*. Churchill Livingstone, Edinburgh.

Fisher, C., Ramsay, A. D., Griffiths, M. and McDougall, J. (1985) An assessment of the value of electron microscopy in tumour diagnosis. *Journal of Clinical Pathology*, **38**: 403–408.

Gatter, K. C., Falini, B. and Mason D. Y. (1984) The use of monoclonal antibodies in histopathological diagnosis. In: *Recent Advances in Histopathology 12*, Anthony, P. P. and MacSween, R. M. M. (eds.), Churchill Livingstone, Edinburgh, pp. 35–67.

Robbins, S. L. and Kumar, V. (1987) Neoplasia. In: *Basic Pathology*, Fourth Edition, W. B. Saunders, Philadelphia, pp. 182–212.

Sklar, J. (1985) DNA hybridisation in diagnostic pathology. *Human Pathology* **16**: 654–658.

Taussig, M. J. (1984) Neoplasia. In: *Processes in Pathology and Microbiology*, Second Edition, Blackwell Scientific Publications, Oxford, pp. 689–809.

6 | Staging and Investigation of Cancer

C. J. WILLIAMS

Choice of treatment for cancer is based on a knowledge of the natural history of that particular tumour and information on the extent of its spread. Staging, at a specific time (usually at diagnosis), is an attempt to define the exact extent of the tumour and its metastases (if any). It is a key component of treatment decision-making. An additional, and crucial, rationale for staging classifications is that they allow comparisons between results in different institutions. The need for unified classifications was recognized as early as the 1920s, and a group of gynaecologists, supported by the League of Nations, devised a staging system for carcinoma of the cervix. Since World War II a number of international bodies have developed a wide variety of staging classifications; unfortunately there are now often several different classifications for a single tumour site. The main bodies concerned with staging are the International Union Against Cancer (UICC), American Joint Committee for Cancer Staging and End-Results Reporting (AJCCS) and the International Federation of Gynaecological Oncology (FIGO). The problem of multiple classifications is highlighted by laryngeal cancer; in 1970 Vermund presented data on the role of radiotherapy using no less than seven staging classifications!

Recently, the UICC and AJCCS have co-operated to unify their approach and classifications. The UICC has stated that their objectives for staging are:

- to aid the clinician in planning treatment
- to give an indication of prognosis
- to assist evaluation of end results
- to facilitate the exchange of information between treatment centres
- to assist in the continuing investigation of cancer

Although the approach to staging has to be based on the particular characteristics and natural history of each type of cancer, a common system has been developed for most solid tumours. This is known as the TNM system:

T = extent of the primary tumour
N = condition of the regional lymph nodes
M = presence or absence of distant metastasis

The exact state of the cancer can be accurately recorded using the following technique (see Figure 1 for an example):

- The use of a series of subscripts to indicate ascending degrees of involvement (e.g. T_1, T_2, etc., N_1, N_2, etc., M_0, M_1).
- Grouping of several TNM assignments into a smaller number of clinical stages (usually four). In this way up to 50 TNM categories can be placed into a small number of stages so that the system becomes practical.
- Staging can be defined as clinical, or pathological when it is based on histological findings from tissue obtained at surgery.

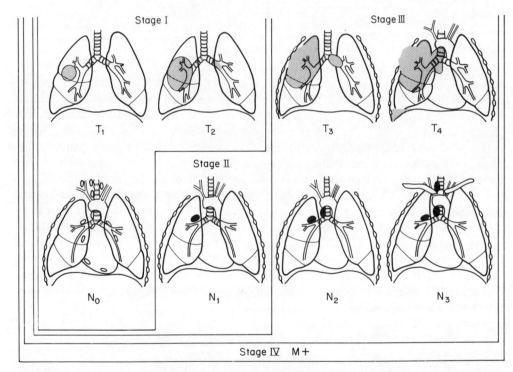

Figure 1. Anatomical staging for lung cancer. Tumour (T) categories: Size and confinement to lung are the major considerations in the progression of non-oat cell cancers: T_1 vs. T_2 depends on the mass being less or more than 3 cm. The depth of invasion is reflected by extension through the pleura (T_3). Invasion of the mediastinum, heart, great vessels, trachea, oesophagus, vertebral body, carina or a malignant pleural effusion is designated T_4. Node (N) categories: Location within the lung hilar (N_1) or mediastinal (N_2) indicates the common progression. Supraclavicular nodes are N_3. Stage grouping emphasizes the early resectable stages confined to a lobe or lung (T_1 and T_2) with and without hilar disease (N_1) as I and II respectively. Advanced disease (T_3), pleural invasion and mediastinal nodes are stage III, with metastases reflecting stage IV. Modified from AJS *Task Force on Lung Cancer*. Chicago, 1978, based on *UICC TNM classification*, Fourth edition, Geneva. 1987. Reproduced by permission

- Some staging systems also use histological tumour grade when this is likely to influence treatment choice and prognosis.

It is beyond the scope of this chapter to discuss in detail the description (oncotaxonomy) of the TNM system. Simplified staging systems are given in the sections on individual tumours. Although sometimes clumsy, staging is essential in the process of choosing treatment and often gives an accurate guide to prognosis (Figure 2).

Stage Migration

This is also known as the 'Will Rogers phenomenon' after the American comedian who said 'when the Okies left Oklahoma and moved to California, the IQ rose in both states'. This same process occurs in staging, when more sensitive techniques are developed. Figure 3 shows an example of how this effect operates. Basically, more sensitive staging tests will ensure that only patients with the most minimal disease are classified as having early stage disease. As a consquence patients who would have, in the past, been classified as having early disease, are with the new tests, found to have advanced disease. This has the effect of making the advanced disease a more favourable group. Although, as in the example, treatment may have remained unchanged and the results for the entire groups are the same, it appears that the results in each stage have improved.

Because of this phenomenon, it is always unwise to compare current data with a historical control, especially when staging techniques have been refined.

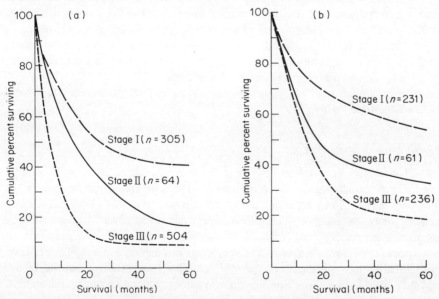

Figure 2. Survival according to TNM stage grouping. Squamous carcinoma of the lung (a) clinically staged and (b) surgically staged. (Reproduced by permission from AJS Task Force on Lung Cancer. Chicago 1978)

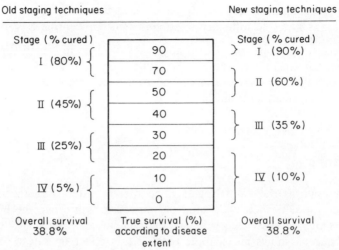

Figure 3. Stage migration. In this example, even though treatment is unchanged and the overall survival rate is the same, there appears to be improved survival for each stage after introduction of more sensitive staging techniques

Investigations Used to Stage Cancer

Decision making in staging is initially based on the findings of a thorough history and physical examination, together with a knowledge of the histological tumour type. For patients with a small localized lesion, say breast cancer, without extension into surrounding tissues, the regional draining lymph nodes should usually be evaluated next. If there is no nodal spread, further complicated investigation for distant metastasis is probably not indicated as the chances are high that all will be normal; in this case a chest X-ray and routine chemistry and full blood count are adequate. However, some malignant tumours tend to spread early and an examination for distant spread is indicated even when the tumour is apparently small. Examples of such tumours include small cell lung cancer and non-Hodgkin's lymphomas.

Recent improvements in diagnostic imaging have revolutionized the process of staging, as described below.

Computed Tomography (CT)

Current CT scanners can define detailed anatomy with a precision undreamed of 10 years ago. They do, however, have limitations and can give both false negative and false positive results. For instance, metastatic tumour may not cause sufficient nodal enlargement to be detected by CT; alternatively, nodes enlarged by an inflammatory process might be wrongly interpreted as tumour (Figure 4). Interpretation of CT images requires considerable expertise, experience and a good knowledge of radiological anatomy; ideally they should only be evaluated by those trained in the technique. Despite such problems, CT scans are an important way of defining the extent of a primary cancer (T), the involvement of draining lymph nodes (N) and spread to distant organs (M). CT scanning is, however, relatively expensive, it can be time consuming,

(a)

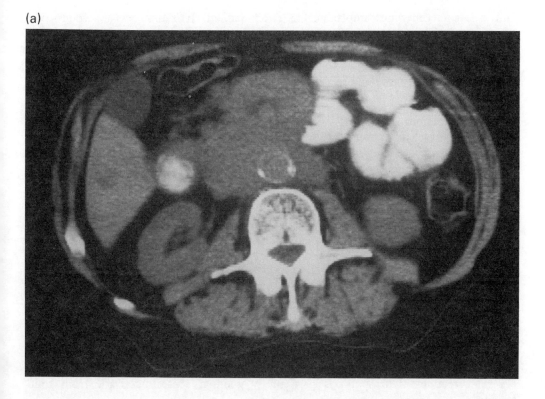

(b)

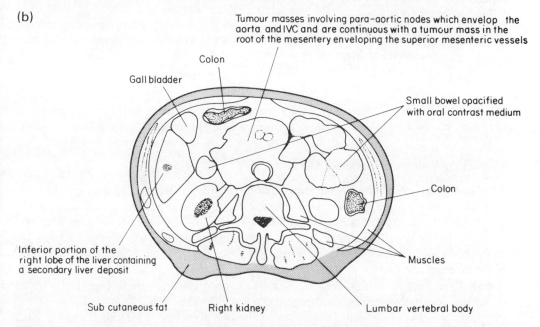

Figure 4. (a) CT image of the abdomen. (b) Schematic representation of (a) outlining the anatomical structures

and it is sometimes uncomfortable for a sick patient. It is unnecessary when other simpler techniques can define the presence and extent of tumour.

It is important that patients with known tumour masses, who are not candidates for local therapy, do not undergo unnecessary CT scans or other tests which delay therapy, burden imaging services and are expensive. Before considering CT imaging examine whether it is likely to be useful. Possible uses of CT include:

- detection of previously unrecognized disease
- accurate definition of known disease in order to facilitate surgery or radiotherapy planning
- establishment of a baseline for future estimation of response to therapy

If CT fulfils none of these criteria it is probably redundant. These criteria apply to most clinical tests—in general an investigation is only worth performing if it is going to influence management of the patient.

Ultrasound Imaging

This technique, which was first introduced 30 years ago, has been considerably refined in the past decade. The image depends on the echoes created at the interfaces of tissues which have different elasticities (Figure 5). Its chief advantage is that it is quick, inexpensive and non-invasive. In addition, because the operator can freely orientate the plane in which he is examining, a suspect area can be examined from several directions. Ultrasound is particularly good at separating cystic from solid lesions.

Disadvantages include:

- Ultrasound echoes cannot be obtained from areas behind bone or gas-filled loops of bowel.
- Its resolving power in the abdomen is generally not as good as CT imaging.

Although it is most commonly used to examine the abdomen and pelvis, ultrasound may also be used to look at specific organs such as the breast, thyroid and testes.

Magnetic Resonance Imaging (MRI)

This is a new (1973) and so far experimental technique which depends on the fact that nuclei with an uneven number of particles (protons and neutrons) spin at random. If a patient is placed in a strong magnetic field some of the nuclei will align with the magnetic field. Most imaging is done using hydrogen ions because they are numerous in the body and are easy to image. When (hydrogen) protons are bombarded by pulses of electromagnetic energy of the appropriate wavelength they will adopt an antiparallel state with respect to the magnetic field. This makes them unstable and when the pulse ends they revert to equilibrium, becoming parallel to the magnetic field. In doing so, they emit a signal of the same frequency as the one absorbed. This signal can be used to construct a computer-derived image of the location of hydrogen in that section of

(a)

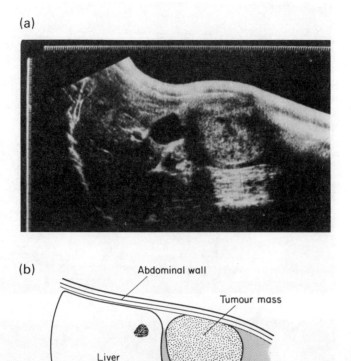

(b)

Figure 5. (a) Ultrasound image of the upper abdomen. (b) Schematic representation of (a) showing the anatomical structures

the body (Figure 6). The signal is also influenced by the physical and chemical environment in which the protons reside; this gives additional parameters which can be manipulated to give the maximum amount of information.

MRI has several potential advantages over other current imaging techniques:

- Whilst information obtained by other techniques is from one parameter the MRI signal depends on four parameters that can be manipulated to enhance the image.
- Patent blood vessels can be seen without contrast.
- There is no biological hazard associated with the test.

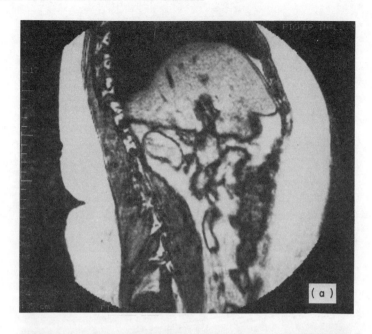

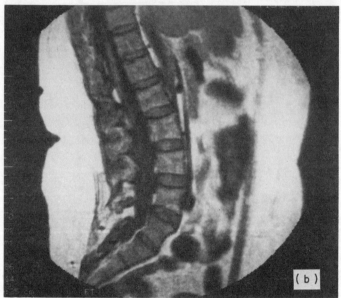

Figure 6. MRI of the thorax (a) and abdomen (b).

However, the anatomical detail it provides at a number of important sites outside the CNS is still inferior to CT. Scanning takes longer than CT and is even more expensive.

Although a potentially exciting tool MRI is only just becoming available and its true value has yet to be defined. Promising areas in cancer investigation include:

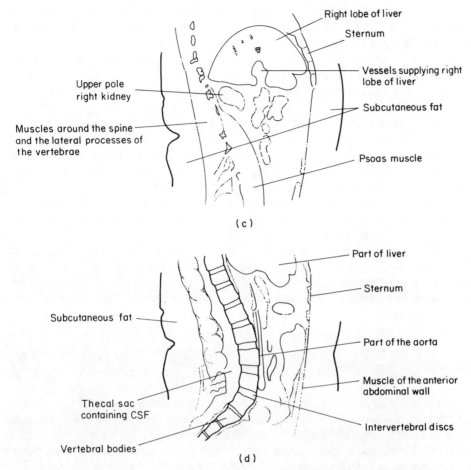

Figure 6 (c),(d): Schematic representation of the anatomical structures present in (a) and (b)

- tumours in the brain and spinal cord and meninges
- tumours in soft tissues or adjacent to bone
- examination of the pelvic organs
- examination of the head and neck, including thyroid and larynx

For the future, magnetic resonance spectroscopy holds promise in the study of tumour differentiation and invasiveness. A technique called proton chemical shift imaging is just being developed; since this can be done at lower magnetic field strengths, many simultaneous studies can be performed. Tumour-specific monoclonal antibodies bound to para-magnetic metals may also be developed. Clearly, there is still much to learn and it is important that MRI is properly compared with other techniques and that images are compared with pathological and autopsy findings.

Isotope Imaging

Small doses of radioisotopes are injected intravenously during these tests. By choosing the appropriate vehicle and isotope, localization at specific sites can be achieved. For instance, technetium-99m-labelled sulphur colloid is taken up by Kuppfer and endothelial cells in the liver; tumours fail to take up the isotope and show up as 'cold' areas within the liver (Figure 7).

Skeletal metastases are particularly well demonstrated by isotopic imaging, and this is the investigative technique of choice. Technetium-labelled phosphate compounds are rapidly taken up into bone. Since metastases generally have an increased blood flow and osteoblastic activity they appear as 'hot' areas of increased activity (Figure 8). Multiple myeloma, where osteoblastic activity is minimal, is an exception. However, because the mechanism is non-specific any other condition causing increased bone activity (fracture, arthritis, etc.) will potentially give a false positive result (Figure 8). Experience is therefore required in interpreting isotopic bone images, and check X-rays may be necessary when there are isolated abnormal areas.

Brain scans have been largely replaced by CT imaging. Special isotopic imaging techniques, such as gallium scans, for collections of pus and certain tumours, have been developed but are not in general use.

Currently there is a lot of interest in the use of radiolabelled tumour-specific monoclonal antibodies as a technique for localizing tumours. Although such studies are in their infancy and there are many potential problems, they are of special interest as such antibodies may provide a way of delivering high doses of radiation or toxins directly to the tumour.

Radiological Contrast Studies

Many of the traditional X-ray contrast studies are useful in the diagnosis or staging of cancer, but discussion of them is unnecessary here since their use is well known and they are utilized in many branches of medicine. Lymphography is, however, mainly restricted to the staging of cancer. Radiographic contrast is injected into the lymphatics on the dorsum of each foot and during the next 24 hours X-rays are taken which show opacified lymph nodes in the pelvis and abdomen. These glands will remain opacified for 6 or more months. The advantages of lymphography are:

- Tumour involvement of normal sized lymph nodes can be recognized by the abnormal pattern of filling (lace-like in lymphoma and holes in carcinoma).
- A simple plain film of the abdomen is all that is required for routine follow-up for as long as the glands remain opacified.

There are, however, a number of disadvantages:

- The test itself is time-consuming and needs a skilled operator.
- The para-aortic nodes are only filled to the level of the renal hilum. This leaves coeliac, splenic hilar, porta hepatis and mesenteric lymph nodes unopacified.
- Large nodes obliterated by tumour may not opacify at all. For this reason an IVP is done with the abdominal film to make sure that there are no unopacified nodes displacing the ureters.

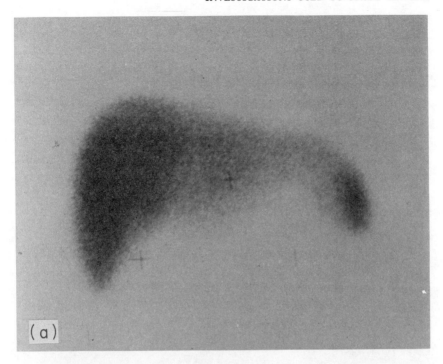

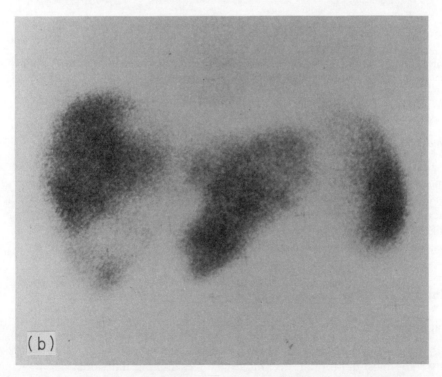

Figure 7. (a) Isotopic image of a normal liver. (b) Isotopic image of a liver containing metastatic cancer (cold areas of decreased uptake)

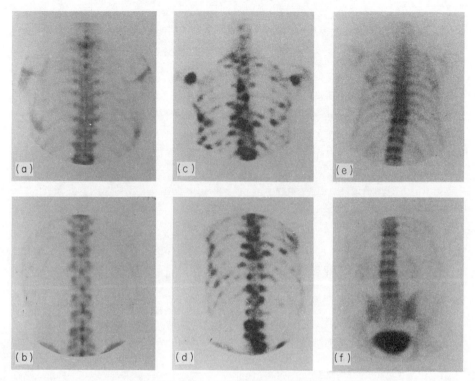

Figure 8. Normal isotopic bone image of the thorax (a) and abdomen (b). Isotopic bone image of the thorax (c) and abdomen (d) of a man with extensive prostatic cancer metastatic to bone (hot areas of increased uptake). (e), (f): Isotope bone images of a patient with osteoporosis and vertebral collapse. Although multiple areas of increased uptake are seen in the vertebrae these are homogeneous in their appearance and symmetrical in their pattern of distribution

Guided Biopsy

The wealth of anatomical information now available through various radiological techniques means that many areas of the body previously inaccessible, except by surgery, can now be reached by percutaneous needle biopsy under local anaesthetic.

The technique can be applied safely to most sites in the thorax and abdomen, for the diagnosis of primary or metastatic tumour, and can save the patient the discomfort and expense of exploratory surgery.

Evaluating Imaging Techniques

The appropriate use of any investigation requires that the doctor ordering it knows:

- the natural history of the disease being studied
- the most appropriate technique(s) for examining individual organs

- the sensitivity of the test (the proportion of positive tests in abnormal tissues)
- the specificity of the test (the proportion of negative tests in normal tissue)
- that there is appropriate expertise in performing and interpreting the test—some techniques, such as ultrasonography, rely heavily on the skill of the operator

Surgery in the Staging of Cancer

Surgery has generally been used in an attempt to completely remove a tumour with the intention of cure, or palliatively to relieve symptoms. Occasionally now, it is used as part of the staging process in several tumours.

- This approach is best exemplified by the use of staging laparotomy in some patients with Hodgkin's disease (Chapter 20). Because the choice of treatment may lie between radiotherapy and chemotherapy it is of paramount importance that the extent of disease is accurately known. Only then will it be possible to see if radiotherapy is feasible and, if it is, to plan the extent of the fields needed. Such operations, done only to define the extent of disease, are uncommon in other tumours and are only rational if there are various therapeutic approaches capable of successful treatment of disease at different stages. A single approach capable of curing disease at all stages would, of course, obviate the need for such painstaking staging.
- Surgical staging is often done during an operation to remove a primary cancer. Whilst the operation is being done a careful examination of all accessible sites at risk should usually be undertaken. Ovarian carcinoma is managed this way; up to 30% of patients with apparently localized disease are upstaged if careful staging is carried out (Chapter 15).
- Biopsies are often used to make the diagnosis of cancer. Sometimes they are used to give additional information for staging. This may include biopsy of lymph nodes, skin nodules, the liver or perhaps most commonly bone marrow biopsy and aspiration. The introduction of ultrasound and CT scanning has also opened up the possibility of biopsy of less easily accessible sites, such as intra-abdominal lymph nodes, lung masses and the pancreas. Endoscopic techniques, with biopsy have had the same effect.

Tumour Markers

Some tumours produce substances which can be detected in the blood or urine. Because the levels of these substances are often related to the bulk of active tumour their presence may be used to help diagnose, monitor response to therapy and detect relapse. Unfortunately, few if any, markers of human tumours have completely fulfilled the ideal requirements for a really useful clinical test. These are:

- the marker should be specific for the tumour
- it should be produced by all tumours of that type
- it should be easy to measure
- it should be a sensitive indicator of tumour mass
- it should be able to detect very small tumour volumes
- its production in metastases should parallel that in the primary

Lastly, though not a property of the marker, there must be an active therapy for the tumour concerned—a 'perfect' marker for an advanced cancer will be useless if there is no treatment available.

Because of these stringent requirements tumour markers have generally made little impact on the management of most cancers. Table 1 lists the markers which are currently used; more detail on their utility is given in the relevant chapters. Most potential markers fail because they are not specific for the tumour concerned and there is no treatment available for advanced disease if it is present. At present, β-HCG and AFP are the tumour markers which are nearest to the ideal and because of this the most clinically useful (Figure 9).

Conclusions

- Staging gives a useful guide to prognosis.
- Staging plays an important part in the process of choosing treatment; remember, extensive staging is only justified if

Table 1. Commonly used 'useful' tumour markers

Marker	Tumour
Beta-human chorionic (β-HCG) gonadotrophin	Choriocarcinoma and germ cell tumours
Alpha-fetoprotein (AFP)	Teratoma and hepatoma
Carcinoembryonic antigen (CEA)	Tumours of the GI tract and breast
Alkaline phosphatase	Marker of bone or liver involvement with tumour and some bone cancers
Prostatic acid phosphatase	Prostate cancer
Monoclonal antibodies to tumour antigens	Currently these are mainly used in ovarian carcinoma, with some success
Ectopic hormone production (calcitonin, ACTH, ADH, MSH)	Rare syndrome of hormone production — medullary thyroid tumours, carcinoid, small cell lung, for example
Quantitative immunoglobulin levels in plasma and urine	Multiple myeloma and, rarely, non-Hodgkin's lymphoma

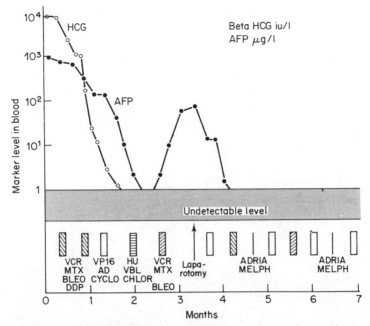

Figure 9. Response to chemotherapy with subsequent relapse and complete remission after surgery in a patient with anaplastic germ cell tumour of the testis metastatic to para-aortic nodes. From Bagshawe (1983) *Clinics in Oncology*, **2**: 176, W.B. Saunders; reproduced by permission

there is an active therapy available for advanced disease or if a 'toxic' treatment is planned for early disease.

- Internationally accepted staging systems are essential for the comparison of results between different centres.
- Remember that the introduction of more sensitive staging techniques is likely to cause 'stage migration'—comparison of results with historical data becomes very suspect.
- 'Appropriate' staging requires a thorough knowledge of the natural history of the cancer concerned together with detailed information on the utility of the tests.

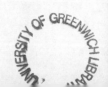

7 | Principles of Cancer Management

C. J. WILLIAMS

Ideal care for a cancer patient is not simply a matter of selecting the best techniques with which to treat the tumour. Therapy must be seen in the context of the individual and his or her family. Whilst every attempt at cure or tumour control should be made, this must be accompanied by attention to symptom control and emotional support. One of the crucial questions in patient care that is often ignored or muddled is just what is the *goal of treatment*. Any therapeutic choice must balance the chances of benefit against the discomfort or dangers of treatment: such a choice can only be made if the doctor has decided what goals are achievable. For instance:

- Very advanced testicular cancer is curable with chemotherapy and this should be the goal. In this instance both the young patient and his doctor will find acceptable a treatment with multiple severe side-effects.
- On the other hand, advanced malignant melanoma is incurable with chemotherapy and the goal is symptom control, so that even moderately toxic treatment is very hard to justify.

So, in order to make this fundamental decision the clinician needs to have a thorough knowledge of:

- the natural history of the disease
- the extent of tumour spread
- the patient's general health and fitness for treatment
- the effectiveness of the available treatments
- the toxicities associated with these therapies

Only when this information is available can the clinician decide whether treatment is *curative* or simply *palliative*.

Cancer management has become increasingly complicated and technical. This means that good co-operation between those caring for the patient is essential. Most cancers will need hospital treatment and will potentially involve:

- Surgeon to take a biopsy and possibly excise the cancer.
- Pathologist to interpret the biopsy specimen.
- Radiologist, ultrasonographer and nuclear medicine consultant to organize and interpret diagnostic staging techniques.
- Radiotherapist and radiographer.
- Medical oncologist and chemotherapy nurses.
- Specialist nurses (such as mastectomy nurses) to counsel and support patients and their families.
- Hospice doctors and nurses for home or in-patient care of the dying.
- The patient's general practitioner who can help support them and their family, manage some of the treatment and act as the patient's friend.

Each of the principals in this list will be supported by a team of other doctors, nurses and secretarial staff. Clearly, cancer care really is a team effort. This chapter discusses some of the basic principles of management for each of the major treatments available. The discussion here is simple since the management of individual tumours is covered in Part 2.

Surgery

The surgeon occupies a unique position in cancer management as over 90% of patients with malignancy will have some form of operation. This may be done in order to:

- make the diagnosis or stage the cancer
- excise the tumour (as primary therapy)
- manage complications of the cancer
- prevent cancer (rarely)

Diagnosis

Most patients who have cancer will be referred initially to a surgeon. At this stage cancer may be suspected or just part of the differential diagnosis associated with the patient's complaints. The surgeon often bears the responsibility of making the diagnosis—for this he will need a good knowledge of the natural history of the various common cancers. Eventually a tissue diagnosis will be obtained; even if the characteristics of a palpable lump or radiological mass appear to be those of an obvious cancer, histology is *always* required. If this is omitted non-cancerous lesions will occasionally be treated inappropriately.

- Always obtain histological proof of cancer. Sometimes, the cancer will only become available for biopsy at a formal operation—frozen section may be used to prove the diagnosis before proceeding to radical surgery.

- Occasionally, surgery will be used to stage cancer. Operations designed solely to look for cancer spread are rare. Normally, staging laparotomy to stage Hodgkin's disease (page 376), is the only instance when this type of operative staging is employed.

Because the surgeon is so often the doctor who makes the initial diagnosis it often falls to him to break the news to the patient and their family. Choosing a good surgeon is not just a case of selecting an adept operator; the patient will need a good diagnostician and, in the case of cancer, a sympathetic doctor who can explain the situation sensitively and honestly. It is not possible to make rules about how to tell patients bad news, though guidelines can be given:

- Try to see the patient together with a close relative or friend.
- In general, the great majority of patients will appreciate honesty.
- Try to get a feel as to what the patient already knows—many patients already suspect cancer, possibly because of the attitude of staff and what they have overheard. If the patient already has a good idea it may be easier to have a frank discussion.
- Explain what was found and what was done at the operation and why.
- Use the word cancer in the discussion. Employing euphemisms or even the word tumour sometimes results in the patient thinking that they have a benign condition. Try to explain the situation as clearly as possible.
- Give the patient time to ask questions and allow them to go over old ground as much as they need.
- Do not force the pace.
- If there are positive, but realistic, things to say, make sure that you say them; if the tumour is potentially curable make sure that the patient understands.
- If more treatment is needed explain why and what it consists of.
- Do not press the patient to make any treatment decisions immediately. Give them time to consider the situation and to ask any further questions they may have.
- Do not try to play God by giving a clear-cut prognosis. Even if you know the median survival is 6 months for a cancer of this stage do not tell the patient they have 6 months to live. Since your estimate is a median figure half will die before this and half after this time. Patients and their families will take your estimate to heart and such pronouncements can be very destructive.

- Even if the cancer is incurable do not give the patient the impression that the situation is hopeless and that you have given up. Patients in this position can always be helped and it can be amazing what patients can achieve even in the face of an incurable disease—but they need to know that their doctors will do all they can to support and help them.
- View every patient as an individual and try to temper honesty with sensitivity.

Surgery as Primary Therapy

Nearly three-quarters of cancer patients will be considered as candidates for surgical resection of their cancer in an attempt to achieve cure. The appropriateness of such an operation will depend on a knowledge of:

- the natural history of the malignancy
- the results of staging

Surgery will normally only be undertaken if staging shows that the cancer is apparently localized. However, some tumours are rapidly growing and widely spread even when clinical staging procedures suggest a localized cancer. For instance, small cell lung cancer is very rarely cured by resection of lung tissue even when it appears to be surgically operable.

Surgical excision in an attempt to achieve cure should be reserved for localized tumours of histological type likely to be confined to the primary site. Despite this many patients whose tumour has been completely resected will eventually have tumour recurrence, either locally or at distant sites (Table 1).

Table 1 shows that an alarmingly large number of patients have unrecognized tumour at the time of surgery. This has led to the hypothesis that cancers frequently metastasize at an early stage, with occult microscopic metastases becoming clinically evident after

Table 1. Relapse rates for some common solid tumours treated surgically*

Site of tumour	Relapse rate (%)
Breast	60
Colon	50
Rectum	40
Stomach	80
Oesophagus	80
Pancreas	90
Malignant melanoma	50
Non-small cell lung cancer	70
Ovary	50

*Relapse rates will vary with the stage of the disease at presentation.

the primary cancer has been excised. Because of this the early use of systemic therapy (adjuvant) has been tested extensively in the past two decades.

The requirements of a curative operation are:

- complete excision of the tumour with a margin of normal uninvolved tissue
- in some instances, resection of draining lymph nodes, preferably *en bloc*

The utility of this long accepted approach has to be examined in properly controlled trials since in some circumstances less radical operations may produce results equivalent to extensive surgery (see Chapter 15 on breast cancer).

Palliative Surgery

Even though the potential for surgical cure in many solid tumours is low, excision of the primary is often helpful to the patient since unpleasant problems can be avoided. For instance, excision of an extensive Dukes C colon cancer may carry a high risk of relapse but the patient, even in the event of relapse, will have benefited since obstruction of the bowel is likely to have been prevented. In some instances surgery may be planned to deal with a complication of the cancer even when there is no hope of cure. Judicious use of such an approach can help patients, but careful assessment of the pros and cons of such surgery is needed (Figure 1).

Preventive Surgery

Very occasionally, surgeons will be called upon to remove an organ which is at great risk of becoming malignant. Despite the trauma of surgery and its possible mutilation this is justifiable in certain circumstances. Such operations are most commonly done to remove the large bowel, for instance when the risk of cancer approaches 100% in the case of familial multiple polyposis coli and chronic ulcerative colitis.

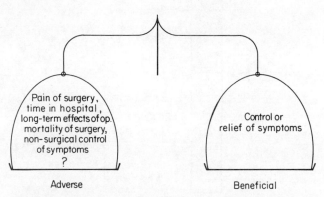

Adverse   Beneficial

Figure 1. Weighing the pros and cons of palliative surgery

Radiotherapy

Radiotherapy involves the use of ionizing radiation to treat cancer. The radiation used is of very high energy and short wavelength. Figure 2 shows the electromagnetic spectrum from radio waves, through visible light to the very short wavelength X-rays. Ionizing radiation is capable of displacing electrons from their orbit around the nucleus of atoms. This creates unstable (ionized atoms) and the free electron is often captured by nearby atoms, which also become unstable because of their additional negative charge. When living tissue is exposed to ionizing radiation cellular destruction can be initiated. Because the characteristics of the radiation can be manipulated the radiotherapist is able to control the amount of cellular damage.

Following Roentgen's discovery of X-rays in 1895 and Curie's discovery of radium in 1898, radiation was used, often disastrously, to treat various illnesses. Although some cancers seemed to respond temporarily to irradiation, severe side-effects were common and cure was rare. In 1934 Contard showed that radiotherapy was more effective if the radiation was delivered in multiple small doses (fractions) over a long time period. This dose-time relationship remains a major factor in modern radiotherapy. In the past 30 years there have been major improvements in the types of radiation available and in the ways it can be used.

Biological Basis of Radiotherapy

Ionizing radiation results in the production of free electrons which react with water to form highly reactive free radicals. These interact with surrounding biological molecules, especially DNA, causing strand breaks. This damage may be sublethal and reparable

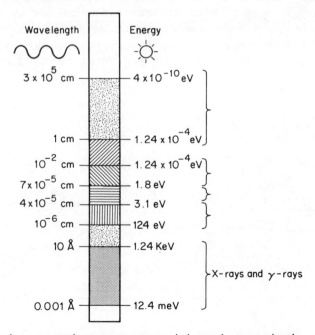

Figure 2. The electromagnetic spectrum: energy is inversely proportional to wavelength

or may cause death of the cell. The radiation sensitivity of a tissue or tumour therefore depends both on the amount of damage sustained by its cells, and their ability to repair sublethal damage. There is a wide variation in sensitivity of normal tissues and tumours. Even within a tumour, sensitivity may vary depending on the oxygenation and pH of different parts of the cancer: poorly oxygenated tumour is less sensitive to irradiation. Since large tumours frequently have poorly oxygenated areas this may be one explanation for failure of tumour control. An additional problem may be that tumour stem cells could be less radiosensitive; a few residual stem cells may then be capable of repopulating a malignant tumour despite its apparent destruction.

The discovery that repeated low doses of radiation appeared to be the most effective and safest way to give radiotherapy has led to the delivery of radiation in multiple fractions over a time period of up to 1–2 months. Experimental studies of the effects of radiotherapy on tissues suggest that at relatively low doses sublethal damage occurs. This is shown as a 'shoulder' on the dose-response curve (Figure 3). The less sensitive the tissue is to radiation the broader is the shoulder on the curve. Since the shoulder may represent sublethal damage, repeated fractions of radiation before repair can be completed cause further damage, which may become lethal. Should normal tissue be able to repair damage more quickly than cancer cells then a therapeutic advantage would be gained by using a dosage scheme of repeated small fractions (Figure 4).

Current ideas on the delivery of curative radiation therapy can be summarized thus:

- Multiple fractions should be given over a relatively protracted time course.
- Small fractions will cause much sublethal damage.
- Normal tissues may repair this sublethal damage more quickly than tumours can.

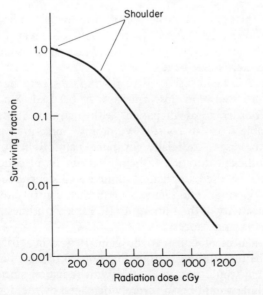

Figure 3. Cell survival (on a semi-logarithmic plot) versus radiaton dose yields a plot with an initial sloping curve ('shoulder') at low dose, evolving into a straight line at higher doses

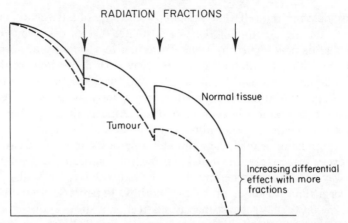

Figure 4. Fractionation of radiotherapy resulting in enhanced cytotoxicity compared to normal tissue as the tumour repair of sublethal damage is slower than the normal tissue. From Duncan, N. and Nias, A. (1977) *Clinical Radiobiology*. Churchill Livingstone, Edinburgh. Reproduced by permission

- Repeated small fractions will therefore reduce toxicity to normal tissues, allow a maximal dose and will give good tumour cell kill.
- Other theoretical advantages of fractionation include: improvement in tumour oxygenation as treatment progresses and the tumour shrinks; improved well-being of the patient and better treatment tolerance; flexibility in treatment planning so that, for instance, the radiation field can be reduced in size as the tumour shrinks.

One exception to fractionation is the use of intracavitary radioactive sources. These are, in the case of uterine or cervical cancer, used to deliver a high dose in a short time period. This is made possible by the relative lack of radiosensitivity of the normal local tissue, i.e. the uterus (see page 312).

When radiotherapy is being used to treat symptoms with no expectation of long-term disease control a short low-dose course may be used. Since repeated visits for radiotherapy are a burden to an ill patient with incurable cancer, a short course of treatment is preferable if it can control symptoms. Sometimes a single fraction or a few fractions may be used, especially for bone pain. Relief of pain will often be temporary but of sufficient duration to help a terminally ill patient.

The dose that can be used to treat a tumour will depend upon the tolerance of surrounding normal tissues. The chances of disease control are therefore related to this dose and the sensitivity of the tumour itself. Table 2 outlines the relative sensitivity of some normal tissues and cancers.

An idea of the chances of cure can be gained by using Table 2 to compare the radiosensitivity of the tumour and surrounding normal tissues. For instance, malignant melanoma in the lung would not be curable with radiation since the cancer is radio-insensitive and the lung would be so severely damaged by the dose required to control the cancer that radiation could not be used safely.

Table 2. Relative sensitivity to radiation of some normal tissues and malignancies

Radiation sensitivity*	Normal tissue	Malignant tumour
Sensitive	Bone marrow Gonads Lens of eye Lymphatic tissue Mucosa of bowel	Ewing's sarcoma Leukaemia Lymphoma Seminoma Some childhood tumours
Moderately sensitive	Bowel wall Breast Liver Lung Kidney Neural tissue Skin	Adenocarcinoma at various sites (breast, bowel, ovary) Small cell lung cancer Squamous carcinoma at various sites (gynaecological, head and neck, skin)
Insensitive	Bone Muscle	Connective tissue tumours Malignant melanoma

*In general, the most sensitive tissues and tumours are those dividing and growing most rapidly.

- All tumours can be eradicated by radiation if a high enough
     dose is used.
- Since the dose that can be delivered safely is governed by the
     sensitivity of normal tissues and tumour, curability depends
     on the relative sensitivities of both tissues.

Radiation Damage to Normal Tissues

Radiotherapy causes acute effects, which depend on the site being treated and the size of the field. They may include:

- malaise
- nausea and vomiting
- inflammation of the normal tissues causing symptoms such as
     cough, dysphagia, diarrhoea and frequency of micturition
     and dysuria, depending on the organ being treated.

Long-term effects do not develop for several months and may gradually progress for years. They are nearly always due to damage to the microvasculature and are usually permanent. They include:

- sclerosis and scarring of the irradiated area
- poor healing and occasionally necrosis
- weakening and fracture of bone
- stenosis of hollow organs (gut, bladder, etc.)
- bleeding (bowel, bladder)
- nerve palsies and radiation myelitis

Other long-term effects that need to be considered include:

- Carcinogenicity: data from Hiroshima and follow-up of irradiated patients have shown that radiation does induce cancer in a small proportion of those exposed. Acute myelogenous leukaemia is the induced second malignancy seen most commonly in irradiated patients.
- Teratogenicity: exposure of the foetus to irradiation during the first two trimesters of pregnancy carries an unacceptable risk of serious malformation.
- Mutagenicity: theoretically, exposure of germ cells to irradiation may cause mutations which could result in abnormality of future offspring. However, most mutations in germ cells appear to be lethal and there has not been an increased incidence of abnormal offspring of men who have been irradiated.

Cure and Palliation

Although radiotherapy is frequently used palliatively, it is also used as primary curative therapy in several tumours, provided they are at a relatively early stage: examples include cervical and laryngeal cancer. Radiation may also be used to gain long-term control of disease even though it is not itself necessarily curative. Radiation to the chest wall following mastectomy or for local recurrence of breast cancer is an example of such a use—it reduces the risk of local relapse or controls recurrent disease, but does not influence survival, which is dependent upon the presence or absence of distant metastases. When radiotherapy is used to obtain cure or long-term survival, prolonged courses with multiple fractions are often used. Alternatively intracavitary treatment may be used to deliver a high local dose. If the aim of treatment is symptom control, shorter, less complicated treatments are usually preferred so that the patient's life is disrupted as little as possible.

Chemotherapy and Hormone Therapy

There has been a clear need for effective systemic treatments of cancer: many patients die because surgery and/or radiotherapy fail to control distant metastases, in spite of eradicating the primary. Systematic staging at diagnosis will frequently detect disease which has already spread to distant sites (Table 3). Even when such staging tests are normal some of these patients will prove to have microscopic metastases which only become evident later, when the patient relapses. Recently monoclonal antibodies directed at tumour determinants have been used to demonstrate small collections of malignant cells in the bone marrow of patients otherwise apparently free of metastases.

Other types of cancer, such as leukaemia and lymphoma, are never amenable to surgery and often not to radiation, so that a systemic therapy is the only possible treatment for these conditions.

Table 3. Sites of metastatic disease in small cell lung cancer

Site*	Proportion of patients with metastases (%)
Liver	24
Bone	21
Supraclavicular lymph nodes	21
Bone marrow	17
Cervical lymph nodes	14
CNS metastases	4
Skin metastases	4

*Other sites, such as adrenal, are commonly involved but were not looked for in this series of 100 consecutive patients treated in Southampton.

Nitrogen mustard was the first cytotoxic drug to be developed in the mid 1940s, though some hormonal drugs had been available prior to this. Since then new drugs have been developed steadily (Figure 5).

Although a detailed knowledge of the pharmacology, mode of administration, toxicity and effectiveness of anti-cancer drugs is needed by chemotherapists and radiation oncologists, such information is superfluous at an undergraduate level. Not only is this area of medicine highly specialized, it is also changing very rapidly with the development of new drugs and new ways of using them. However, a broad understanding of the principles of cytotoxic therapy is useful for the non-specialist.

The Cell Cycle

Since most anti-cancer drugs interfere with cell division, an understanding of the cell cycle is important. The cell cycle has been defined as the interval between the mid point of mitosis in a cell and the mid point of the subsequent mitosis in one or both daughter cells. Four phases of the cell cycle have been described (Figure 6). During the S-phase there is synthesis of nucleic acids. The M-phase signifies the process of mitosis. The G1 and G2 (G = gap) phases are associated with biochemical activity, but little morphological change. Cells which are not prepared for or undergoing division—resting cells—are described as being in G0.

- Drugs that affect cells whether they are in G0 or in cell cycle are called non-cycle active drugs.
- Drugs which only affect cells in a particular phase of the cell cycle are described as phase-specific drugs.
- Drugs that exert their effects only when cells are in cycle, but at no specific phase, are called cycle-specific drugs.

Cell Kinetics

Tumours are heterogeneous, being made up of a mixture of cells which have different patterns of behaviour. Three theoretical compartments have been described:

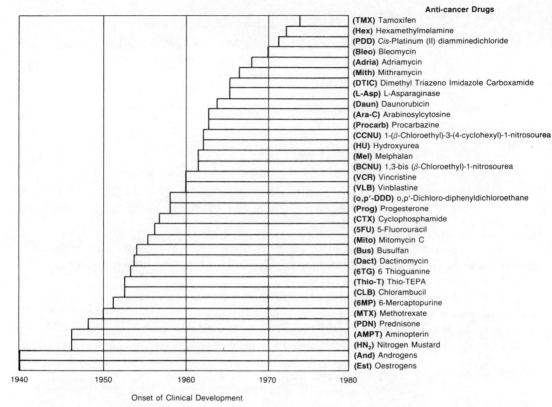

Anti-cancer Drugs

(TMX) Tamoxifen
(Hex) Hexamethylmelamine
(PDD) *Cis*-Platinum (II) diamminedichloride
(Bleo) Bleomycin
(Adria) Adriamycin
(Mith) Mithramycin
(DTIC) Dimethyl Triazeno Imidazole Carboxamide
(L-Asp) L-Asparaginase
(Daun) Daunorubicin
(Ara-C) Arabinosylcytosine
(Procarb) Procarbazine
(CCNU) 1-(β-Chloroethyl)-3-(4-cyclohexyl)-1-nitrosourea
(HU) Hydroxyurea
(Mel) Melphalan
(BCNU) 1,3-bis (β-Chloroethyl)-1-nitrosourea
(VCR) Vincristine
(VLB) Vinblastine
(o,p'-DDD) o,p'-Dichloro-diphenyldichloroethane
(Prog) Progesterone
(CTX) Cyclophosphamide
(5FU) 5-Fluorouracil
(Mito) Mitomycin C
(Bus) Busulfan
(Dact) Dactinomycin
(6TG) 6 Thioguanine
(Thio-T) Thio-TEPA
(CLB) Chlorambucil
(6MP) 6-Mercaptopurine
(MTX) Methotrexate
(PDN) Prednisone
(AMPT) Aminopterin
(HN₂) Nitrogen Mustard
(And) Androgens
(Est) Oestrogens

1940   1950   1960   1970   1980

Onset of Clinical Development

Figure 5. Development of new cytotoxic drugs and hormones 1940–1980. There has been a steady increase in the number of clinically useful agents introduced into standard practice

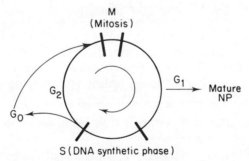

Figure 6. The cell cycle. M $\equiv$ Mitosis (prophase/metaphase/anaphase/telophase). G $\equiv$ Gap. S $\equiv$ DNA synthesis. $G_0 \equiv$ Resting phase. $G_1 \equiv$ Early growth phase. $G_2 \equiv$ Later growth phase. NP = Non-proliferating

- cells undergoing active division—those in cell cycle
- cells that are capable of entering cell cycle, but as yet are not doing so (G0)
- end-stage cells that have left cell cycle and cannot return—cells that die a natural death

The number of cells in any one compartment varies within an individual tumour, between each type of cancer, from patient to patient and with time. The proportion of the tumour in cell cycle is referred to as the *growth fraction*. The growth fraction is the chief mechanism whereby the tumour grows. Tumours may also increase in size more rapidly by shortening the cell cycle time or by decreasing cell loss. However, many tumours do not seem to be able to shorten cell cycle time (most tumours have longer cell cycle times than many normal tissues), and cells that die a natural death often exceed half the tumour mass.

Apart from some haematological malignancies many tumours are relatively slow growing, have large numbers of cells destined to die and rather low growth fractions. This explains much of the lack of success of chemotherapy in the slower growing solid tumours: indeed, in the face of such a situation it is surprising that cytotoxic therapy has any useful effect. Clearly, the effectiveness of such treatment does not depend solely on rapidly growing tumour cells being damaged more than normal cells by cytotoxics.

Doubling Times and Cell Turnover

The doubling time of a cancer is the time it takes for a tumour to double its cell numbers. This is not the same as the cell cycle time—only if the growth fraction is 100% would the cell cycle time be the same as the doubling time. The *in vitro* cell cycle time of many normal and neoplastic cells is between 15 and 72 hours.

Some normal tissues (mucosa of the GI tract and bone marrow) have a high growth fraction, short cell cycle time and consequently short doubling times. These tissues are especially susceptible to the effects of cycle or phase-specific drugs. Fortunately, their rapid growth allows rapid recovery following exposure to cytotoxic drugs.

The doubling times of many solid tumours are long (>100 days) though some haematological cancers have doubling times as short as 4 days. These figures must be contrasted with normal myeloblasts, which double their number in 60 hours. Although malignant tumours appear relatively slow growing compared with certain normal tissues there is a clear correlation between doubling time and 'curability' using current chemotherapy (Table 4).

Table 4. Correlation between doubling time and 'curability' for various human tumours

Tumour	Doubling times (days)	Regime inducing 'cure'
Burkitt's lymphoma	1.0	Single agent*
Choriocarcinoma	1.5	Single agent†
Acute lymphoblastic lymphoma	3–4	Drug combination
Hodgkin's disease	3–4	Drug combination
Testicular teratoma	5–6	Drug combination
Breast carcinoma	60	None
Colon carcinoma	80	None
Non-small cell lung cancer	100	None

*Drug combinations are always used now.
†Drug combinations are used for patients with adverse prognostic features.

Tumour Burden

Tumour size is often a limiting factor in cancer chemotherapy. This may be for a number of reasons:

- A high proportion of cells in large tumours may be in a non-proliferative state (G0).
- Vascularization of large tumours is heterogeneous; some areas are avascular or necrotic. Drug entry is often erratic.
- Large numbers of cells require more courses of treatment to eradicate them. Chemotherapy seems to follow first-order kinetics—i.e. a given treatment will kill a constant proportion of cells rather than a constant number (provided the growth fraction and cell cycle time remain constant). Because of this it takes as long to lower a tumour burden from 10^6 to 10^3 cells (loss of 1 mg of tissue) as it does to lower the cell number from 10^9 to 10^6 (loss of 1 g of tissue).
- When numerous repeated courses of cytotoxics are needed the chances of resistance developing are markedly increased.

Duration of Treatment

At the time of diagnosis as many as 10^{12} malignant cells may be present. Successful chemotherapy may kill as many as 99.9% of all cells with a single cycle of treatment (3-log kill); however, this will still leave 10^9 cells surviving. This number is barely detectable clinically and a 'remission' will be recorded (Figure 7). It is, of course,

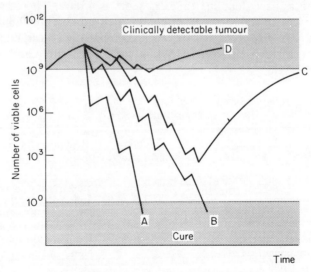

Figure 7. Schematic representation of the variability of response to cytotoxic chemotherapy. Patient A is cured by three cycles of treatment; patient B is cured by six cycles; whereas patient C responds well initially but after the sixth cycle resistant disease grows back; patient D has little or no response

necessary to continue therapy; fortunately, the cell kill rate may increase after the first treatment as more cells enter the growth fraction, a phenomenon known as recruitment.

The correct duration of treatment is still difficult to estimate: it requires assumptions to be made about:

- total tumour burden
- rate of tumour cell kill
- the proliferation of surviving malignant cells
- recovery time of normal tissues.

In practice, there is little evidence that prolonged combination chemotherapy increases the chances of cure: most adult patients receive a maximum of six to nine treatments.

Drug Resistance

Some tumours appear to be primarily resistant to cytotoxic chemotherapy (renal cell carcinoma, for instance), whilst in others resistance may appear to be acquired. If a proportion of cells in the original tumour are resistant to a cytotoxic drug they will re-establish the tumour after the drug-sensitive cells have been killed. Alternatively, drug-sensitive cells may become resistant during treatment. The use of combinations of drugs having different mechanisms of action may help overcome the problem of resistance. Although resistance to one or more of the drugs may be present or develop these cells may remain sensitive to the remaining drugs. Known mechanisms of resistance include:

- insufficient uptake of the drug
- decreased activation of the drug
- increased deactivation of the drug
- increased concentration of target enzyme by induction or gene amplification
- decreased requirement of a specific metabolic product
- increased use of alternative (salvage) biochemical pathways
- increased DNA repair
- increased active transport of drug out of cells

The choice of drugs for combination chemotherapy has been largely empirical and broad rules have been formulated:

- Only drugs known to be active by themselves are used.
- The individual drugs should have different mechanisms of action.
- Their dose-limiting toxicities should be dissimilar.
- They should if possible be synergistic (more than additive anti-tumour effects)—such combinations should be sought, though care is needed that there is not also synergy for toxicity.

Host Factors

Determinants of response to chemotherapy and other therapies are often related to the host as well as the cancer cells. Although a simple concept, the general status of the patient's health is often the best indicator of tumour responsiveness and outcome. Scales of 'performance status' are used in trials in an attempt to measure the patient's fitness for treatment. An additional and crucial role of such scales is for the comparison of trial results. A trial only admitting patients of high performance status is almost certain to have better results than one containing a majority of patients of low performance status, regardless of treatment.

Host factors may have an effect on tolerance of treatment, and part of the prognostic effect of performance status may be related to this.

Toxicity of Cytotoxic Drugs

All anti-cancer drugs have harmful side-effects. Though each drug has its own spectrum of toxicity all have one common property: they cannot distinguish between normal and malignant cells.

The rate of cellular proliferation varies enormously between different normal tissues, but generally the effects of cytotoxics are seen most acutely in those tissues with the highest proliferative activity:

- bone marrow—pancytopenia (reversible)
- mucosa of mouth and GI tract—mucosal ulceration, diarrhoea (reversible)
- hair follicles and skin—hair loss, skin and nail changes (reversible)
- sperm production—azoospermia (transient or permanent depending on the drugs used)

The extent to which these systems are affected varies greatly from drug to drug.

Individual drugs also have direct biochemical effects which result in specific organ toxicities not directly related to an anti-proliferative effect. These include:

- nausea and vomiting—one of the major subjective problems for the patient; very dependent on the drug being used
- peripheral neuropathy—principally a problem with the vinca alkaloids and cisplatin
- cardiomyopathy—principally caused by the anthracycline drugs
- pneumonitis—mainly a problem with bleomycin but lung infiltrates can occur with a wide variety of anti-cancer drugs
- renal toxicity—often a problem in patients receiving cisplatin and, less commonly, high-dose methotrexate
- bladder inflammation—most often seen in patients receiving ifosfamide or cyclophosphamide
- hepatic damage—not especially common though it can occur with long-term methotrexate
- damage to local tissues when some drugs extravasate

Toxicity affecting the kidney and liver is of great potential importance since this may delay drug metabolism and excretion thus potentiating toxicity. Safe drug administration requires a good knowledge of the pharmacology and toxicity of the drugs being used. No one unfamiliar with cytotoxic compounds should administer them since they are potentially lethal. Before giving any cytotoxic make sure that:

- the blood count is adequate
- there is no dysfunction in the major organ of excretion
- the patient is tolerating the treatment
- the patient is responding adequately to the treatment
- the methods of handling and administering the drug and any potential acute effects are fully appreciated
- the drug dose can be calculated accurately according to the patient's surface area
- the patient is advised to contact a doctor (preferably the one giving the treatment) if they become febrile or ill during treatment. Neutropenic sepsis is potentially fatal within hours. Febrile patients with a low granulocyte count should be admitted to hospital to receive intravenous broad-spectrum antibiotics once appropriate cultures have been taken.

Testing New Treatments

Because anti-cancer drug therapy still requires much improvement and because new compounds are rapidly becoming available, clinical trials of these drugs have formed a major part of medical oncology.

- Phase I studies are the first use of a new drug in man. Treatment is started at a low dose and, dependent upon patient toleration, is gradually increased until the *maximum tolerated dose* (MTD) is found.
- A dose just below this level is then used in a Phase II trial, which is designed to test whether the drug has any useful activity.
- Interesting drugs are then used in Phase III studies, where they will be compared with standard treatment to see if they represent an improvement in care.

Patients in Phase I and II trials have usually failed all conventional therapy and their chances of a major response are poor.

Hormones

Beatson was the first to show that some tumours were sensitive to their hormonal environment: in 1896 he reported that the advanced breast cancer of some patients regressed after oophorectomy. Hormones appear to bind to receptors in the cytoplasm of cells and sterically alter the shape of the protein receptor which, following transport to the nucleus, interacts with DNA initiating messenger RNA and protein synthesis.

There are now a large number of hormones and 'anti-hormones' which can be used, and operations to remove the source of endogenous hormones (oophorectomy, for instance) are common. These hormones are not without toxicity although they are generally better tolerated than chemotherapy.

Conclusions

Having made a histological diagnosis of cancer and having assessed the extent of spread the clinician must then ask the key question: what is the realistic goal of therapy? If the goal is 'cure' attitudes towards the unpleasantness and morbidities of treatment will be very different compared to a case in which only palliation is achievable. In this situation the balance between benefit and adverse effects must be carefully weighed.

In order to select appropriate therapy the clinician needs to have a thorough knowledge of cancer biology and of the natural history of cancer. This must be allied with mastery of the pharmacology, radiobiology and side-effects of the therapies that may be applied.

8 Paraneoplastic Manifestations of Cancer

C. J. WILLIAMS

Some cancers produce indirect effects on different organs in the body. These are not due to the presence of the cancer in that tissue: often they are mediated by hormones or other substances produced by cancer cells. Such syndromes can affect any organ system and may produce profound illness. Sometimes they may occur up to several years before a cancer is detected. For the sake of simplicity they will be discussed by major organ system—coverage is brief and is intended as a reference source.

Neurological Complications

Most neurological problems in cancer patients are caused by direct involvement of the brain, spinal cord, meninges or nerves. Less common, though equally devastating in their consequences, are the non-metastatic neurological disorders.

Though the CNS can be affected by infections, vascular disorders, metabolic abnormalities and the effects of treatment for cancer, this section concentrates on the so-called 'remote effects' of cancer. These are classified as follows:

- Brain and cranial nerves
    Dementia (limbic encephalitis)
    Bulbar encephalitis
    Subacute cerebellar degeneration*
    Optic neuritis
- Spinal cord
    Amyotrophic lateral sclerosis
    Subacute motor myelopathy
- Peripheral nerves and roots
    Subacute sensory neuropathy*

Sensorimotor peripheral neuropathy
Acute polyneuropathy
Autonomic neuropathy
● Polymyositis and dermatomyositis*
Myasthenic syndrome
Myasthenia gravis
Neuromyotonia

*These disorders may precede the diagnosis of cancer. Their presence is strongly suggestive of malignancy.

Brain and Cranial Nerves

Limbic Encephalitis. This is a rare disorder which presents with dementia. Its features are given in the box.

Loss of recent memory
Agitation
Hallucinations
Dysarthria
Seizures

Clinical findings are shown in the box.

The CSF is usually normal
EEG may show slow waves in the temporal regions
Pathologically there is extensive neuronal loss and astroglial
    proliferation

It is most commonly seen in patients with lung cancer.

Bulbar Encephalitis. This is also most commonly seen in patients with bronchogenic carcinoma. Its features are given in the box.

Dystonia
Central hypoventilation
Ophthalmoplegia
Seizures

Subacute Cerebellar Degeneration. This syndrome has been reported in the following malignancies: lung, ovary, breast, stomach and lymphoma. Clinically the following manifestations are seen (see box).

Subacute development of ataxia of upper and lower limbs
Dysarthria
Dysphagia
Motor weakness and reflex changes are less common

These changes may precede the diagnosis of cancer by up to 2 or more years. The syndrome tends to be progressive; major findings are given in the box.

CSF shows mild pleocytosis and increased protein.
Pathologically there is panhemispheric loss
    of the Purkinje cell layer; this affects the molecular and granular
    layers of the cerebellum, spinocerebellar tracts and the pyramidal
    and dorsal columns.

Optic Neuritis. This is a rare paraneoplastic effect. The findings are given in the box.

Decreased vision
A central scotoma
Papilloedema

It is important to differentiate this disorder from secondary involvement of the optic nerve by tumour.

Spinal Cord

These syndromes are uncommon.

Amyotrophic Lateral Sclerosis. This is occasionally associated with cancer; its main features are given in the box.

Fasciculations with muscular atrophy
Weakness secondary to denervation
Hyperreflexia
Loss of lower motor neurones in the anterior horn region of the
spinal cord

Subacute Motor Myelopathy. This is most often associated with lung cancer. Clinically it is recognized by the following (see box).

Its fulminating ascending motor and sensory deficit
Degenerative changes in both white and grey matter

Peripheral Nerves

These are the commonest of the paraneoplastic effects on the CNS. Two major groups of sensory neuropathies have been described:

- A mild symmetrical peripheral sensory loss which occurs late in
    the disease course.
- A subacute severe sensory motor neuropathy which may
    precede the diagnosis of cancer. Its course may be
    fluctuating.

Pure sensory neuropathy is frequently a precursor of cancer. Major findings are given in the box.

CSF—a mild pleocytosis and elevated protein
Loss of dorsal root ganglion cells
Loss of both myelin and axis cylinder
Tendency to progress
Ataxia
Sensory loss
Normal power

The syndrome is irreversible. It is associated with lung cancer, thymoma, lymphoma and oesophageal, ovarian and laryngeal carcinoma.

Occasional cases of acute ascending polyneuropathy (Guillain-Barré syndrome) have been reported in cancer patients. The syndrome is indistinguishable from the usual illness and may be coincidental.

Polymyositis and Dermatomyositis

These syndromes are associated with cancer in adults, and any patient presenting with them should be assessed for an underlying neoplasm. Cancers of the lung, ovary and stomach predominate. The features of dermatomyositis are given in the box.

Weakness, pain and oedema of proximal muscles of the limbs
Ptosis and diplopia
Necrosis and phagocytosis of muscle fibres with inflammatory
    infiltration of perivascular tissues

Steroids may ameliorate the symptoms.

Myasthenic Syndrome (Lambert-Eaton). This is characterized by the following features (see box).

Muscle weakness and fatigability—especially in the pelvic girdle and
    leg muscles
Diplopia, ptosis
Dysarthria
Paraesthesia
Lack of response to Tensilon
Potentiation of the muscle potential on repetitive stimulation

---

It is particularly associated with lung cancer, especially the small cell variety. It may precede diagnosis by 1 or more years. Although it is not usually reversible, despite response of the underlying tumour, remissions have been reported.

Hormonal Complications

Cancers secrete a wide variety of hormones. Although many of these are biologically inert some can produce profound metabolic consequences. Some of the hormones produced by cancer cells are shown in the box.

ACTH	Hypophosphataemic factors
Calcitonin	Neurophysins
Chorionic gonadotrophin	Osteoclast activating factor
Corticotrophin releasing	Parathyroid hormone
hormone	Prolactin
Erythropoietin	Prostaglandins
Gastrin	Secretin
Glucagon	Somatomedins
Growth hormone	Somatostatin
Hypoglycaemic factors	Vasopressin

Some of these hormones are only rarely produced by tumours so that discussion will be limited to the commonest syndromes of ectopic production related to cancer.

ACTH

The syndrome of ectopic overproduction of ACTH is named after Cushing, who was the first to describe such a hormone syndrome related to cancer. The great majority of cases (more than 85%) are found in association with tumours of six types:

- Carcinoma of the lung—55% of cases (especially small cell)
- Carcinoma of the thymus—10% of cases
- Carcinoma of the pancreas—10% of cases (includes islet and carcinoid)
- Neural crest tumours—5% of cases (neuroblastoma, phaeochromocytoma, etc.)
- Bronchial adenoma—5% of cases (includes carcinoid)
- Medullary carcinoma of thyroid—5% of cases

Although the finding of clinically evident cushingoid features is uncommon (2%), raised levels of ACTH may be found in up to 50% of patients with small cell lung cancer. The clinical features of ectopic ACTH overproduction are often different from classical Cushing's syndrome. They are given in the box.

Hyperkalaemia
Glucose intolerance
Hypertension
Muscle weakness

Tests to confirm the diagnosis are given in the box.

High-dose dexamethasone does not suppress the plasma cortisone
  level
Plasma ACTH levels will be raised
High molecular weight prohormones may be detectable

Treatment is of the underlying tumour. As a temporary measure, whilst this is being attempted, blockade of adrenal production of cortisol may be undertaken. Drugs that can be used include Metyrapone and aminoglutethimide (alone or in combination).

Inappropriate ADH

This syndrome (SIADH) was first reported in 1957 and since then has come to be recognized as one of the commonest hormonal syndromes associated with cancer. Findings are shown in the box.

Hyponatraemia
Renal sodium loss
Hypervolaemia
Inappropriately high urine osmolality

Clinically the syndrome does not usually become obvious until the serum sodium falls below 120 mmol/l, when the patient becomes confused and drowsy. It is most commonly associated with small cell lung cancer, up to 50% of cases showing ectopic production of ADH. Hyponatraemia in this tumour appears to be associated with a poorer response to therapy.

The treatment of choice is that applicable to the underlying tumour—usually chemotherapy in the case of small cell lung cancer. Whilst this is being started water restriction can be used temporarily to correct the hyponatraemia. An alternative is demeclocycline, which may make the distal tubule unresponsive to ADH. Ultimately, as in most hormonal syndromes associated with cancer, long-term control depends on the effectiveness of the anti-neoplastic treatment.

Hypercalcaemia

The features and management of this complication of cancer are discussed more fully on page 142. Although hypercalcaemia may in some instances be caused by extensive bony destruction, it is often caused by ectopic production of a parathormone-like substance, osteoclast activity factor (OAF) or possibly prostaglandins.

A wide variety of cancers may cause hypercalcaemia and their mechanism of doing so varies from one to another. An approximate distribution of types of cancers causing hypercalcaemia is given in Table 1.

It seems likely that most solid tumours causing hypercalcaemia do so by producing a biologically active substance which is similar to parathormone (PTH). In the case of haematological malignancies, the data favour the cause of hypercalcaemia as being production of osteoclast activating factor (OAF).

Gynaecomastia due to Gonadotrophin Secretion

Although rare, this syndrome is especially important as the underlying malignancy is often curable, even when the patient presents at an advanced stage. Until recently it was thought that human chorionic gonadotrophin (HCG) was only produced by trophoblastic cells of the placenta, choriocarcinoma, teratomas and seminoma. However, data now show that HCG can be produced by a wide variety of carcinomas.

Despite this, nearly all clinical cases of gynaecomastia associated with cancer in men are due to teratomas. The finding of extensive tumour in a young man with recent onset of gynaecomastia is highly suggestive of an HCG-secreting teratoma. Treatment of the underlying tumour (page 339) is usually all that is required; the gynaecomastia subsides after the level of HCG has fallen.

Haematological Complications

Anaemia

This is an extremely common finding in advanced cancer. It is often the result of a number of factors, some of these being secondary to the cachexia caused by the malignancy. Frequently it is a result of blood loss from the gastrointestinal tract. In other patients features of 'anaemia of chronic disease' develop (see box).

Table 1. Approximate incidence of hypercalcaemia in various cancers

Cancer/site	Incidence of hypercalcaemia
Kidney	14%
Squamous lung	13%
Leukaemia	13%
Breast	12%
Lymphoma	12%
Urogenital	7%
Gynaecological	7%
Liver	6%
Oesophagus	4%
Miscellaneous	12%

Initially normochromic/normocytic (subsequent hypochromasia 30%)
Less prominent microcytosis than Fe deficiency
Bone marrow Fe stores normal
Sideroblasts in bone marrow reduced
Serum Fe reduced
Transferrin levels reduced (cf. raised in Fe deficiency)

This syndrome is still poorly understood but frequently no treatment is needed. An autoimmune haemolytic anaemia may complicate some haematological cancers.

Polycythaemia

This is an uncommon complication of cancer. It is caused by ectopic production of erythropoietin. The commonest tumours associated are renal in origin (Table 2).

Most of the renal tumours are hypernephromas; the liver tumours are hepatomas; and the CNS tumours are cerebellar haemangioblastomas. Uterine tumours are usually leiomyosarcomas, though fibroids may also be associated with erythropoietin secretion.

The polycythaemia of malignancy is, in contradistinction to polycythaemia rubra vera, usually not accompanied by a rise in white cells or platelets.

Treatment of the underlying malignancy, if possible, is the treatment of choice; symptomatic venesection can be used but is rarely required. Disappearance of the erythrocytosis has been clearly demonstrated when the underlying tumour is resected.

Microangiopathic Haemolysis (page 164)

This refers to destruction of red cells as they pass through partially occluded small blood vessels affected by tumour. It is a common feature of diseases associated with vascular endothelial damage or fibroid deposition. Mucin-producing adenocarcinomas, especially of the stomach, are the malignancies most commonly associated with this condition.

There is often simultaneous evidence of active *disseminated intravascular coagulation* (DIC) with thrombocytopenia and hypofibrinogenaemia. Microangiopathic haemolytic

Table 2. Incidence of polycythaemia in various cancers

Tumour/site	Incidence
Kidney tumours	52%
Liver	18%
CNS	14%
Uterus	7%
Adrenal	3%
Miscellaneous	6%

anaemia may also be found with the 'haemolytic-uraemic syndrome' or 'thrombotic thrombocytopenia purpura' (TTP). This consists of haemolytic anaemia, thrombocytopenia, renal disease, fluctuating neurological signs and fever.

The treatment of microangiopathic haemolytic anaemia in cancer patients essentially involves dealing with immediate complications and reversing the underlying condition. Transfusion requirements may be high. Intravascular coagulation may require heparin and coagulation factor replacement. DIC is a particular problem in patients with promyelocytic leukaemia. Treatment of TTP is contentious and there is no agreed management.

Migratory Thrombophlebitis

Deep venous thrombosis in association with cancer was first noted by Trousseau, after whom the syndrome is named. Though it is classically associated with pancreatic cancer it is seen in a wide variety of carcinomas. Some patients also show fibrin deposition on heart valves (*murantic* or *non-bacterial thrombotic endocarditis*). The clinical features of deep venous thrombosis in association with cancer are somewhat different from the usual deep venous thrombosis (see box).

May precede the diagnosis of cancer (month–years)
Migratory and recurrent
Unusual sites—arms and neck
May be resistant to heparin treatment

Hyperviscosity (page 162)

This is a collection of clinical findings which occur when the viscosity of blood rises to high levels. It may occur in polycythaemia (red cells), leukaemia (white cells), myeloma and Waldenström's macroglobulinaemia (proteins). Its features are shown in the box.

Fatigue, anorexia, weight loss
Vascular—epistaxis, bleeding from mucous membranes, bruising, plethora, priapism
Ophthalmic—blurred vision, retinal haemorrhages, exudates, venous dilatation
CNS—headache, dizziness, drowsiness, tinnitus, poor hearing, unsteadiness

---

Treatment is, of course, that of the underlying cause. When the hyperviscosity is due to hyperproteinaemia, plasmapheresis may be of temporary benefit whilst anti-cancer treatment is instituted.

Renal Complications

The kidney may be affected by cancer in many ways:

- Direct effect
  obstruction
  infiltration by tumour
  infiltration by tumour products
- Metabolic consequences
  uric acid nephropathy
  hypercalcaemia
  'tumour lysis' syndrome
- Treatment effects
  anti-cancer drugs
  radiation nephropathy
- Remote effect of cancer
  nephrotic syndrome

Of these only nephrotic syndrome can be described as a paraneoplastic effect. The association of nephrotic syndrome with cancer was only described as recently as 1966. Nephrotic syndrome may predate the diagnosis of cancer by up to several years. The cancer is most commonly an adenocarcinoma though this syndrome has been reported in association with Hodgkin's disease.

Skin Complications

Indirect cutaneous manifestations of malignancy are relatively common, and a number of characteristic dermatological conditions are highly suggestive of an underlying cancer. Their treatment is that of the associated malignancy.

Acanthosis Nigricans

This can occur in various forms, including familial forms. The variety associated with cancer is characterized by hyperpigmented velvety thickening of the skin of the neck and axillae. The syndrome may predate diagnosis of cancer by years. The cancer is nearly always an adenocarcinoma (stomach or colon) and the outlook is generally very poor.

Acquired Ichthyosis

This is a scaly dermatosis which is associated with lymphoma, especially Hodgkin's disease. It usually occurs after diagnosis of the malignancy.

Dermatitis Herpetiformis

This is a highly pruritic subepidermal bullous disease in which small groups of vesicles erupt symmetrically on the body. It is linked with gluten-sensitive enteropathy and to intestinal lymphoma.

Dermatomyositis

This is a skin and muscle disease that is linked in some adults to internal malignancy. The muscle disease manifests itself as proximal symmetrical weakness that progresses. Electromyography and muscle biopsy may be characteristic, and muscle enzymes are usually raised.

The skin lesions (which differentiate dermatomyositis from polymyositis) are a heliotrope rash (violaceous periorbital oedema), Gottron's papules (violaceous lesions over bony prominences), poikiloderma, periungal telangiectasia and a photosensitive rash. About 25% of adults with dermatomyositis turn out to have malignancy.

Erythema Gyratum Repens

This is a rare eruption characterized by persistent erythematous bands that form a serpiginous pattern. They form a pattern said to resemble 'grains of wood'. An underlying cancer is almost invariably found.

Hypertrichosis Lanuginosa

This is an uncommon condition in which there is excessive growth of fine lanugo hair; although there are other associations (endocrinopathies and porphyria) cancer of any type may be associated and be diagnosed later.

Multiple Seborrhoeic Keratosis

In this condition, also known as the *Leser-Trélat sign*, there is a sudden appearance of multiple seborrhoeic keratoses. It is usually associated with an underlying cancer.

Necrolytic Migratory Erythema

This is also known as the glucagonoma syndrome, since glucagonoma is the tumour with which it is usually associated. It consists of erythematous angular patches with an active border. The trunk is usually involved and annular polycyclic lesions develop. Other features include angular stomatitis, weight loss and glucose intolerance.

Nodular Fat Necrosis

This is usually associated with an underlying pancreatic malignancy.

Pyoderma Gangrenosum

This is characterized by necrotic ulcers with an overhanging border. It develops rapidly, spreading concentrically with necrosis and ulceration. It is occasionally associated with multiple myeloma.

Inherited Conditions

The skin may also give a clue to patients who are genetically predisposed to develop cancer. These inherited conditions are summarized in Table 3.

Muscle and Joint Complications

Dermatomyositis and polymyositis have been mentioned in the section on skin.

Hypertrophic Pulmonary Osteoarthropathy

This is a condition almost exclusively associated with lung cancer. The periosteum of the ends of the long bones becomes raised, thickened and inflamed. New bone is laid above the periosteal surface and joints become swollen and inflamed. Its cause is unknown, though it may regress on resection of the primary cancer.

Table 3. Inherited skin conditions associated with cancer

Condition	Associated malignancy/site
AUTOSOMAL DOMINANT	
Tylosis (hyperkeratosis of soles and palms)	Oesophagus
Gardener's syndrome (colonic polyps, skin and bone lesions)	Colon
Cowden's syndrome (multiple hamartomas)	Breast, thyroid, colon
Peutz-Jeghers syndrome (intestinal polyps, melanotic macules of mouth and lips)	Intestine, stomach
Torre's syndrome (sebaceous gland tumours)	Colon
Neurofibromatosis (*café au lait* spots of skin, neurofibrosarcoma)	Leukaemia, neurofibrosarcoma
AUTOSOMAL RECESSIVE	
Ataxic telangiectasia (telangiectases of neck, face, elbows and knees)	Lymphoma
Bloom's syndrome (characteristic facies, light-sensitive rash)	Leukaemia, lymphoma and carcinoma
Wiscott Aldrich syndrome (eczema, purpura, pyoderma)	Lymphoma
Fanconi's anaemia (patchy hyperpigmentation)	Leukaemia
Chédiak-Higashi syndrome (defective skin and hair colour)	Lymphoma

Conclusions

- There are a wide variety of indirect, or paraneoplastic, effects of cancer.
- Although the pathogenesis of some is clear (ectopic ACTH production in Cushing's syndrome, for example) it is unknown in many others.
- The treatment of choice in all cases is that of the underlying malignancy.
- Symptomatic treatment often fails if the underlying cancer is uncontrolled.
- Some of these syndromes may precede the diagnosis of cancer by months or years; a judicious search for an occult primary should be made in such circumstances.
- Paraneoplastic effects may sometimes delay the diagnosis of cancer by suggesting pathology in another system.
- Because they complicate diagnosis, symptoms and management of cancer, knowledge of the types of paraneoplastic phenomena is desirable.

9 Cancer Emergencies

J. SWEETENHAM

Patients with cancer may develop various emergency conditions during the course of their illness. These can arise:

- as complications of the underlying disease
- as complications of its treatment
- for reasons completely unrelated to cancer

The third of these is clearly important, although this chapter deals exclusively with the first two. It should not be forgotten, however, that common medical or surgical emergencies will occur and may have no relationship to the patient's malignant disease.

The emergencies described here are not necessarily unique to patients with cancer, but the presence of malignant disease may profoundly influence their management. For example, acute renal failure developing in the terminal phase of advanced malignant disease is usually best left untreated.

Two important principles clearly underlie the management of cancer emergencies:

- Appropriate management of an emergency in a cancer patient requires knowledge of the likely long-term prognosis for that patient.
- The most important aspect of treatment of any cancer-related emergency is the treatment of the underlying malignant disease.

It is important to remember to take time to think and plan management. Emergencies in cancer patients rarely require an 'instant treatment', so that a few minutes spent in thought may result in optimal care.

Cardiovascular Emergencies

Cardiac Tamponade

This is a state of low cardiac output caused by poor filling of the heart during diastole. It occurs because the intrapericardial pressure is raised, for one of two reasons:

- fluid in the pericardium—pericardial effusion
- increased stiffness of the pericardium—pericardial constriction

The commonest cancer-related cause is pericardial effusion.

The causes of cardiac tamponade are listed in Table 1. Small insignificant pericardial effusions are a common incidental finding in cancer patients. Progression to tamponade can, however, be very insidious. The clinical features of pericardial effusion and constriction vary and are therefore considered separately.

Pericardial Effusion.   The symptoms are non-specific and the onset can be very gradual. Once tamponade is established, rapidly progressive circulatory collapse may occur. Common symptoms include:

- dyspnoea
- dizziness
- precordial pain
- palpitations

The physical signs are summarized in Table 2.

Two investigations of major importance are:

- Chest X-ray—this will show a large heart shadow with the normal contours obliterated.
- Echocardiogram—this is by far the best investigation. An

Table 1. Cancer-related causes of cardiac tamponade

Cause	Comments
Pericardial effusion	Due to tumour involvement of the pericardium
Secondary tumours (common)	e.g. Bronchial carcinoma Breast carcinoma Leukaemia Hodgkin's disease Non-Hodgkin's lymphoma
Primary tumours (rare)	e.g. Mesothelioma Sarcomas
Malignant infiltration of the pericardium	Produces a thickened pericardium
	Causes as for pericardial effusion
Radiation pericarditis	Radiotherapy to the pericardium may cause a latter constrictive pericarditis

Table 2. Physical signs of pericardial effusion

Sign	Comments
Raised jugular venous pressure	Easily overlooked. Pressure wave is almost normal. Must be examined very carefully
Pulsus paradoxus	Classical sign of tamponade. Pulse diminishes in volume or disappears on inspiration. Can be accurately determined with blood pressure cuff
Faint heart sounds	Due to distension of pericardial sac with absent apex beat fluid
Pericardial rub	Often heard. Even in the presence of large effusions
Signs of congestive cardiac failure	These are often present

echo-free space will be seen and the ventricular function can be accurately assessed.

Malignant Pericardial Infiltration. This is much less common in cancer patients. It produces a pattern of pericardial constriction, the most prominent symptom being dyspnoea. The characteristic physical signs are listed in Table 3. Investigations are:

- Chest X-ray—this may be normal, although the heart may be slightly enlarged with a straight left border. The superior vena cava may be dilated.
- Echocardiogram—this will demonstrate the restricted ventricular mobility.

Radiation Pericarditis. This produces the same clinical picture as malignant pericardial infiltration.

Treatment

- *Pericardial aspiration* is the most important single measure in patients with life-threatening tamponade due to a pericardial effusion. It should be undertaken only by those experienced in the technique, and preferably with ultrasound guidance.
- *Radiotherapy* can be used subsequently, or primarily in patients without life-threatening signs if they have a particularly

Table 3. Physical signs of pericardial constriction

Sign	Comments
Raised jugular venous pressure	The pattern is abnormal. Prominent X and Y troughs
Ascites	With little or no lower limb oedema
Massive hepatomegaly	
Atrial fibrillation	Common

radiosensitive tumour (e.g. breast cancer, lung cancer, Hodgkin's disease).

- *Chemotherapy* should be used in the same circumstances for chemosensitive tumours (e.g. small cell lung cancer, widespread lymphoma or Hodgkin's disease).
- *Surgery* may be required for recurrent effusions. A pericardial window is constructed to allow fluid to drain into the pleural cavity. A pericardiectomy is sometimes required for radiation pericarditis.

Superior Vena Caval Obstruction

The superior vena cava (SVC) is a thin-walled blood vessel lying within the rigid thoracic cage and closely related to the contents of the mediastinum. Because of this it is very susceptible to compression or infiltration by tumours. Obstruction is almost always the result of *extrinsic compression* by enlarged mediastinal lymph nodes. The resulting syndrome may be due to the compression itself, or consequent thrombosis of the SVC. Occasionally the SVC will be directly infiltrated. The more common malignant causes of SVC obstruction are shown in Table 4.

The symptoms of SVC obstruction are characteristic:

- Facial and neck swelling are common early symptoms. A frequent complaint is of apparent tightening of clothes around the neck. The cause is increased venous back pressure.
- Swelling of chest and upper limbs may also result from the increased back pressure.
- Other consequences of the raised venous pressure include headaches and hoarseness, a rare complaint associated with laryngeal oedema.

Other less specific symptoms include dyspnoea, cough and chest pain. The major physical signs are listed in Table 5. They are all due to increased venous back pressure. Investigation of SVC obstruction depends upon the clinical circumstances. The diagnosis can be made on the basis of the clinical features alone and any investigation will be used to search for the cause of the obstruction. Although SVC obstruction has, in the past, been considered to be a life-threatening emergency there is little evidence to

Table 4. Malignant diseases causing SVC obstruction

Small cell bronchial carcinoma (about 80% of all cases)
Non-small cell bronchial carcinoma
Non-Hodgkin's lymphoma
Hodgkin's disease
Breast carcinoma
Teratoma

Table 5. Signs of superior vena caval obstruction

Sign	Comment
Venous distension	Of the superficial neck veins, chest veins and upper limbs
Fixed elevation of JVP	Even in the upright position
Plethora and oedema	Of the face and upper limbs
Papilloedema and dilated retinal vessels	
Horner's syndrome	Rare

support this. Treatment should, where necessary, be withheld until an accurate histological diagnosis has been made. When patients present initially with SVC obstruction empirical treatment with radiotherapy or chemotherapy should be avoided since this can make it difficult to subsequently arrive at the diagnosis. The following investigations should be performed:

- Physical examination may help; e.g. widespread lymphadenopathy might indicate a malignant lymphoma.
- Radiography is essential: a chest X-ray will show a mediastinal mass in most cases, and may show a bronchial primary; CT scanning is rarely needed unless surgery is being considered, when operability can be assessed.
- Cytology and histology are essential: sputum cytology is positive for malignant cells in about 60% of patients with SVC syndrome. A bronchial primary may also be seen and biopsied at bronchoscopy.
- Surgery should be considered to obtain adequate tissue if other diagnostic measures fail. There is no evidence that surgery is dangerous in the presence of distended mediastinal veins and it should be done if a tissue diagnosis is required.

Treatment.   Although not life threatening, SVC obstruction can be very distressing and treatment should therefore be initiated as soon as possible after a tissue diagnosis has been obtained, or immediately in patients with an established diagnosis. The most important principle of therapy is to *treat the underlying tumour*, with chemotherapy or radiotherapy:

- Chemotherapy is used for tumours such as small cell bronchial carcinoma, non-Hodgkin's lymphoma, Hodgkin's disease and teratoma.
- Radiotherapy is the treatment of choice for all other causes of malignant SVC obstruction.

With either form of treatment, symptoms usually start to improve within 72 hours. Signs of obstruction may persist for weeks though some cases are permanent, since thrombosis within the SVC may not resolve.

Complications of SVC obstruction are very rare and the prognosis is that of the underlying malignancy.

Respiratory Emergencies

Upper Airways Obstruction

This is a rare, but life-threatening complication of some forms of cancer. The trachea is an unusual site for malignant obstruction for two reasons:

- Primary tumours of the trachea are rare.
- The trachea is relatively rigid and is resistant to malignant invasion by other primaries.

Causes of upper airways obstruction are shown in Figure 1.

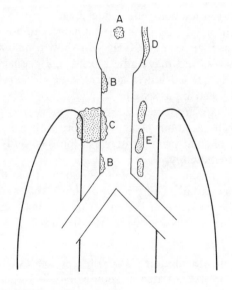

A. Primary malignant tumor of larynx or hypopharynx	Rare
B. Primary malignant tumours of the trachea	Rare
C. Malignant infiltration from surrounding organs	e.g. carcinoma of bronchus; carcinoma of oesophagus; carcinoma of thyroid
D. Laryngeal oedema	e.g. retropharyngeal haemorrhage due to thrombocytopenia; drugs; ? SVC obstruction
E. Compression by enlarged lymph nodes	e.g. carcinoma of bronchus; Hodgkin's disease; non-Hodgkin's lymphoma

Figure 1. Causes of upper airways obstruction

Symptoms usually develop gradually and the patient is therefore usually able to compensate for the respiratory embarrassment over a long period of time. Typical symptoms include:

- dyspnoea
- cough
- wheezing
- stridor
- orthopnoea

Acute decompensation and severe respiratory difficulty can occur, especially if another respiratory problem, such as a chest infection, develops.

Physical signs are listed in Table 6.

The following investigations will usually delineate the site of obstruction and help determine the cause:

- Chest X-ray will often reveal a cause such as primary lung
    cancer or enlarged lymph nodes within the chest.
- Penetrated chest X-ray—this gives more detail of the trachea
    and cancer and may demonstrate the obstruction.
- Lateral neck X-rays—these may be used to localize an
    obstructing mass.
- Computed tomography—this is particularly useful if the
    situation is not too pressing. It will often indicate both the
    site and extent of the obstructing lesion as well as a primary
    site of the tumour.

Emergency bronchoscopy should be avoided since manipulation of the head and neck, or trauma to an obstructing lesion can result in oedema or bleeding, and produce complete stenosis.

Treatment. This is dependent very much on the cause. Treatment options are listed in Table 7.

Table 6. Physical signs of upper airways obstruction

Sign	Comments
Dyspnoea	Can be severe. Patient may be very distressed and anxious. Cyanosis may be present
Stridor	Common. Typically more pronounced during inspiration
Reduced breath sounds	All lung fields. Commonly obscured by transmitted stridor
Signs of primary tumour	e.g. Generalized lymphadenopathy in lymphoma

Table 7. Treatment of upper airways obstruction

Treatment	Comments
Emergency laryngotomy/ tracheostomy	Rarely necessary since symptoms usually develop slowly. No use for tracheal lesions unless very high
Steroids (e.g. dexamethasone)	Often produce rapid improvement by reducing oedema. Should always be used as first-line therapy
TREATMENT OF CAUSE	
Surgery	Rarely possible or useful. Can be used for limited primary tracheal lesions
Radiotherapy	Frequently useful. Best modality for most tumours. Steroids should be given since radiotherapy may cause oedema and symptoms may worsen initially
Chemotherapy	For chemosensitive tumours, e.g. lymphoma, small cell bronchial carcinoma
Laser therapy	Obstructing endotracheal lesions can be removed under direct visualization. Can be used alone or with photosensitizing drugs, e.g. haematoporphyrin

Metabolic Emergencies

Hypercalcaemia

This is a common metabolic consequence of cancer. The mechanisms by which it is thought to occur are shown in Figure 2, and the malignancies most commonly causing hypercalcaemia are listed in Table 8. As Figure 2 shows, several polypeptide hormones have been implicated as humoral factors producing hypercalcaemia. Parathyroid hormone (PTH) itself is rarely elaborated by tumours, although related polypeptides appear to be responsible for many cases of hypercalcaemia.

Hypercalcaemia produces hypercalcuria, and calcium in the urine provokes an osmotic diuresis, with resulting dehydration. Dehydration is the cause of many of the symptoms, which are:

- thirst—often in association with a dry mouth
- polyuria—with consequent dehydration
- lethargy and weakness—if left untreated may progress to stupor or coma
- anorexia, nausea and vomiting—all of which add to the problem of dehydration
- constipation

Physical signs are non-specific and are the signs of dehydration, or of the underlying malignancy.

Treatment. This depends on three major factors:

- Calcium level—mild elevations require only very simple measures if the patient is well.

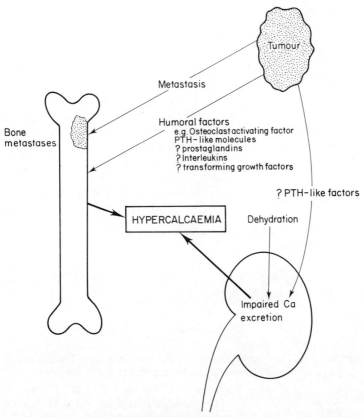

Figure 2. Schematic representation of mechanisms causing hypercalcaemia in cancer

- The patient's general condition—the serum calcium does not
  always correlate well with the patient's symptoms and signs.
  This can be influenced by the speed at which hypercalcaemia
  develops. If it develops over a long period symptoms may be
  minimal and treatment is less urgent.
- Long-term prognosis—in a patient with a very poor long-term
  prognosis it may be appropriate to leave hypercalcaemia
  untreated and allow the patient a relatively comfortable,
  distress-free death.

Treatment options are listed in Table 9.
The most important investigation is the serum calcium. It is important to remember
that the serum calcium must be corrected for serum albumin according to the formula
shown in Figure 3.

Syndrome of Inappropriate Antidiuretic Hormone Secretion (SIADH)

This is a common problem in patients with cancer, which is occasionally severe and
may then present as an emergency. It occurs because certain tumours are able to

Table 8. Malignant causes of hypercalcaemia

Cause	Comments
Haematological malignancies	Hypercalcaemia secondary to tumoral factors; e.g. myeloma, non-Hodgkin's lymphoma, acute leukaemia
Solid tumours with bony metastases	Breast carcinoma★, bronchial carcinoma
Solid tumours without bony metastases	Produce humoral factors — ? prostaglandins, ? PTH-like molecules; very rarely PTH. e.g. bronchial carcinoma, head and neck cancer, cervical cancer

★Hypercalcaemia may be a result of 'tumour flare' in association with the onset of treatment (either hormonal or chemotherapy) for breast cancer.

Table 9. Treatment of hypercalcaemia

Treatment	Comments
(1) Treat the underlying malignancy	The most important measure, but not always immediately effective in emergency
(2) Hydration	Symptomatic patients are ALWAYS dehydrated. If symptoms are mild and hypercalcaemia not severe use oral rehydration. For all other patients use vigorous and prompt intravenous rehydration. Use normal saline — sodium and potassium excretion parallel each other
(3) Corticosteroids	Useful only for tumours which are normally steroid-sensitive (e.g. lymphoma, leukaemia, myeloma)
FOR RESISTANT CASES:	
(4) Calcitonin	Inhibits bone resorption. Given as intravenous infusion
(5) Diphosphonates (e.g. etidronate)	Pyrophosphate analogues. Inhibit osteoclast bone resorption. Given intravenously
(6) Mithramycin	Inhibits osteoblast activity. Effect lasts for several days. Toxic and rarely necessary
FOR VERY REFRACTORY CASES:	
(7) Inorganic phosphate	Produces reciprocal fall in serum calcium. Can be given intravenously — may cause hypertension, renal failure + ectopic calcification. Orally — used chronically — produces diarrhoea
(8) Haemodialysis	Consider only for those with good long-term prognosis. Rarely necessary

Assume that 'ideal' serum albumin = 40 g/l

Correct serum calcium by 0.02 mmol/litre for every g/l of serum albumin above or below 40

E.g. if albumin is 30 g/l correct calcium by −0.2
E.g. if albumin is 50 g/l correct calcium by +0.2

Figure 3. Formula for correction of serum calcium

produce and secrete antidiuretic hormone (ADH), inappropriate to the plasma osmolality. The effect is, therefore, to produce *water overload*.

Important cancer related causes are shown in Table 10. It is most commonly seen in small cell lung cancer. Excess water is distributed between the intracellular and extracellular fluids. This means that the osmolality of both is reduced. Thus, there is no osmotic gradient and oedema is *not* a feature. Swelling of the cells occurs, which is particularly dangerous in the brain.

The symptoms are mainly due to water overload in the brain. They are:

- anorexia, nausea and vomiting
- headache
- drowsiness, fits and coma

There are no specific physical signs.

A mild degree of SIADH is frequent in patients with bronchial carcinoma. The diagnosis is usually made when routine electrolyte measurement shows a low serum sodium. Occasionally, severe SIADH can be the first presenting symptom of lung cancer.

Only two investigations are usually necessary.

- serum sodium—this is reduced, and may be as low as 105 mmol/l
- plasma osmolality—this also is low

Treatment. Because it is frequently asymptomatic, the most appropriate treatment, where possible, is to treat the underlying tumour. Other measures may be necessary for symptomatic patients, who may die if their water overload is not corrected.

Table 10. Malignancies causing SIADH

Bronchial carcinoma (especially small cell)
Bronchial carcinoid tumours
Hodgkin's disease
Non-Hodgkin's lymphomas
CNS metastases from any tumour
Others (very rare) e.g. carcinomas of prostate, larynx; thymoma; mesothelioma

- Fluid restriction—to a daily fluid intake of about 1 litre. This is usually all that is required.
- Hypertonic saline infusion—this can be used in small volumes for severe cases (serum sodium <115 mmol/l) as a short-term measure. Normal saline is of NO use—the sodium is rapidly excreted through the kidneys.

Acute Tumour Lysis Syndrome

This is a rare but potentially fatal complication of treatment of some malignant diseases which are highly sensitive to chemotherapy. It occurs after cytotoxic therapy, especially if the tumour burden is high. Numerous metabolites are released from tumour cells, which lyse as a result of treatment, and produce a condition which can result in acute renal failure and cardiac arrhythmias or arrest. The commonest tumours in which it occurs are:

- high grade non-Hodgkin's lymphomas—Burkitt's or Burkitt's-like lymphoblastic lymphoma

- acute lymphoblastic leukaemia ⎫
- acute myeloid leukaemia   ⎬ Especially if the initial mobile cell count is high (indicating a large tumour burden)

Metabolic features of the syndrome are listed in Table 11 and represented schematically in Figure 4.

Note that certain factors prior to treatment predispose to development of the syndrome. Many large tumours outgrow their blood supply and necrosis of cells occurs releasing urate and phosphate. Renal impairment may therefore exist prior to chemotherapy and this may be exacerbated in lymphomas by ureteric compression from abdominal lymph nodes.

Table 11. Metabolic features of acute tumour lysis syndrome

Feature	Comments
Hyperuricaemia	Urate is released from lysed cells and deposited in kidneys. Causes renal impairment. Urate in joints may produce gout
Hyperphosphataemia	Inorganic phosphate is released from tumour cells. Phosphate deposition in kidneys is very common. In some cases, phosphate crystals are present
Hypocalcaemia	A result of hyperphosphataemia. Increases myocardial excitability
Elevated urea and creatinine	A result of urate and phosphate deposits in kidneys
Hyperkalaemia	Due to release of intracellular K^+ and reduced K^+ clearance by kidneys

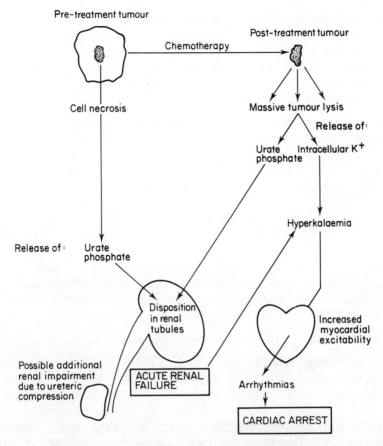

Figure 4. Events in the acute tumour lysis syndrome

Management. This should be aimed at prevention, rather than treatment of an established syndrome, and should be undertaken in all patients with the aforementioned tumour types. Management comprises the following:

- Measure serum urate, phosphate, calcium, urea and electrolytes prior to initiating chemotherapy.
- Commence allopurinol at *least* 12 hours prior to chemotherapy. This is a xanthine oxidase inhibitor which will prevent production of further uric acid.
- Establish adequate intravenous hydration. This produces a diuresis which enhances excretion of urate and phosphates. The patient should pass at least 100 ml/hour of urine before treatment commences.
- Alkalinize urine if urate is elevated—oral sodium bicarbonate is usually adequate and alkalinization enhances uric acid excretion. It should be given until the uric acid is normal but *stopped* when chemotherapy is commenced since, if the

urine remains alkaline, phosphate deposition in the kidneys will occur. *If possible treatment should be delayed until the urate level is normal.*

- Commence calcium resonium—this can be given orally or as an enema. It chelates potassium in the gut, reducing its absorption.

Most problems from acute tumour lysis will occur in the first 12 to 24 hours after chemotherapy. It is essential during this period (and prior to treatment) to monitor the following:

- ECG
- serum K^+
- urea and creatinine
- calcium and phosphate
- urate

If hyperkalaemia develops it should be managed as shown in Table 12. Remember that if hyperkalaemia or renal failure develop and are refractory to the above, measures of haemodialysis should be commenced. The prognosis of the tumour concerned is usually good and dialysis is therefore entirely appropriate in the short term.

Neurological Emergencies

Spinal Cord and Nerve Root Compression

Early diagnosis and treatment of compression of the spinal cord is essential since it can progress rapidly to paraplegia with loss of sphincter control. Even in patients with a poor long-term prognosis, cord compression should usually be actively investigated and treated since the resulting loss of sphincter control and inability to walk can make the patient's remaining life very distressing.

Neoplastic causes of cord or root compression are shown in Figure 5. Extradural metastases are by far the commonest cause. The effect may be due to direct compression from a deposit, or vertebral collapse from lung metastases. Some tumours (e.g.

Table 12. Treatment of hyperkalaemia

Treatment	Comments
Measurement of arterial blood gases	Severe acidosis makes hyperkalaemia difficult to correct
Intravenous sodium bicarbonate	If patient is severely acidotic
Intravenous calcium chloride	If ECG shows hyperkalaemic changes
Dextrose/insulin infusion*	Shifts extracellular $\rightarrow$ intracellular K^+
Haemodialysis	If all of the above measures fail

*This does *not* reduce total body potassium. It shifts it into the cells. Haemodialysis may be required to clear the potassium.

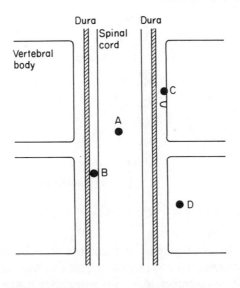

A.	Intramedullary (within spinal cord)	Rare e.g. ependymoma; astrocytoma
B.	Extramedullary (within dura mater)	Rare e.g. neurofibroma; meningioma
C/D.	Extradural*	(i)Primary tumours (rare) e.g. meningiomas; sarcomas

(ii)Secondary tumours (common)

Breast	Thyroid
Prostate	Kidney
Bronchus	Myeloma
Lymphoma	Leukaemia

*Effect may result from vertebral collapse, especially in myeloma and breast cancer.

Figure 5. Neoplastic causes of cord or root compression

lymphomas) extend from paravertebral lymph nodes through the intervertebral foramina, producing root or cord compression by direct extension. The frequency at which various levels of the cord are affected is shown in Figure 6. Compression is usually from the anterior aspect of the spinal cord.

Symptoms of cord or root compression are highly characteristic, although often insidious in onset, and therefore easily misdiagnosed. The characteristic symptoms are as follows:

- Back pain—this is almost always the earliest symptom. It may precede the others by many weeks or months. Pain is typically in the central back, often radiating in a band-like fashion to the front of the trunk on one or both sides as a result of nerve root irritation.

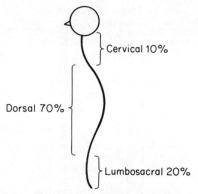

Figure 6. Frequency with which various levels of cord are affected by compression

- Weakness—the exact pattern of weakness depends upon the level of compression; again, the symptoms may develop insidiously. Remember that cord compression may occur in bedridden patients, and the patient may therefore be unaware of increasing weakness. Initial symptoms often include difficulty with balance and unilateral or bilateral weakness, sometimes with foot drop. Such symptoms may progress rapidly to paraplegia.
- Sensory loss—this is very common. Complaints of numbness and tingling below the level of compression are the symptoms most often reported.
- Sphincter disturbance—constipation is a common symptom. Loss of bladder sphincters may take the form of incontinence, retention or both. It usually precedes frank paraplegia by 12 to 24 hours and if present requires very urgent correction.

The importance of back pain cannot be overemphasized. In any cancer patient with back pain, spinal cord compression *must* be considered in the diagnosis.

Physical signs are highly variable, often very subtle and depend upon the level of compression. They are summarized in Table 13.

Investigation of cord compression requires two important tests:

- Plain X-rays—of the vertebral column to show areas of vertebral collapse.
- Myelography—serves two functions: to confirm the diagnosis and to determine the level of compression and allow treatment to be properly directed.

It is important to remember that in some tumours, notably breast carcinoma and lymphoma, compression may be due to multiple lesions at various levels and it may be necessary, if there is a complete block on lumbar myelography, to undertake cervical myelography as well. This will delineate the upper and lower extent of the disease, which is important if radiotherapy is being considered. Myelography should ideally be

Table 13. Signs of spinal cord/nerve root compression

Sign	Comments
Weakness	Characteristically upper motor neurone with hypertonia, hyperreflexia and extensor plantar responses. The pattern of weakness and reflex changes may indicate the level of compression
Sensory loss	Any sensory modality may be affected. Examination of cutaneous sensation often indicates a sensory level. As with the motor level, this may be several segments below the true level of compression
Reduced anal tone	A patulous, atonic anal sphincter is characteristic
Palpable bladder	May be present as a result of retention

performed in a specialized neurosurgical centre since neurological deterioration may occur during myelography and an emergency laminectomy will then be necessary.

Treatment.   For the cancer patient with cord compression the major treatment decision to be made is whether or not to undertake surgery. This will depend upon the clinical circumstances. If cord compression is a presenting feature of a tumour, surgery is essential to obtain material for histology. For patients who are known to have chemosensitive or radiosensitive malignancies, surgery is often not necessary. Treatment options are summarized in Table 14.

Prognosis.   This depends primarily on the pretreatment state:

- 60–80% of patients who are ambulatory before treatment remain so. 35% of paretic patients regain the ability to walk.

Table 14. Treatment of spinal cord/nerve root compression

Treatment	Comments
INITIAL — PRIOR TO MYELOGRAM	
Dexamethasone	Cord oedema often worsens neurological deficit. Commence dexamethasone as soon as the diagnosis is suspected. Continue until definitive treatment commences. If patient has radiotherapy, continue during its commencement
SUBSEQUENT TREATMENT	
Surgery	Laminectomy is the standard operation. Removal of tumour allows the cord to bulge and thereby relieves pressure. Most compressive lesions are anterior and a posterior laminectomy usually does not allow complete excision
Radiotherapy	May be used after surgery *or* instead of surgery for patient known to have a radiosensitive tumour
Chemotherapy	Will produce rapid relief of compression in chemosensitive diseases; e.g. lymphoma, leukaemia, teratoma

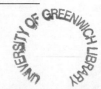

- Few if any of those who are paraplegic before treatment will subsequently walk again.

Other features also affect the prognosis:

- Speed of onset of symptoms—patients with a rapidly progressive compression do badly.
- Site of compression—the prognosis is better for posterior lesions (which are rare)—they are more easily removed.
- Presence of bony involvement—vertebral collapse carries a poor prognosis.

Fits

Fits are a fairly common problem in cancer patients, and may be due to a number of different factors. The fits are most commonly grand mal seizures, although focal fits may occur, especially with a focal lesion in the brain. The various causes of fits in cancer patients are listed in Table 15.

The commonest of these causes is intracranial tumour, which is most frequently due to metastatic spread from primaries such as bronchial carcinoma. They may present as an emergency if they are long-lasting and resistant to standard therapy, i.e. status epilepticus—this is a highly dangerous situation since prolonged fits may lead to cerebral anoxia. A detailed account of the investigation and treatment of epilepsy is not appropriate here. The most important principle of treatment in the short term is to control the seizures prior to commencing investigations as to their cause. In the long term, treatment is aimed at preventing further seizures, the most important principle being that of *treating the underlying tumour*.

Emergency Management.

- This should aim at controlling fits. A benzodiazepine should be given intravenously (diazemuls is one of the most commonly

Table 15. Causes of fits in cancer patients

Cause	Comments
Intracerebral tumour	Most commonly metastases from extracranial primaries. Primary brain tumour relatively rare
Intracerebral infiltration	Occurs in leukaemias or lymphomas. No discrete mass lesion present
Meningeal infiltration	Especially in leukaemia or lymphoma
Meningitis	May occur as a result of cancer or treatment-related immunosuppression
Electrolyte abnormalities	e.g. hypocalcaemia, hypomagnesaemia — may be related to chemotherapy
Intracranial haemorrhage	May occur into cerebral tumours, or due to thrombocytopenia
Drugs	e.g. cisplatin (very rare)

used—it is in a lipid-based diluent and penetrates the central
nervous system quickly).

- Phenytoin can be given intravenously in resistant cases, but
  requires constant monitoring of the heart for arrhythmias.
- Intravenous chlormethiazole (Heminevrin) can be given by
  continuous infusion in status epilepticus. It has a very short
  half-life and the rate of infusion can be accurately titrated
  until the fits cease.
- Dexamethasone should be given if intracerebral tumour or
  infiltration is suspected—it reduces cerebral oedema, which
  may be responsible for the fits.

Long-Term Management.   Once status epilepticus has been controlled, management is
aimed at determining the cause, and preventing recurrence of fits. Briefly, the
investigations should be as shown in Table 16.

Long-term control of fits depends upon the cause. Low serum Na, Ca or Mg should
be corrected, and platelet support given for thrombocytopenic patients. For patients
with intracranial tumour, the tumour itself must be controlled. This may be by:

- Radiotherapy—to the cranium with or without the spinal cord.
- Intrathecal drugs—methotrexate and cytosine arabinoside may
  be given directly into the theca at lumbar puncture. They
  are only of use when the tumour is likely to be sensitive to
  chemotherapy.
- Systemic chemotherapy—can be used for chemosensitive
  tumours, although penetration of drugs into the brain can be
  erratic.
- Surgery—may be feasible for some primary brain tumours and
  very occasionally for metastatic tumours.

Table 16. Summary of investigations of fits in cancer patients

Investigation	Comments
Computed tomography of head	Most important single investigation. Reveals intracranial metastases, haemorrhage and often infiltration. May show cerebral oedema. *Essential* prior to lumbar puncture
Isotope brain scan	Useful if CT is not available, but less accurate
Lumbar puncture	*Do not* perform in presence of papilloedema, or if CT indicates raised intracranial pressure. Cytology or CSF may reveal malignant cells. Xanthochromia may indicate haemorrhage. Also exclude meningitis
Full blood count	Haemorrhage more frequent with thrombocytopenia
Electrolytes, calcium and magnesium	Look for low serum levels of Ca, Mg and Na

Definitive treatment of the cause may not always control seizures since the residual scarring may lead to an excitable focus in the brain from which fits may continue. Standard anticonvulsants, such as phenytoin or carbamazepine are effective.

Remember that in a patient with severe seizures and a widespread incurable malignancy, sedation to control fits may be the only appropriate 'active' measure.

Renal Emergencies

Acute Renal Failure

There are several potential causes of acute renal failure which can be related to cancer and its treatment; these are shown in Table 17. Most are dealt with in other parts of this book. This section deals specifically with renal failure due to ureteric obstruction. Symptoms and signs of renal failure from ureteric obstruction are non-specific. They include general malaise, anorexia, nausea and vomiting, confusion, stupor or even coma.

Patients with obstructed ureters may complain of pain due to ureteric colic. This pain, which characteristically starts in the loin, may radiate to the groin and is episodic in nature. Anuria is unusual since both ureters must be obstructed. It does, however, occur with very large retroperitoneal masses, or with pelvic tumours such as carcinoma of the cervix.

Investigations.   These have two functions:

- To confirm the diagnosis; the important investigations are:
  measure urea, creatinine and electrolytes—the urea will be
  elevated; potassium levels may also be high.

Table 17. Cancer-related causes of acute renal failure

Cause	Comments

Obstructive uropathy	Extrarenal obstruction is common.
	Caused by:
	(a) Retroperitoneal lymph nodes —
	    lymphoma
	    testicular tumours
	(b) Retroperitoneal tumours —
	    sarcomas
	(c) Pelvic tumours —
	    cervical carcinoma
	    bladder carcinoma

Hypercalcaemia	See page 142
Tumour products	Paraproteins in myeloma, Waldenström's macroglobulinaemia, Acute tumour lysis syndrome — see page 146
Direct renal infiltration	Rare, e.g. leukaemia, lymphoma
Nephrotoxic drugs	e.g. cisplatin, antibiotics (aminoglycosides), antifungals (amphotericin), antivirals (acyclovir)

- To determine the cause:
    renal and abdominal ultrasound—this is the investigation of
        choice to demonstrate ureteric obstruction. It will show
        hydronephrosis and may give a clue to the level of
        obstruction. In addition, it may show enlargement of kidneys
        due to renal infiltration. Nodal masses or other
        retroperitoneal tumours causing obstruction and pelvic
        masses are also likely to be shown.

Other investigations, such as intravenous urography or retrograde pyelography, are
rarely needed.

Treatment of Ureteric Compression.   As with other cancer emergencies, the decision to
treat at all depends upon a reasonable prognosis. Death from renal failure is usually
pain free and the patient is rarely distressed. If renal failure develops in the face of
an incurable disease, it may be inappropriate to try to treat it.
    Treatment is primarily that of the underlying tumour. It may therefore require:

- Chemotherapy—this is appropriate for disease likely to respond
    very promptly to chemotherapy, such as lymphoma or
    teratoma. Renal failure will be rapidly reversed and the
    metabolic disturbances will often be corrected without
    further treatment.
- Radiotherapy—will help for some retroperitoneal and pelvic
    tumours, such as cervical carcinoma. However, responses are
    not usually very rapid and other measures may be required
    in the short term; these include:
- Nephrostomy tubes—a nephrostomy is a tube which is
    introduced percutaneously into the dilated renal pelvis under
    ultrasound guidance. It allows urine to flow, relieving back
    pressure on the kidneys. The obstruction can be bypassed
    until definitive treatment, such as chemotherapy or
    radiotherapy, becomes effective.
- Acute haemodialysis—may also be needed sometimes to correct
    metabolic disturbances until treatment of the underlying
    tumour takes effect.

Gastrointestinal Emergencies

Bowel Obstruction

Bowel obstruction due to cancer may occur at any level from the oesophagus to the
rectum. The symptoms and signs will obviously vary according to the level of
obstruction. They are summarized briefly in Table 18. The most appropriate
investigations will also vary widely according to the suspected site of obstruction. The
most useful ones are shown in Table 19.

Table 18. Summary of symptoms and signs of gastrointestinal obstruction according to site

Site	Symptoms/signs
Oesophagus	Progressive dysphagia for solids, then liquids. Aspiration may produce cough, pneumonia or even lung abscess. Weight loss is very common. Dysphagia may become complete, even for saliva
Stomach/duodenum	Pain after meals with epigastric fullness. Progresses to vomiting — often effortless and undigested food particles visible. Dehydration common. Palpable mass or succussion splash often present
Small intestine	Nausea, vomiting and constipation. Abnormal distension with tympany. Hyperactive bowel sounds
Large intestine	Classical symptoms: colicky abdominal pain; vomiting, abdominal distension. Absolute constipation. Palpable mass and abdominal distension with hyperactive bowel sounds. Dehydration frequent

Table 19. Investigation of gastrointestinal obstruction

Suspected site of obstruction	Primary investigations
Oesophagus	Chest X-ray — may show primary pulmonary lesion responsible for obstruction. Barium swallow. Oesophagoscopy (with or without biopsy)
Stomach and duodenum	Gastroscopy is investigation of choice
Small intestine	Plain abdominal film shows dilated small bowel loops. Abdominal ultrasound may show a mass
Large intestine	Plain abdominal film shows distended large bowel. Caecum often distended also. Abdominal ultrasound may show a mass

The causes of malignant obstruction of the gastrointestinal tract are numerous. In the oesophagus and stomach, the obstructing lesions are almost always primary carcinomas of those organs. Only a very small proportion of cases of small intestinal obstruction are due to primary carcinomas. Most arise due to compression, direct extension from an adjacent tumour mass, or volvulus of the small intestine around areas of abdominal carcinomatosis. Ovarian carcinoma is a common malignant disease which produces small or large bowel obstruction due to the above mechanisms.

Large bowel obstruction is frequently due to a colonic or rectal carcinoma, although it too may arise because of infiltration, compression or volvulus related to other intra-abdominal primary tumours. Pelvic malignancies, such as bladder cancer, may infiltrate and obstruct the rectum.

Treatment.   The main principles of immediate treatment of gastrointestinal obstruction are:

- decompress the obstructed gut
- rehydration

The relative importance of these two varies according to the site of obstruction (e.g. there is no obstructed bowel to decompress in oesophageal obstructions, but rehydration is critical). Very large volumes of fluid are secreted into the stomach and intestine, and even when large fluid losses are not evident as vomitus, the patient may be severely dehydrated.

In all but very high obstructions, the bowel can be effectively decompressed by a nasogastric tube. Intravenous hydration, with careful monitoring of the electrolytes, should commence immediately. Large amounts of potassium will be secreted into the bowel, and potassium-supplemented i.v. fluids are frequently necessary. Subsequently treatment is complex and depends upon the cause and site of obstruction. It is usually surgical, although this may be inappropriate in certain circumstances. This is especially true of patients with advanced abdominal carcinomatosis; the patient has incurable disease and surgery is unlikely to improve the situation. In these circumstances, the patient should be rehydrated intravenously and have a nasogastric tube if vomiting is distressing. Symptoms will sometimes settle spontaneously over the next few days. If they fail to settle, surgery can be considered, although if the disease is very far advanced it may be more sensible simply to relieve distress and not undertake further treatment.

In patients with ovarian cancer, chemotherapy may produce some palliation of symptoms.

Bowel Perforation

Perforation of part of the gastrointestinal tract is a recognized presenting feature of some cancers, particularly of the stomach. The other circumstance in which it may occur is in patients with very chemosensitive tumours, such as lymphoma, which involve the full thickness of the bowel wall. When chemotherapy is given, tumour necrosis may produce perforation. This is a particular problem in patients with lymphoma since perforation may occur at multiple levels. It usually occurs within 12 to 24 hours after the start of treatment.

Important symptoms are:

- sudden onset of abdominal pain
- fever
- shock

The classical physical signs are:

- 'board-like' abdominal rigidity
- absent bowel sounds

The diagnosis can be confirmed by plain abdominal X-ray, which shows free gas under the diaphragm.

Treatment.   This is primarily surgical. Prior to surgery, it is important to give:

- adequate fluid and electrolyte support
- antibiotics (including cover for anaerobic organisms, e.g. metronidazole)

Remember that patients receiving large doses of steroids may not develop the normal complex of symptoms and signs. This may occur in lymphoma, where steroids are frequently used. Thus, if sudden fever and hypotension develop in a lymphoma patient shortly after commencing chemotherapy, consider bowel perforation, even if bowel involvement has not been diagnosed prior to treatment.

Fever in Neutropenic Patients

Infection in cancer patients is common. There are numerous predisposing factors; see Table 20. The infective complication which most commonly presents as an emergency in a cancer patient is fever with neutropenia. Infection in a patient with neutropenia is a life-threatening emergency. Patients may deteriorate very quickly, and progress from being well to collapse and death within a few hours.

Risk Factors

Two major factors determine the risk of infection in a neutropenic patient:

- Degree of neutropenia—the risk becomes significant with neutrophil counts below $1 \times 10^9/l$. Infection is almost inevitable with a count of $0.1 \times 10^9/l$ or less.
- Duration of neutropenia—the risk is directly proportional to the duration. It is relatively uncommon with short-lived episodes, which occur with some types of chemotherapy, but very common when neutropenia persists for 5 days or more.

In cancer patients reversible neutropenia most commonly occurs as a consequence of chemotherapy. The time course is predictable, beginning within 7 to 10 days from the onset of chemotherapy. In these circumstances the factors which determine the degree and duration of neutropenia are:

- Dose of drugs—thre is a clear correlation between the dose of myelosuppressive drugs and degree of neutropenia.
- Previous treatment—the severity of neutropenia with a given drug or combination tends to become worse with successive courses of treatment. Patients who have had multiple courses of chemotherapy or radiotherapy are particularly at risk.
- Bone marrow infiltration—patients with extensive bone marrow infiltration have relatively few normal marrow elements

Table 20. Factors predisposing to infection in cancer patients

Factor	Comments
Disruption of mechanical barriers to infection	e.g. skin — surgery, i.v. cannulae, tumour ulceration Mucous membranes — indwelling catheters, mucositis secondary to chemotherapy or radiotherapy
Neutropenia	Drug induced. Radiation induced. Infiltration of bone marrow by tumour (e.g. lymphoma, leukaemia). Hypersplenism.
Abnormal cell-mediated immunity	e.g. lymphoma. Drug-induced — steroids
Hypogammaglobulinaemia	e.g. chronic lymphocytic leukaemia. Myeloma.
Splenectomy	e.g. in staging for Hodgkin's disease

remaining. Since the bone marrow has so little functional reserve, neutropenia is likely to be severe and prolonged. This is particularly true for patients with acute leukaemia.

Causes

Numerous organisms can cause neutropenic fever. Many cases are probably viral, since no pathogen is ever isolated, and a few may be fungal or protozoal. However, many are bacterial. The common infecting bacteria are listed in Table 21. But remember, fever in a neutropenic patient may arise from other causes:

- underlying tumour (lymphoma, sarcoma)
- drugs (bleomycin)
- blood or platelet transfusion

Symptoms and signs may be very non-specific. The most important are:

- Fever—suspect the diagnosis if a fever of 38°C or more develops in a patient who is at risk of neutropenia. Remember that patients will often NOT complain of fever, but will say they feel cold or 'shivery'.
- Malaise—any degree may be present, progressing to collapse.
- Localizing symptoms/signs—these may be present, for example, in skin sepsis or chest infections. However, localizing symptoms and signs rely on an adequate inflammatory response and, often, on the formation of pus. Neutropenic patients often have insufficient neutrophils to form pus and localizing signs of infection may therefore be absent.

Table 21. Common bacterial causes of neutropenic fever

Escherichia coli
Pseudomonas aeruginosa
Klebsiella pneumoniae
Staphylococcus aureus
Bacteroides spp.
Multiple infections with the above are common

Investigations

In the presence of neutropenic fever, investigations should not delay treatment. The investigations listed in Table 22 should be done immediately, and broad-spectrum antibiotics started *before* the results of investigations are available.

Treatment

Treatment should commence without delay and should use at least two bactericidal antibiotics given intravenously. At least one of the two antibiotics should be an effective anti-*Pseudomonas* agent. Antibiotic choices vary enormously: a 'standard' regimen includes a semisynthetic penicillin, such as azlocillin or piperacillin, and an aminoglycoside, such as gentamicin or tobramycin.

If localizing signs are present other antibiotics may be added. For example:

- For skin sepsis—include an anti-staphylococcal penicillin, such as cloxacillin.
- For perineal or dental infection, anaerobes are often present and metronidazole should be included.

In penicillin-sensitive patients, cephalosporins, such as cefotaxime, can be substituted.

If a causative organism is identified once antibiotics have commenced, then specific antibiotics can be introduced later. In any event, antibiotics should continue for a minimum of 7 days once the temperature has returned to normal, or until the granulocyte count is above 1×10^9/l.

Table 22. Investigations in neutropenic fever

Investigation	Comments
Thorough clinical examination	Look for evidence of local sepsis: e.g. i.v. cannulae, perineal infection, skin sepsis, dental sepsis
Blood cultures	If central venous line is present, take cultures from central and peripheral lines. Include anaerobic cultures
Throat swab	
Midstream urine specimen	
Chest X-ray	
Culture of cannula tip if suspected	

If the temperature fails to settle rapidly after commencing these antibiotics consider anaerobic or staphylococcal infection. Systemic fungal infection can also occur with neutropenia and may require intravenous antifungal treatment, such as amphotericin. The risk of fungal infection increases with the duration of neutropenia.

Haematological Emergencies

Thrombocytopenia

Along with neutropenia (see above) this is a common haematological consequence of chemotherapy for cancer. It may present as an emergency with bleeding, which is often difficult to control. It usually occurs together with neutropenia. Cancer-related causes are listed in Table 23.

Spontaneous bleeding is a serious emergency. Fortunately it is rare unless the platelet count is below $20 \times 10^9/l$. However, severe bleeding can occur with higher platelet counts if the patient is infected, or using drugs such as aspirin or alcohol, which inhibit platelet function. Bleeding due to thrombocytopenia characteristically occurs in the skin and retina. The classical signs are:

- purpura
- spontaneous bruising
- retinal haemorrhages

When any of these occur in the setting of thrombocytopenia, urgent treatment is required, since more life-threatening bleeding may occur, particularly intracranial haemorrhage, or haemorrhage into the gut. Patients with severe thrombocytopenia should be examined twice daily for evidence of fresh purpura, retinal haemorrhage or haematuria.

Treatment.   The most important emergency treatment is platelet transfusion. Indications for such transfusions are listed in Table 24. Standard platelet transfusion consists of 6 units, but more can be given if this fails to stop bleeding. Transfusions are usually given with steroids to minimize allergic reactions. When many transfusions are required

Table 23. Cancer-related causes of thrombocytopenia

Cause	Comments
Bone marrow infiltration	Leukaemias, lymphoma
Chemotherapy	Especially nitrosoureas (CCNU, BCNU), carboplatin
Hypersplenism	Occurs in lymphoma/leukaemias with enlarged spleen
Disseminated intravascular coagulation	
Idiopathic thrombocytopenia	Anti-platelet antibodies produced in some tumours, e.g. lymphoma

Table 24. Indications for platelet transfusion in thrombocytopenia

Indication	Comments
Obvious haemorrhage	If platelets $<20 \times 10^9/1$ or higher with injection, drugs, etc. If platelet count $>20 \times 10^9/1$ consider other causes for haemorrhage
Fresh purpura or retinal haemorrhage	
Prior to transfusion of other blood products	The additional red cells will dilute the patient's own circulating platelets
Prior to surgery	
Prophylaxis	In patients with infection. Patients with very prolonged thrombocytopenia, e.g. undergoing induction treatment of acute leukaemia

over many weeks, it may be necessary to use platelets which are matched for tissue type to reduce antibody formation. Other types of treatment include:

- Splenectomy or splenic radiotherapy—for hypersplenism. Splenectomy is also occasionally necessary for immune thrombocytopenia.
- Steroids—should be used in idiopathic thrombocytopenia.
- Treatment of underlying tumour—especially in the lymphomas; often resolves idiopathic thrombocytopenia or hypersplenism.

Hyperviscosity States

The viscosity of whole blood depends upon the numbers of the various blood cells, and the viscosity of the plasma. There are two important cancer-related causes of hyperviscosity:

- Hyperleucocytosis—a vast increase in the number of circulating white blood cells, as is seen in leukaemia.
- Paraproteinaemia—high levels of paraprotein are seen in myeloma and may also produce the syndrome of hyperviscosity.

Hyperviscosity is regarded as an emergency since it can produce serious neurological consequences (e.g. cerebrovascular accidents or fits) and may lead to impaired vision. If patient has symptoms and signs of hyperviscosity, they require urgent treatment.
The symptoms are non-specific and include:

- lethargy
- general malaise
- confusion
- loss of visual acuity
- dyspnoea

Important clinical features and associated signs are listed in Table 25.

Investigations.   In a patient with known malignant disease, only two investigations are generally required to confirm a diagnosis of hyperviscosity. These are:

- Full blood count—hyperviscosity is only likely to be the cause of the symptoms if the white cell count is $150 \times 10^9/l$ or over in acute leukaemia, or $200 \times 10^9/l$ or over in chronic leukaemias. If the white count is below these values, another cause for symptoms should be sought.
- Immunoglobulins, paraprotein measurement and serum electrophoresis—in emergency situations, the first of these (or the total protein) is usually sufficient.

Measurement of whole blood viscosity is rarely necessary. Other investigations should be dictated by the underlying malignancy.

Treatment.   This depends to some extent upon the severity of symptoms and the rate at which they develop. Symptoms which are rapidly progressive require urgent treatment. In the short term, the most rapidly effective treatment is plasmapheresis. In this way it is possible to remove a large proportion of the circulating paraprotein, or white cells, and thereby temporarily reduce the viscosity. This may need to be repeated on several occasions whilst definitive treatment is commencing.

Once again, the most important therapeutic manoeuvre is to treat the underlying malignancy. Treatment should commence as early as possible, and if plasmapheresis is being considered it should start at the same time. Steroids should be started for tumours which are likely to respond (such as myeloma or acute lymphoblastic leukaemia).

Table 25. Clinical features of hyperviscosity

Clinical features	Examples
Signs of underlying malignancy	Hypercalcaemia or bony disease in myeloma. Cytopenias in leukaemia
Neurological disorders	Encephalopathy. Peripheral neuropathy. Cerebrovascular accidents. Seizures. Subarachnoid haemorrhage
Bleeding disorder	Epistaxis. Gingival and mucous membrane bleeding. Retinal haemorrhage. Purpura
Ocular manifestations	Retinopathy. Venous congestion. Haemorrhage with impaired vision
Cardiovascular disorders	Congestive cardiac failure. Anaemia (secondary to expanded plasma volume)

Chemotherapy, if indicated, should also commence as soon as possible, remembering, in the case of the leukaemias, the problem of acute tumour lysis (see page 146).

- Red cell transfusion should be avoided in hyperviscosity—a low haemoglobin is often seen with hyperviscosity, due to haemodilution. High plasma protein levels draw fluid into the intravascular space because of the high osmotic pressure. Red cell transfusions may worsen hyperviscosity and should be withheld until the acute phase of the disease is over (when the haemoglobin may return to normal anyway).

Disseminated Intravascular Coagulation (DIC)

This is a highly complex condition which occasionally presents as an emergency in patients with cancer. A detailed account is not possible, but broad outlines for diagnosis and treatment are given.

Coagulation abnormalities of various types are very common in patients with cancer. Many of these are attributable to DIC. In DIC, an exaggerated response to tissue injury appears to occur. Thromboplastin-like material is released from tumour cells. This generates the production of thrombin from prothrombin, and coagulation of blood occurs. There are three consequences of this:

- Levels of normal clotting factors are depleted.
- Platelet consumption may occur in the formation of clots.
- Accelerated fibrinolysis occurs in an attempt to compensate for increased coagulation.

The balance of these three will determine the form which DIC takes. It may remain *balanced*, when the rate of clot formation and clot lysis due to fibrinolysis are the same. It may be *thrombotic*. However, the situation which most commonly presents as an emergency is *haemorrhagic DIC*.

Consumption of clotting factors and platelets results in severe haemorrhage, which may or may not be associated with thrombocytopenia. Haemorrhagic DIC occurs in about 10% of all patients with cancer, usually in a very mild form. Severe haemorrhage, presenting as an emergency is rare, though it is common in patients with one type of acute myeloid leukaemia (promyelocytic).

Investigations.   In a patient with cancer and severe haemorrhage, a full blood count is the most important investigation since thrombocytopenia is by far the commonest cause. When DIC is suspected, measure the fibrin degradation products (FDP). One feature of DIC is accelerated fibrinolysis, which results in increased production of breakdown products. Other tests of clotting may also help, but FDP is the most useful assay.

Treatment.   Treatment of DIC is very difficult, and haemorrhagic DIC has a very poor prognosis. Important measures are listed in Table 26. Treatment is highly specialized, and the advice of a haematologist should be sought immediately.

Table 26. Treatment of disseminated intravascular coagulation

Therapy	Comments
Treat underlying malignancy	Start treatment as early as possible. DIC usually cannot be controlled unless underlying disease is effectively treated
Heparin	Since the primary defect is coagulation, this is important, even in the face of haemorrhage. It is potentially very dangerous
Replacement of clotting factors	These become depleted. Fresh frozen plasma is the best source
Platelet transfusion	To restore the consumed platelets

Summary and Checklist of Symptoms

Most of the common cancer-associated emergencies have been dealt with in this chapter. However, it is important to emphasize the principles of management, which are listed below:

- The importance of long-term prognosis should not be forgotten—this will often profoundly influence emergency treatment in a cancer patient. To make a sound judgment about treatment requires a knowledge of the treatment options after the emergency has been successfully managed, and the likely length of survival. If any uncertainty exists, always seek advice from someone experienced in treating malignant disease. Once you have decided to give active treatment, however inappropriately, it is very difficult to withdraw this at a later stage.
- Remember that the treatment of the underlying tumour is fundamental to the management of all cancer-related emergencies.
- Remember that the emergency may be unrelated to the tumour, although its presence may still alter management.

A checklist summarizing common emergency symptoms in cancer patients, with a list of possible diagnoses, is given in Table 27 (page 166).

Table 27. Checklist of symptoms and possible cancer-related causes

Symptom	Possible causes
Dyspnoea	Chest infection Pulmonary embolism Upper airways obstruction Cardiac tamponade Severe metabolic acidosis, e.g. renal failure
Chest pain	Pulmonary embolism Cardiac tamponade Cord/nerve root compression/irritation
Abdominal pain	Gastrointestinal obstruction Gastrointestinal perforation Cord/nerve root compression/irritation Ureteric obstruction Chest infection
Drowsiness/confusion/coma	Cerebral metastases with raised intracranial pressure Meningitis Renal failure Hypercalcaemia SIADH Intracerebral bleeding (e.g. with thrombocytopenia) Hyperviscosity Overwhelming sepsis

Weakness	Focal – Cerebral metastases
	      Cerebral haemorrhage
	      Cord compression or nerve, root compression
	Generalized – Paraneoplastic symptoms
	      Cause of drowsiness/confusion/comas (see above)

Haemorrhage	Thrombocytopenia DIC Hyperviscosity
Headache	Raised intracranial pressure Cerebral haemorrhage Meningitis SVC obstruction
Fever	Infection Transfusion of blood products Underlying tumour

10 Symptomatic Care of Advanced Cancer

R. HILLIER

CONTROL OF PAIN

Controlling symptoms and supporting patients with advanced cancer are among the most rewarding tasks in cancer medicine. This chapter deals with pain and related symptoms about which all students and doctors need to know.

Research indicates that despite media reports of bad management and poor quality of life in cancer patients, good symptom control can be taught. Indeed, the practical details are easily learned, although it may take a little experience to turn this knowledge into really effective care.

The Extent of the Problem

Each year about 132,000 people in Britain die of cancer. More than half (excluding those with skin cancer and early cervical neoplasia) are known to have incurable disease at the time of diagnosis. Others will develop local recurrence or distant metastases at a later date.

Thus, a family doctor with an average list of 2000 patients will have approximately five patients with advanced cancer on his list at any one time; surgeons, physicians and cancer specialists will see many more. Expert symptom control and an understanding of the psychosocial problems of these patients are now an integral part of cancer medicine and can no longer be simply relegated to the GP with the words 'nothing further can be done'. In fact this is seldom, if ever, true.

It is only now that some medical schools are setting questions in final examinations on care of the dying; this creates an immediate and pragmatic reason for students to know more about it.

Preliminary Considerations

Despite recent advances in cancer management and a more open attitude to the disease by doctors, the media and the general public, the spectre of cancer still looms large over patients and those who fear it. The following comments by a doctor whose wife had been vaguely unwell for about 10 days may serve as an example. As he lay in bed one night he describes what happened in the following words:

'Then came the worst moment of my life. Suddenly, with horrible clarity everything fell into place and I knew what was wrong. She had leukaemia. Why hadn't it occurred to me before? The more I thought about it the more convinced I became. For the first time I was thinking the unthinkable.'

These explosive words are those of a wise and experienced physician. It could be argued that doctors know what to expect and, perhaps because of that, have more to fear. But knowledge often provokes less anxiety than do the vague imaginings of the frightened patient and his family. The reality may be awful, but the myths and fears which surround that reality may make it infinitely worse. Although patients often hide their true feelings behind a stoical exterior, it is important to identify their anxieties and deal with them in a competent and supportive manner.

The Patient

Most patients who present with symptoms of cancer, such as haemoptysis or a lump in the breast, have already considered the possibility that they may have malignant disease. Recognition of this will help in dealing with the patient's anxiety and his or her possible misapprehensions.

Despite greater public awareness of cancer, the following misapprehensions among patients remain common:

- Cure is difficult if not impossible—this may explain the late presentation of symptoms by some patients. If it is incurable why bother with hospital and treatments which may be unpleasant?
- Pain and suffering inevitably occur at the end, even if the patient is symptom-free now—the comment 'I am not in pain *yet*, doctor' often points to this belief.
- Cancer is commonly hereditary—this is a complex subject but in the sense that patients mean it, it is usually untrue.
- Incontinence and dementia are common terminal symptoms whilst haemorrhage, choking and suffocation are thought to be common modes of death—patients seldom volunteer these anxieties; they must be elicited by direct questioning and the patient reassured. They are uncommon if the disease is properly managed, although dementia may occur in those with cerebral tumours.
- They will eventually become a burden to their families who will then fail to cope.

- When admission to hospital is necessary a bed may not be available.
- Doctors and hospitals will use them as experimental guinea pigs.

In practice continuing care specialists will hear each of these fears voiced at least once a week. It is therefore important to seek them from the patient, deal with the anxieties they cause and reassure whenever possible.

Reassurance does not consist of bland statements that all will be well, that no-one need suffer pain or that there is no cause for worry. True reassurance is to listen sensitively to the fears, elicit the reasons for them and then discuss them openly and honestly in a realistic, practical and compassionate way. The facts should be explained as optimistically as they will allow and the patient must be reassured of the doctor's continued interest, reassessment and support.

The Family

Patients are often easier to help than their relatives. Anyone working with cancer patients is familiar with the anger, bitterness and resentment that relatives often express. Although this may reflect their feelings of impotence and grief in the face of advancing disease, it often presents as antipathy towards the medical and nursing staff who, understandably, find this behaviour threatening and difficult to cope with.

Relatives and friends may feel under an obligation to protect the patient and to withhold information about 'the bad news'. Consequently as well as sharing many of the anxieties of the sick person, they will have additional concerns of their own:

- Should the patient be told the diagnosis or prognosis?
- Have the doctors really done everything possible? Should a second opinion be sought; should alternative medicine be tried?
- What if something unexpected happens, e.g. 'collapse', a fit, sudden uncontrollable pain, bleeding or sudden death?
- Where do I go for help in an emergency?
- Will the children cope?
- Supposing I become exhausted and cannot cope? What if I fail?

Families tend to be more overt in their anxieties and concerns than patients, but require equal if not greater time to be heard, advised and supported. This is especially important if the patient is at home for it is often on relatives and friends that successful management depends.

On the positive side, the expectations of patients and families, however great they may seem, are often less than those of the doctors and nurses who attend them. Therefore try to identify the families' needs with precision and do not make assumptions.

Doctors

Although care of patients with advancing disease is rewarding it may also be stressful for doctors in the following situations:

- A poor relationship exists with the patient or family.
- Needless pessimism—studies show that doctors' estimates of the curability of different cancers are almost always too pessimistic.
- Concern that narcotic analgesics are dangerous.
- The fear of missing a potentially curable disease—though a worthy goal, it may, if taken to extremes, initiate unnecessary admission, investigation and distress; good clinical judgment is essential.
- Belief that death is a failure—rationally, we all know that this is not the case, but emotionally it often feels like it and to pretend otherwise is to be unreasonable. To combine a natural sadness at the impending death of a patient with a positive approach to the particular patient's problem may not be easy.

Symptom Control

Assessment

In patients with early disease, attempts to control or palliate by anti-cancer therapy will also tend to make the patient feel better. As cancer advances, there may be a conflict between symptom control and side-effects of treatment, and the judgment of the clinician may be sorely tested if he is to alleviate symptoms without doing harm.

In the face of uncontrolled symptoms of advanced cancer, the following steps are essential:

- Take an accurate history and note the patient's perception of his problem.
- Perform a limited but appropriate examination, every step of which is designed to answer a relevant question.
- Inaugurate simple investigations provided they are relevant.
- Weigh the evidence, which may be incomplete, and make a presumptive diagnosis.
- Discuss the findings with the patient, outline a treatment programme and ensure that he understands. Encourage him to ask questions and to repeat what he believes you have said.
- Initiate treatment while watching for unwanted effects and promise continued support.
- Review, review and review again.

In patients with pain, a history of previous attempts at analgesia, especially the drugs used, is essential. Future treatment options will become clear if the following questions are asked about analgesics which have been tried before:

- Did they have *any* effect on the pain?
- Did they relieve or only reduce it?

- For how long were they effective?
- Did they have unpleasant side-effects? If so, what?
- Which was the patient's favourite analgesic and which did he dislike?

The answers may be surprising. Analgesics thought to have been effective, may only reduce the pain to tolerable levels and then only for short periods. Weak analgesics may be preferred to strong ones because sufficient attention has not been paid by the prescriber to unwanted or frightening side-effects. All these issues should be fully pursued; this will not only allow use of appropriate measures but also has the advantage of indicating the clinician's competence to the patient.

The Nature of Pain

The sensation of pain has two components. The first is nociception—the perception of the painful stimulus. The second is the emotional response to that perception. Put simply, a patient with indigestion will view his pain quite differently to the patient who has terminal abdominal cancer.

The incidence of severe unrelieved pain in cancer patients is approximately 9%, but as death approaches this figure rises to almost 60%. However, it should never be forgotten that patients with cancer may also have non-malignant pains which require quite different management (Table 1).

Table 1. Common pains of non-malignant origin in cancer patients

RELATED TO TREATMENT
Postoperative
Radiation fibrosis
Oesophagitis
Tracheitis

RELATED TO DEBILITY
Constipation
Infection
Stiff joints
Myalgia
Bed sores
Post herpetic neuralgia
Pulmonary emboli
Urinary retention

OTHERS
Musculoskeletal
Tension headaches
Pains of past illnesses

Cancer Pain

Cancer pain differs from both acute and chronic pain:

- It neither diminishes with time nor has the gross psychological components characteristic of those patients with chronic back pain who are referred to pain clinics.
- It becomes worse as the tumour extends.
- It becomes purposeless and demoralizing.
- It is influenced by past experiences.
- It may occupy the patient's whole attention and cause isolation from friends and society.
- It ends in death.

Principles of Pain Control

Once the pain has been diagnosed and assessed, several strategies may be used (see box).

Explanation

Limit the pathological process by surgery, radiotherapy, chemotherapy or other measures.

Disrupt nerve pathways by neurolytic procedures or neurosurgery.

Lower pain threshold by drugs or management.

Rest or immobilize the affected part.

Choice of treatment is governed by the type of pain and its cause, the severity of the illness, the likely outcome and possible adverse affects. The extent of disruption to the patient's life must also be considered. For example, a relatively fit man would be able to wait for, and cope with, a neurosurgical procedure in a way which would be impossible for a severely ill man with pain from widespread bone cancer who lives a considerable distance from a major hospital. In this situation, lowering the pain threshold may be the treatment of choice. It is simple, may be applied in the home and works quickly.

In the following section, the use of analgesic drugs is described. But before considering these, Table 2 lists factors which modulate the pain threshold, irrespective of the specific pain relieving measures that are used. It cannot be emphasized too strongly that failure to recognize the effect these symptoms have on physical pain is a common reason for failed pain control in many patients.

Table 2. Factors that lower or raise the pain threshold

Threshold-lowering factors (i.e. more pain)	Threshold-raising factors (i.e. less pain)
Fatigue	Rest
Insomnia	Sleep
Anxiety	Understanding + anxiolytic
Fear	Reassurance
Depression	Counselling + antidepressant
Discomfort	Symptom control
Inappropriate drug	Beneficial drug

Principles of Analgesia

- Pain is what the patient says it is—when in doubt about the amount of pain, this is a useful maxim. Much treatment failure is due to disbelieving or belittling pain complaints in patients with cancer.
- Continuous pain requires continuous relief—treatment only when required (PRN dosage) is irrational, inhumane and synonymous with underdosage.
- The dose for each patient is individually determined—be prepared to titrate rapidly upwards until pain is controlled.
- When weak analgesics fail, change to a stronger drug, not one of similar potency.
- Use oral drugs when it is possible—they produce better pain control, less tolerance, fewer side-effects and are more convenient; only use suppositories or the parenteral route in those who are vomiting or cannot swallow.
- Most opioid analgesics cause constipation and nausea—most patients require a laxative and some need antiemetics.
- Respiratory depression is rare and is no excuse for using inadequate analgesia.
- Drug tolerance is not a practical problem—re-emergence of pain is usually due to advancing disease and thus requires a higher dose.
- Cancer patients in pain and taking oral narcotics do not become psychologically dependent—physical dependence occurs after 10–14 days but does not prevent dose reduction if pain lessens.
- Is adjuvant therapy required? Pain caused by tumour involving bone, brain, nerves, perineum, pleura or posterior abdominal wall may not respond well to opioids alone. In these situations adjuvant therapy (see later) or physical methods of pain control may be required.

The Analgesic Ladder

Pain may be usefully described as mild, moderate or severe. The appropriate drug for each of these constitutes a so-called 'analgesic ladder' consisting of weak, moderate or strong drugs. Even with mild pain, the dose required should be sufficient to remove the pain for the duration of action of the drug so that the next dose is given before the previous one has worn off. Despite a plethora of analgesics on the market, many in combination, it is wise to use a few drugs and know them well (Table 3).

Practical Considerations in Pain Control

Diamorphine and Morphine

Diamorphine is rapidly deacetylated in the gut wall and liver to morphine and 6-monoacetyl morphine (itself analgesic). Because of this and because diamorphine (heroin) is the main drug of abuse, morphine alone is the drug available in many countries. Studies in the United Kingdom show that for practical purposes there is little difference between the two drugs and they are therefore regarded as interchangeable, with diamorphine being the prodrug for morphine. In practice, almost all heroin abuse is conducted through illegal trafficking and not theft from hospital or community pharmacies. Recent attempts in the USA to have heroin legalized have failed: emotional bias is considerable.

Despite these observations, it is wrong to assume that a prodrug is the same as the drug to which it is metabolized, for the simple reason that drug transport to the site of action is important. Indeed, there are minor advantages in using diamorphine related to its greater solubility; this gives the following benefits:

- It is more rapidly absorbed.
- Because of quicker transit through the gut, nausea is less common in some patients (although the mechanism of drug-induced emesis is mainly through the chemoreceptor trigger zone in the midbrain).
- Diamorphine (100 mg dissolves in 0.2 ml of water) is always used for injection in preference to morphine sulphate or hydrochloride (100 mg dissolves in 4 ml of water). In a cachectic patient, an i.m. injection of 4 ml every 4 hours is inhumane.

However, diamorphine is less stable than morphine and although degradation is slow and practically unimportant, its shelf life is regarded by most pharmacists as 2 weeks, unless stored in a refrigerator.

Prescribing. Diamorphine can be made up at the required strength in chloroform water to 5 or 10 ml. High doses make the solution bitter but sweeteners or syrups should not be used in the mixture as these shorten the half-life. They may be taken at the time of ingestion however. The initial dose of diamorphine is 5 mg 4-hourly

Table 3. Analgesics for mild, moderate and severe pain

Type of pain (analgesic group)	Analgesic	Usual adult dose	Dose interval (hours)	Available routes	Comments
Mild (Non-narcotics)	Aspirin	600 mg	4	Oral	Also effective for bone pain
	Paracetamol	1 g	4	Oral	
Moderate (Weak narcotics)	Codeine	30–60 mg	4	Oral / Injection	Constipation common
	Co-proxamol { dextropropoxyphene 32.5 mg / paracetamol 325 mg	1–2	4	Oral	Less constipating / Safe in terminal cancer
Severe (Strong narcotics)	Diamorphine	2.5–100 mg (or higher)	4	Oral / Injection	POTENCY RATIOS / Morphine 7.5 mg oral ≡ Diamorphine 5 mg oral (1.5 : 1)
	Morphine	5–150 mg (or higher)	4	Oral / Injection / Suppository	Diamorphine 5 mg oral ≡ Diamorphine 2.5 mg i.m. (2 : 1)
					Morphine 7.5 mg oral ≡ Diamorphine 2.5 mg i.m. (3 : 1)
					No ceiling effect
	Morphine sulphate Continus MST	10–100 mg (or higher)	12	Oral	Twice daily dose increases compliance / Stabilize on above then change to MST

and of morphine 10 mg 4-hourly because of the difference in potency (see Table 3). The following description refers to diamorphine.

The diamorphine dose is increased by 5 mg steps to 20 mg; then by 10 mg steps to 60 mg, and by 20 mg steps thereafter. Patients should be advised that initial drowsiness will wear off and that drug dependence and tolerance do not occur. It is wise to use a laxative: lactulose (10–15 ml t.i.d.) with Senokot tabs (2 b.d.) is a useful combination. Half of all patients require an antiemetic. The least sedative is haloperidol (0.5 mg t.i.d. or 1.5 mg nocte); more anxiolytic is prochlorperazine (5 mg 4-hourly) while a sedative antiemetic is chlorpromazine (12.5–25 mg 4-hourly).

Patients who are afraid of diamorphine may need to start on an almost homeopathic dose in order to gain their confidence. The word 'heroin' is emotive and should not be used.

Slow-Release Morphine

The duration of action of most opioids is about 4 hours, requiring six doses per day. Many cancer patients have had little or no medication in the past and find this dosage schedule unacceptable. The advent of morphine sulphate continus (MST) has introduced a preparation which, because of its packaging, allows morphine sulphate to leach out of the tablet over a period of 12 hours. Although not pharmacologically different from the parent drug, this is a definite practical advantage.

The normal starting dose for the frail elderly is 10 mg b.d. Less ill patients may start on 30 mg b.d. In patients with moderate but continuous pain which is known to be responsive to soluble opioids, it is possible to use MST as the first strong analgesic. However, it is wise to stabilize patients on soluble diamorphine or morphine initially in the following situations:

- Those with evidence of impaired drug absorption.
- Patients with a past history of poor pain control.
- Existing severe unrelieved pain or variable pain of considerable intensity.
- Patients who are distressed or anxious.

Drugs to Avoid

It has already been suggested in this chapter that a few drugs should be used in order to know them well. However, a number of drugs in common use are missing from the list shown and this requires explanation:

- Methadone—has a duration of action of up to 72 hours; it is therefore cumulative and may cause overdosage.
- Pethidine and Dextromoramide—have a duration of action of $1\frac{1}{2}$ –2 hours. This frequency of dosage is socially unacceptable. Moreover, pethidine taken orally is a poor analgesic and confers no advantage in patients with colic as was once supposed.
- Pentazocine—has a high incidence of psychomimetic side-effects; these are more common in the elderly.

- Buprenorphine—the theoretical advantage of this for nauseated patients is outweighed by the nausea, vomiting and nightmares that the drug induces. Furthermore, because it binds more powerfully to opioid receptors than diamorphine it theoretically displaces more effective drugs if used concurrently. It has a ceiling effect of 2.0 mg per day and should not be prescribed with other opioids.

There will always be new drugs developed which are said to have theoretical advantages. Unfortunately, in practice they often confer little benefit to patients with advancing cancer and should be used only after extensive trials and proven results.

Adjuvant Medication

Diamorphine and morphine are excellent analgesics which induce few serious side-effects. They are most effective for soft tissue and visceral pain, and when used correctly they have the advantage of considerable efficacy with no 'ceiling' to the dose. However, there are a number of situations where adjuvant medication in the form of co-analgesics or other drugs are required. Co-analgesics are drugs with a different mode of action which produce improved pain control and fewer unwanted effects. Table 4 shows pains which may require additional drugs to control them.

Alternative Routes of Administration

Analgesics and other drugs are usually prescribed orally. They can also be given by the rectal route or by injection in patients who are vomiting, dysphagic or very weak. Intravenous infusion is appropriate for short periods only (e.g. for postoperative pain) but because it requires careful monitoring and cannot be safely used at home except in special circumstances, it is not indicated in those with long-term cancer pain. Considerable, but so far unsuccessful, efforts are being made to introduce a safe, effective and convenient pump at a reasonable cost for continuous i.v. infusion at home or when the patient is ambulant. In the meantime the best alternative is continuous subcutaneous infusion by a small electrically powered syringe driver. However it is indicated only when other routes are inappropriate (Table 5).

The syringe driver confers no advantage over oral medication for pain control alone. If the pain is responsive to opioids and the oral dose is insufficient, it should merely be increased. It is a common but erroneous myth that the syringe driver confers improved analgesia. This is only true when there is impaired drug absorption from the gastrointestinal tract.

A number of drugs can be used in the syringe driver but there may be a problem of precipitation or crystallization if very high doses of cyclizine and haloperidol are used. Diazepam, chlorpromazine and prochlorperazine rapidly cause fat necrosis which is painful and causes syringe failure. These drugs are therefore contraindicated.

However, certain drugs may be mixed together and are physically compatible in the syringe (see page 179).

Table 4. Pains requiring specific or additional drugs

Type of pain	Drug	Usual adult dose	Dose interval (hours)	Comments
Bone	Aspirin	600 mg	4	Potent side-effects
	Diclofenac (Voltarol)	75–150 mg	12	Fewer side-effects Long action Suppositories available
Nerve compression	Dexamethasone	2–4 mg	8–12	
Raised intracranial pressure	Dexamethasone	2–8 mg	8–12	
Stabbing or lightning pain	Sodium valporate (Epilim)	200 mg	8	
Muscle spasm	Diazepam (Valium)	5–10 mg	8	
	Baclofen (Lioresal)	10 mg	8	Nausea and drowsiness occur
Infected malignant ulcer	Metronidazole (Flagyl)	400 mg	8	
PAIN ENHANCEMENT				
Anxiety	Diazepam (Valium)	2–10 mg	Nocte or 8	Try one: if ineffective increase dose or change to the other
	Chlorpromazine (Largactil)	10–50 mg	4–8	
Depression	Amitriptyline	10–75 mg	Nocte	Antidepressant of choice
	Mianserin	30–60 mg	12	Less unwanted effects

Table 5. The syringe driver is used when the following routes are impractical for the reasons shown

Route	Reasons
Oral	Vomiting
	Dysphagia
	Weakness
	Coma
Rectal	Diarrhoea/constipation
	Rectal tumour or disease
	Dislike of rectal route
Injection	Cachexia
	Large volume of injection fluid
	Fear of injection
	Long-term parenteral therapy at home

Diamorphine—the analgesic of choice.

Haloperidol—first line antiemetic.

Cyclizine—useful second line antiemetic, especially for terminal intestinal obstruction.

Metoclopramide—second line antiemetic in resistant vomiting; contraindicated in intestinal obstruction.

Dexamethasone—may be used in patients who cannot take medicine by mouth.

In patients who are actually dying, secretions in the throat can cause an unpleasant bubbling known as the 'death rattle'. Hyoscine in the syringe driver prevents these secretions and hence the noise. It can, of course, also be given intramuscularly.

The syringe driver is now widely used in hospitals, and many family doctors have one as part of their practice equipment. They are a useful adjunct to symptom control in selected patients.

To Tell or Not to Tell

No discussion about pain in advanced cancer could ignore the patient's knowledge and attitude towards his illness. Three common situations arise:

- He knows or seriously suspects the diagnosis and can discuss it openly.
- The situation has been explained to him but he lives in a state of 'middle knowledge', i.e. he knows and understands the reality of his diagnosis today, but tomorrow he understands

it differently and this situation may change from day to day.
In this group of patients one must never assume that what
was discussed and agreed yesterday still holds today.

- He has no idea of the diagnosis and prognosis and may even
deny it after being told. Denial is an involuntary
psychological defence against unpleasant truths.

How does one decide whether to tell or not? Patients have the right to know the diagnosis and prognosis but the same right not to know. However, it is now commonplace to tell patients they have cancer when it is diagnosed. This is the time when treatment or palliation can optimistically be offered in all good faith. Furthermore this disconnects the diagnosis from death. Unfortunately in the past the diagnosis and hopeless prognosis were given together and this is partly responsible for the appalling reputation which cancer has today.

If the facts are divulged to patients in a sensitive and compassionate way there are few who will not respond positively. It rapidly becomes apparent during the conversation if one is going too far and this allows an opportunity to 'back-off', for the time being at least. Indeed, if the conversation goes well the patient may tell the doctor his suspicions of the diagnosis and prognosis, and merely seek confirmation. One should always tell the truth but doctors have no right to force it down patients' throats.

If a patient indicates to the medical or nursing staff that he wishes to know more about his diagnosis and prognosis there are four simple rules to remember when discussing it with him (see box).

---

1. Allow 20 minutes without interruption.
2. Remember that when you have divulged the bad news, he will remember little else that you say.
3. Return the following day to answer questions which have arisen overnight.
4. Assure him that whatever happens you will be available for support and advice throughout the remainder of the illness (provided of course that that is true).

When a patient learns from someone that he is going to die, a unique relationship is formed. If this knowledge has been imparted sensitively and well, their gratitude for openness, honesty and compassion may be overwhelming. It is a powerful force towards supporting them throughout the remainder of their illness.

If there are three words which sum up good quality care of patients with advancing disease they are *competence*, *compassion* and good *communication*. If one can achieve these with the dying it enhances one's clinical abilities in all other areas of medicine.

Selected Reading

Doyle, D. (ed.) (1984) *Palliative Care: The Management of Far Advanced Cancer*. Croom Helm, Kent.
Regnard, C.F.B. and Davies, A. (1986) *A Guide to Symptom Relief in Advanced Cancer*. Distributed by Haigh & Hochland, Manchester.
Saunders, C.M. (ed.) (1984) *The Management of Terminal Malignant Disease*. Edward Arnold, London.
Saunders, C. and Baines, M. (1983) *Living With Dying*. Oxford University Press, Oxford.
Twycross, R.G. and Lack, S.A. (1983) *Symptom Control in Far Advanced Cancer: Pain Relief*. Pitman, London.

CONTROL OF OTHER SYMPTOMS

Although localized cancer may cause local problems, recurrent or widespread disease often affects patients generally. Hence, a patient with carcinoma of the breast may develop a single bone metastasis, which causes local pain that is easily alleviated by single fraction radiotherapy. Alternatively, a young patient with rapidly advancing malignant melanoma may have metastases invading many organs throughout the body; as well as causing local symptoms these frequently produce cachexia, lethargy and malaise.

The cause of symptoms must be identified in a manner similar to that used for the causes of pain, as outlined in the first part of this chapter. Sometimes it will not be possible to make a firm diagnosis and here the inconvenience of further investigation must be weighed against a trial and error policy to distinguish different causes. The latter, scientifically approached, may be highly appropriate in patients with late-stage disease because the cause of symptoms is often complex and will often require more than one treatment or drug. The treatment chosen should ideally be rapidly effective, low on toxicity and realistically assessed.

Table 6 shows symptoms recently recorded in 100 consecutive patients dying of cancer at home. There are, of course, many others, but because they are the most common, this list forms the basis for the symptoms to be considered in this chapter.

The Principles of Symptom Control

- Good symptom control requires clearly defined medical leadership.
- Assessment must precede treatment. Many symptoms are caused by multiple factors.
- List all the patient's symptoms and enquire of the carer if any have been omitted.
- Ask the patient and carer to rate these in order of priority.
- Dispense with the bad news first: some of these symptoms will not be amenable to treatment and so the patient should be told.

Table 6. Symptoms recorded in 100
consecutive patients

Symptom	%
Pain	75
Weakness	71
Constipation	49
Depression	46
Anorexia	38
Nausea	28
Vomiting	24
Dyspnoea	21
Painful decubitus	12
Dysphagia	10
Diarrhoea	6
Dry/sore mouth	5

- Concentrate on the good news, namely those symptoms that are treatable.
- Explain in simple terms the underlying mechanism.
- Discuss treatment options with the patient and if possible decide together on the immediate course of action.
- Explain the treatment both to patient and relative.
- Do not limit treatment to the use of drugs.
- Prescribe drugs prophylactically for persistent symptoms.
- Seek a colleague's advice (e.g. anaesthetist, radiotherapist or oncologist) in seemingly intractable situations.
- Never say 'there is nothing more I can do'.

Gastrointestinal Symptoms

There are a wide variety of gastrointestinal symptoms—the most important are discussed in an abbreviated form below.

Dry or Painful Mouth

The causes of this symptom are given in the box.

CAUSES OF DRY/PAINFUL MOUTH:
Drugs
Dehydration
Candida albicans
Ill-fitting dentures

> Aphthous ulceration
> Localized radiotherapy
> Oral tumours

Treatment. Frequently more than one of the possible causal factors are at work. Good oral hygiene is obligatory and will reduce further problems. Regular mouthwashes and dental care are essential and some patients may gain from chewing gum, acid drops and pineapple chunks, all of which increase the flow of saliva. Artificial saliva may be helpful, but needs to be used frequently, especially at meal times.

Unfortunately, many of the drugs used for patients with advanced, progressive cancer also cause a dry mouth. The common ones are the phenothiazines, tricyclic antidepressants, antispasmodics, antihistamines, diuretics, cytotoxic agents and analgesics.

Dehydration is common in the last few days of life. It is important to remember that thirst can be treated as effectively by oral care as it can by increasing fluid intake. Rehydration at this stage of a patient's life is inappropriate and often ineffective. A dry mouth is treated with frequent sips of fluid. Plain water or carbonated water are often best, especially if cool. Sweet drinks are contraindicated becuase they promote dryness. Some patients appreciate crushed ice inserted directly into the mouth.

Oral candidiasis is common in the immunocompromised cancer patient. The classical white plaques of yeast infection which, when scraped off, leave a slightly bleeding mucosa, are not always visible so in any patient with a dry, brick-red mucosa thrush should be assumed and be treated. Oral nystatin is the treatment of choice: 1–2 ml of suspension should be applied to the buccal cavity every 2 hours if the infection is severe, or every 4 hours if it is recent and mild. Alternatively, nystatin pastilles may be sucked. If there is no improvement after 3 days, ketoconazole (200 mg daily) should be prescribed. This is a systemic antifungal agent and although generally not used in fit patients because of liver toxicity, it is perfectly safe to do so in the terminally ill. Amphotericin lozenges may be used, but these dissolve slowly in the mouth leaving a gritty base, and are unpopular.

If a patient cannot eat because of ill-fitting dentures this can be alleviated successfully by the attention of a dentist who may be prepared to visit the patient in their own home. Aphthous ulceration is effectively dealt with by applying Adcortyl in Orabase, a topical steroid containing triamcinolone acetonide, 0.1%, in a base which adheres to moist mucous membranes and thus maintains contact between the drug and the ulcer.

The salivary glands, which are sensitive to radiation, are often rendered ineffective or destroyed by radiotherapy to the oral cavity. In such patients salivary stimulants are often disappointing and frequent drinks of water, or the use of artificial salivas as described above, may be necessary. Advancing oral tumour may further aggravate the situation and all measures so far mentioned need to be meticulously carried out. In addition, debridement with hydrogen peroxide mouthwash 3%, with added lemon juice to taste, and the whole added to 15 mg of warm water, may, if used regularly, keep the tumour relatively clean.

Dysphagia

The following common causes are seen:

- Tumours involving the oral cavity, nasopharynx or supraglottic areas.
- Tumours involving the oesophagus, either primary tumours or those extending upwards from the stomach.
- Tumours in the mediastinum causing external compression and neuromuscular disorders because of involvement of the oesophageal wall or external compression.
- Non-metastatic manifestations of cancer, of which the commonest are disorders of motility.
- Poor oral hygiene, and oesophageal candidiasis (particularly in AIDS, leukaemia and lymphoma).

Treatment. Whenever possible the primary tumour should be treated. This may involve surgery, radiotherapy or more recently laser therapy, which can be used to debulk the tumour. In oesophageal tumours the early passage of celestin or other tube may be more effective than any other treatments. They are usually well tolerated, and provided the patient complies with dietary advice the tube rarely blocks. Fizzy drinks with meals will facilitate the passage of food through the tube. However, if the patient becomes completely dysphagic because the tube is blocked the obstruction can be cleared easily at immediate oesophagoscopy.

Oesophageal candidiasis should be suspected in patients with oral candidiasis, who have dysphagia, oesophagitis and debility. Although it can only be satisfactorily diagnosed by oesophagoscopy it is usually as remediable with treatment as its oral counterpart, and nystatin and ketaconazoles should be used as described previously.

Occasionally relatively small tumours or local fibrosis may involve the pharyngeal or oesophageal wall and so splint the gullet. Perineural spread along the vagus may cause muscular incoordination, and these patients may respond to the use of oral corticosteroids.

It is often distressing for doctors, nurses and the family to observe a patient with dysphagia so gross that he cannot eat and can barely swallow fluids. In relation to this, three questions require consideration:

- *Should the patient be fed by nasogastric tube?*
  1. Although feasible, this is rarely indicated. These patients are often extremely ill and tube feeding prolongs their distress and suffering.
  2. Most patients dislike long-term nasograstric feeding by large bore tubes. Fine bore tubes are more comfortable, but have the disadvantage of requiring an intermittent enteral drip. The latter limits the patient's activity, and at home can cause anxiety in the family—especially when inordinate quantities of fluid are prescribed in the mistaken belief that the patient still requires a normal calorie intake.

3. Once a tube is inserted it requires considerable courage on behalf of the patient—and indeed of the physician also—to remove the tube when the patient and family believe that the inevitable consequence will be death in a few days.

4. Without a tube, it is often surprising to find that fluid sufficient to maintain life may still be ingested.

• *Would a gastrostomy help?*

A gastrostomy is a tube which is internally fixed to the stomach and passes through the stomach wall and abdominal wall to the exterior. At this point it is clamped and may be used either to feed patients or to empty the stomach contents. A gastrostomy for feeding is always contraindicated in terminally ill patients. However, in rare instances where there is complete, inoperable obstruction of the gastric antrum and a formal bypass is impossible, a gastrostomy will allow patients to eat and drink as the fluid drains into a bag. Patients will absorb small quantities of the ingested fluid and may well survive for up to 2 weeks. They are relieved of copious vomiting and distress and carefully selected patients benefit from this procedure.

• *Is total parenteral nutrition (TPN) appropriate?*

This is never indicated in patients who are dying of cancer. It provides no benefit or pleasure to the patient whatever, is extremely expensive, and is bad medical practice.

Anorexia

The reason why patients with advanced cancer become anorexic is complex and obscure. If there is any precipitating cause (e.g. nausea, infection or abdominal distension by ascites) it should be treated. Some tumours cause disordered taste, particularly tumours of the lung and gastrointestinal tract.

Treatment.   The simplest way to promote a good appetite is to offer an aperitif before meals and provide small quantities of food, elegantly prepared, without first negotiating what the patient would like. Often, carers attempt to negotiate each meal. When the patient is ill, weak and anorexic, this is an unwelcome ordeal, but because they do not wish to distress those who look after them, they are often unwilling to say so. A diet that is wisely and imaginatively chosen by the carer will often succeed when negotiation fails.

All the normal rules of feeding may be broken. 'A little of what you fancy does you good', in the words of the old song, is an excellent maxim.

The only effective appetite stimulants are the corticosteroids. In addition to their specific effects, they increase the appetite, promote a feeling of well-being and, by causing fluid retention, induce weight gain. Dexamethasone (2–4 mg daily) or prednisolone (15–30 mg daily) may be used without serious side-effects. Some physicians prescribe an H_2 antagonist to prevent gastric ulceration, but this is no longer thought to be appropriate, except in patients with a previous ulcer history. Corticosteroids occasionally produce euphoria, hypomania or frank psychosis, and if given in the evenings may also prevent sleep. Steroid-induced diabetes may be controlled with insulin.

Nausea and Vomiting

Mechanism.   Figure 1 shows how the various causes of vomiting mediate their effects on the integrative vomiting centres. Clearly, different causes require different treatments so once again the specific cause or causes must be sought (see Table 7).

In patients with advanced cancer, nausea and vomiting may be treated separately. Indeed, they may occur independently or together, and respond differently to medication. Sometimes it will be possible to relieve both. In other situations it may be possible to relieve nausea and only reduce the vomiting; in others the reverse may be true. Both are unpleasant symptoms, which may be more difficult to treat than pain, and may substantially reduce a patient's quality of life by inducing feelings of wretchedness, lack of interest in food or company and embarrassment in front of friends or family.

Treatment.   Table 8 shows the drugs which are effective at different sites.

Drug-Induced Vomiting.   Drugs may cause vomiting by their direct effect on the chemoreceptor trigger zone (e.g. chemotherapy), by causing gastric stasis (e.g. morphine) or by causing gastric irritation (e.g. aspirin).

Uraemia

Although this is a terminal event in pelvic tumours, it is far less common than expected. It may also be more gradual than anticipated, especially since cystectomy with urinary

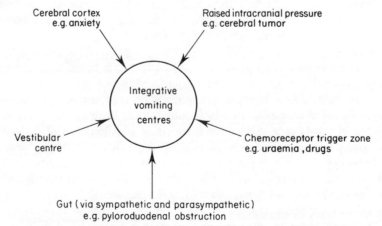

Figure 1. Schematic representation of the various neural mechanisms involved in initiation of vomiting. From Baines (1983) *Antiemetics and Cancer Chemotherapy*, Lazzlo, J. (ed.). Williams & Wilkins, Baltimore. Reproduced by permission

Table 7. Possible causes of nausea/vomiting in advanced cancer patients

Chemical causes
    Drugs
    Uraemia
    Hypercalcaemia
Irradiation
Gastric causes
    Local irritation from drugs, blood, etc.
    External pressure
    Carcinoma of stomach
    Pyloro-duodenal obstruction
Intestinal obstruction
Constipation
Raised intracranial pressure
Vestibular disturbance
Cough-induced vomiting
Psychogenic, especially anxiety

diversion through an ileal loop has become a more common treatment for bladder cancer. However, tumours of the uterus, cervix and prostate still cause postrenal uraemia. Since all drug-induced vomiting affects the chemoreceptor trigger zone, drugs acting at this site may be useful. Unfortunately, the vomiting of uraemia is particularly difficult to control and most patients feel wretched, anorexic and ill. Some claim that the addition of more than one antiemetic may be beneficial, but there is little evidence for this. If intractable and particularly distressing, a sedative antiemetic, such as chlorpromazine, is indicated.

Hypercalcaemia (see Chapter 9)

Although hypercalcaemia occurs in approximately 10% of all malignancies, some studies have shown that transient hypercalcaemia occurs in as many as 30% of patients, but returns to normal without treatment. Consequently, it is important not to treat symptomless hypercalcaemia. Such patients should be monitored regularly for a changing pattern of symptoms and encouraged to maintain their hydration in excess of their normal requirements.

Other patients will develop symptomatic hyercalcaemia irrespective of whether or not they have widespread bone disease. Hypercalcaemia is more common in patients with a large tumour burden, and studies show that it is this, rather than the extent of bone metastases, that determines the likelihood of a raised serum calcium causing symptoms. Occasionally, hyperparathyroidism will be found, but this is rare.

The symptoms of hypercalcaemia include nausea, vomiting, drowsiness, confusion, dry mouth, weakness and anorexia. In patients with a rapid onset of confusion, hypercalcaemia should always be suspected.

Treatment.   A number of agents have been tried in the past but are no longer recommended. These are corticosteroids, calcitonin, a combination of the two and

Table 8. Antiemetic drugs used in patients with advanced cancer.

Antiemetic	Normal adult dose	Site of action*	Comments
Haloperidol	0.5 mg orally t.i.d. OR 3.0 mg orally nocte OR 2.5–5.0 mg i.m. nocte or b.d.	CTZ*	Non-sedative Extrapyramidal symptoms rare at low doses
Prochlorperazine	2.5–5 mg orally 4-hrly OR 5 mg, 25 mg supp.s t.i.d. OR 6.25–12.5 mg i.m. 4-hrly	CTZ	Mildly anxiolytic Extrapyramidal symptoms uncommon
Chlorpromazine	12.5–50 mg orally 4-hrly OR 100 mg supp.s t.i.d. OR 12.5–50 mg i.m. 4-hrly	CTZ	More sedative Anticholinergic Increased sensitivity to sunlight
Promazine	25–50 mg orally t.i.d. OR 12.5–50 mg subcutaneously or i.m. t.i.d.	CTZ	Alternative to chlorpromazine
Domperidone	10–20 mg orally t.i.d OR 30 mg supp.s t.i.d.	Upper bowel + CTZ	Non sedative Improves gastric emptying Low central activity
Metoclopramide	10 mg orally or i.m. t.i.d.	Upper bowel + CTZ	Alternative to domperidone Extrapyramidal effects more common
Cyclizine	50 mg orally or i.m. t.i.d.	VC†	Vomiting on movement Raised ICP Useful adjunct to other antiemetics

*CTZ = chemoreceptor trigger zone.
†VC = vomiting centre.
If a single agent fails the addition of a second drug with a different site of action may be tried. In severe vomiting, parenteral administration for 24–48 hours is obligatory.

mithramycin. The latter may be effective but often precludes the use of further chemotherapy.

The management of hypercalcaemia has been changed since the introduction of the intravenous biphosphonates. A recommended regime for their use is:

- Intravenous fluids—3 litres per day.
- Etidronate disodium—7.5 mg per kg body weight per day infused over 2 hours, daily for 3 days.
- If the serum calcium falls to normal, but at a later date hypercalcaemia occurs again, the treatment may be continued.
- Some workers continue treatment with oral etidronate, but there is little evidence at present that this is beneficial.

Gastric Obstruction and Vomiting

Extrinsic pressure on the stomach from hepatomegaly is said to cause the 'squashed stomach syndrome'. However, late pregnancy and massive ascites rarely cause vomiting, so this concept is suspect. If it does indeed exist, symptoms will be early satiation, flatulence and vomiting soon after food. There is no evidence that flatulence is aided by defoaming agents, but if stomach emptying can be encouraged by the use of a dopamine antagonist, such as metaclopramide, this questionable syndrome might be relieved.

Intrinsic involvement of the stomach from carcinoma may cause severe vomiting even without obstruction. Here again the stomach should be emptied with metaclopramide or cyclizine. A coeliac plexus block may reduce the vomiting as well as any pain. Linitis plastica (the 'leather bottle stomach') turns the stomach into a rigid tube of reduced capacity. Because normal peristalsis cannot occur, vomiting food is common. If the stomach wall is not completely involved by tumour, drugs which empty the stomach— the dopamine antagonists—may be useful. In advanced diseases, however, the patient may become distressed, cachectic and refuse to eat.

If overt obstruction occurs in the stomach, the nausea only may be reduced. In obstruction, the dopamine antagonists become contraindicated as they aggravate the vomiting. Unfortunately in advanced cases surgery is disappointing—many patients achieve no benefit, others receive benefit for a limited period and a number are totally inoperable at laparotomy. It is claimed that corticosteroids may assist by reducing surrounding inflammatory oedema in the stomach wall.

Intestinal Obstruction

Because of the capaciousness of the small and large bowel, obstruction further down the alimentary tract is much easier to manage. A single resectable obstruction should be managed surgically, but in advanced disease there are often large tumour masses, which narrow the bowel at several sites. In such tumours as ovarian carcinoma, the entire gut may be encased in a mass of tumour and fibrotic tissue so that successful surgery is virtually impossible.

Traditionally, the vomiting of obstruction was treated by regular aspiration of the stomach and intravenous fluids (so-called 'drip and suck') If this treatment was unsuccessful at relieving the obstruction after 4 days, surgery was considered. However, there is now good evidence that in this group of patients management of the obstruction by other means can be equally, if not more effective, thus avoiding surgery (which may fail to achieve its objectives anyway). The regime currently favoured is shown in the box below.

Diet—low residue
Drugs—antiemetics
    —cyclizine
    —chlorpromazine if sedation required
Diamorphine—for pain
Docusate—stool softener
Don't use peristaltic agents
Drip and suck only if desperate
Discuss with surgeons if in doubt

It is obviously important in patients with obstruction never to promise that all nausea and vomiting can be relieved. However, the nausea can usually be eradicated, and even in the most intractable cases the vomiting reduced to one or two large vomits per day. By explaining the mechanism of the vomiting, most patients will tolerate this degree of symptoms surprisingly well. Patients may live for several weeks or months, moving from subacute to acute obstruction and back again after successful medical treatment.

Raised Intracranial Pressure

Dexamethasone 16 mg daily should control the vomiting. If not, cyclizine 50 mg t.i.d. is the antiemetic of choice.

Constipation

Most dying patients are constipated, and this may be aggravated by the drugs they take, particularly the analgesics. Weakness, reduced mobility, poor fluid intake, anorexia and a low-roughage diet are common precursors to the problem and may not be easily remedied. Laxatives should be used readily. The aim should be to soften the faeces and promote peristalsis. In current practice the following drugs are used: lactulose (15 mg b.d. or more) combined with senna (either as tablets or liquid and taken in conventional doses). The latter may cause abdominal colic. Docusate sodium may be used as a stool softener alone, particularly in patients with subacute obstruction. Methylcellulose tabs (3–6 b.d.) may be used as a bulking agent and should be taken with a glass of water. It is not popular with patients and should only be used when a bulking agent is required in patients with fluid faeces from a proximal colostomy.

Despite regular laxatives, many patients will require either glycerine or bisacodyl 10 mg suppositories; others will require a Fletcher's or a saline enema.

Unfortunately some patients will present with impacted faeces and this must be cleared from below before the above regime is carried out. This may be achieved by using an aracis oil enema at night to soften the faeces, followed the next morning by a conventional enema to clear the bowel. Sometimes the impaction will be so hard that manual removal of inspissated faeces is necessary. This is clearly very distressing to patients, but should not be omitted due to over-sensitivity on the part of the practitioner or nurse.

Diarrhoea

Causes. The main causes of diarrhoea are:

- Constipation with overflow. The distal portion of impacted faeces eventually liquefies and produces a watery faecal discharge which is often wrongly treated with anti-diarrhoeal agents because the doctor has omitted to examine the rectum. Clearly this is constipation and should be treated as outlined above.
- Subacute obstruction. Approximately one-third of patients develop diarrhoea and the treatment is with antiperistaltic drugs, such as loperamide (2–8 mg daily) or the cheaper and equally effective codeine phosphate (15–60 mg 6-hourly).
- Pancreatic insufficiency, secondary to a large pancreatic carcinoma, produces steatorrhoea and should be treated with Nutrizym (100–150 mg with food). It is essential to give an H_2 antagonist concurrently as pancreatic supplements are rendered inactive in gastric acid.
- Rectal or sigmoid carcinoma.

Patients with carcinoma of the large bowel often present with altered bowel habit; surgery, even if only to give palliation, is the treatment of choice. However, in end-stage disease, patients may have massive tumours which are impossible to remove, debulk or bypass, and may have a rectal discharge of mucus, blood and sometimes pus, which can be distressing.

Some patients will respond to daily prednisolone retention enemas, especially if the diarrhoea has been complicated by recent irradiation. However, these symptoms may be difficult to treat, especially if the anus is distorted by tumour infiltration, when the normal sphincter mechanism is lost. The only practical solution is for the patient to wear incontinence pads and indulge in frequent anal toilet to avoid unpleasant odours.

Respiratory Symptoms

Dyspnoea

This is an enormous, unresearched problem, with a multitude of causes. These can be broadly grouped into:

- Increased ventilatory demand, e.g. respiratory infection in a patient with carcinoma of the lung.
- Decreased ventilatory capacity, e.g. airway obstruction by tumour or loss of lung tissue, either intrinsically due to tumour destruction, or extrinsically by pleural effusion.

It is important to recognize that breathless patients become frightened and often fear suffocation. This anxiety increases the dyspnoea and a vicious circle occurs which may be hard to break.

Management.   When the patient presents with breathlessness a clinical diagnosis is first made and a chest X-ray is commonly required. Checking the haemoglobin, white cell count and blood urea may be needed to identify metabolic causes.

Treatment.   If dyspnoea persists after specific treatment of air-flow problems or infection, the mainstay of treatment is morphine or diamorphine, 2.5–10 mg 4-hourly, orally. Occasionally MST may be useful. Morphine works by reducing the respiratory drive, relieving anxiety, eliminating pain and improving cardiac failure if present. The dose should be titrated against its effect on the dyspnoea, as it is for pain. Despite the teaching that opioids should never be used in asthmatic or breathless patients, the opposite is true in patients with terminal cancer. Respiratory depression is extremely rare—even in patients with gross lung pathology—when the opioids are given by mouth. Fear of respiratory depression should never prevent the use of these effective drugs in the frightened breathless patient.

The corticosteroids in the form of dexamethasone (4 mg/24 hr) or prednisolone (30 mg/24 hr) will relieve bronchospasm, sometimes reduce peritumour oedema or even diminish the size of the tumour itself if it is steroid sensitive. Some believe that steroids are effective in lymphangitis carcinomatosa, when the lymphatics become replaced by tumour. There is no convincing evidence of this, however.

Because the breathless patient is anxious, anxiolytics should be readily available and antibiotics used, not so much to prolong life as to relieve the symptoms, which are frequently aggravated by infection. If a patient has been exposed to many antibiotics in the past, chloramphenicol (250–500 mg q.i.d.) is the antibiotic of choice. Despite its potential side effect of marrow aplasia, it is safe in patients with advanced cancer.

Bupivacaine inhalations by a nebulizer are reputed to relieve dyspnoea by stimulating the j-receptors in the lung. To be effective, particle size must be extremely small. Its efficacy is unknown.

Oxygen is rarely indicated in the dyspnoeic cancer patient. It is more appropriate to explain to the patient what is happening, determine the patient's most comfortable position, encourage him to avoid undue activity, and make practical suggestions about daily living. These may be simple measures like bringing a bed downstairs, or moving to a room adjacent to the lavatory if patients are grossly dyspnoeic on-exertion. It is important to explain that if the symptoms are properly managed, death by suffocation is extremely rare. Even in the patient who develops acute respiratory failure, unconsciousness occurs within a few seconds and their perceived fear of suffocation or strangulation is seen to be quite false. This fact is commonly not appreciated by younger doctors and therefore needs to be emphasized.

Despite this reassurance, some patients will become very breathless indeed, even at rest. How should this be dealt with? It is important to negotiate with the patient whether he wishes to be drowsy, sedated and less dyspnoeic; or alert and breathless. Most patients respond well and clearly to this approach, and often as the staff are becoming distressed by what they see, the patient may wish to remain alert and cope with his breathlessness.

However, there may come a point when 'unacceptable dyspnoea' occurs; when it does it should be treated promptly, vigorously and effectively. This point is identified by the patient stating that despite all the interventions that have been used, they are now so frightened by their breathlessness that they are no longer able to cope. The treatment must now reduce the respiratory drive by increasing the dose of morphine and by relieving anxiety, with either diazepam or chlorpromazine in sufficient dosage. The patient is now on the verge of respiratory failure and the use of these drugs will, as a side-effect, hasten their death.

This is an ethical dilemma which should be considered in advance as it frequently leads to indecisive behaviour in a situation where decisiveness is essential. It is not only bad medicine, but bad ethics to allow a patient to die in terror because of a reluctance to use opiate analgesics to control this symptom and the distress it causes.

Other Treatments.   Occasionally, radiotherapy, blood transfusion, respiratory exercises and physiotherapy will help the dyspnoeic patient. Pleural effusions should be aspirated and this can be repeated if it has previously helped for a reasonable length of time. In late-stage disease, however, pleural effusions may recur within a few days and at this point the use of drugs is usually preferred by patients instead of frequent hospital admissions.

Death Rattle

The so-called 'death rattle' is typically seen as a presager of doom. It is due to the retention of inspissated bronchial secretions in the unconscious patient whose cough reflex is reduced because dying is imminent. It is distressing to relatives and staff, but not to unconscious patients. At the first sign of the death rattle in an unconscious patient, hyoscine (0.4–0.6 mg i.m. or s.c.) should be given. This reduces the bronchial secretions and hence the rattle. It must also always be given with a small dose of diamorphine because although normally a sedative, it occasionally causes agitation and distress. It should not be given to those who are conscious as it produces an unacceptably dry mouth.

Cough

The large number of proprietary preparations available for the treatment of cough indicate that its management remains unsatisfactory. The general rule is that dry coughs should be diminished, but productive coughs encouraged. The latter, together with physiotherapy, may rid the lungs of sputum (which may also be infected) and thus relieve distress.

General management advice.   Patients should stop smoking, live in an environment containing warm, moist air and use a humidifier. Some patients find Benzoin inhalations BPC soothing. Sudden changes in atmospheric temperature should be avoided. Most antitussive and expectorant mixtures have unproven effects, but if a placebo is required, it should at least cause no harm. Mucolytics, drugs which were believed to reduce sputum viscosity and so aid expectoration, are of unproven benefit.

Drugs.   These include linctus BPC (5 mg PRN), codeine or pholcodeine linctus (containing a weak narcotic), and morphine and diamorphine (strong narcotics). Methadone has been used for many years, but has a very long duration of action; it therefore accumulates causing side-effects, of which drowsiness is the most common.

Haemoptysis

The presence of blood in the sputum is another doom-laden symptom in the eyes of the public. In the early part of the century it usually indicated tuberculosis—phthisis—which was then a common cause of death. As the prevalence of lung cancer has increased haemoptysis became linked with cancer—another disease which frightens the general public. Haemoptysis, even in small or infrequent quantities, is viewed by patients with considerable concern. It tends to fluctuate; slight haemoptysis at some time during the illness is no indication that the patient is later likely to have a torrential haemorrhage. The patient may therefore be reassured.

If there is increasing blood in the sputum, such that it becomes distressing, a short course of radiotherapy to the appropriate area of the lung usually prevents further occurrence.

Urinary Tract Symptoms

Urinary Incontinence

Contrary to popular opinion, urinary incontinence is not a common feature of terminal cancer. It will occur, however, in patients with spinal cord lesions secondary to vertebral collapse, in metastatic disease and in some bladder tumours, especially if the bladder remains *in situ*. It occasionally occurs in tumours involving the prostate or urethra, either from primary tumours in these areas or from tumour invasion from adjacent tissues. The constant wetting of clothes and bed, which necessitate frequent changing, washing and drying, is a considerable burden to most families who experience it. Fortunately this is unnecessary. If incontinence is slight, simple padding with incontinence pads may be effective and free from smell. If this fails, a catheter is obligatory.

Two types of catheter are available. One is the condom catheter; this may be attached to the penis and so does not involve urethral catheterization, thus alleviating the risks of bladder sepsis and ascending urinary tract infection. It is particularly useful for patients who require a catheter at night only. In some ill and elderly patients the penis may be too small for this to be effective, and in these situations an indwelling catheter should be used. A urinary drainage bag can be attached to the leg or thigh and the patient can then lead an independent and clean existence. Urine always becomes infected in patients with indwelling catheters, but such infection should not be treated with antibiotics unless there are symptoms of systemic infection.

It is important to recognize that many rules of good medical treatment must be broken to provide good terminal care. The free and liberal use of urinary indwelling catheters is an excellent example of this. Many patients who are incontinent remain so, because the attending doctor tries every means other than catheterization to relieve the problem. This is usually a mistake.

Haematuria

This may be secondary to infection but is normally associated with an ulcerating tumour of the urinary tract. As in bleeding from the lung, radiotherapy should be considered. Intravesical therapy is an alternative. However, the haematuria frequently recurs, especially with bladder tumours, when the urine is often also filled with debris from clots, netrotic tissue and infected material which may block the catheter.

Blocked catheters require a bladder wash-out, but if this fails the catheter should be changed. Subsequently the patients should have daily bladder wash-outs with a uro-trainer containing Suby-G, sodium chloride or mandelic acid 1%.

Other Problems

Fistulae. A small proportion of patients with pelvic malignancy develop fistulae. These can be through an abdominal scar, or they can connect bowel, bladder, vagina and rectum in any combination. Sometimes a fistula can be relieved by a colostomy or by urinary diversion above the lesion. At laparotomy, however, it is more common to find a mass of tumour either adherent to vital structures or so extensive that effective bypass is impossible. There are a number of measures which may be tried:

- Fitting of a colostomy bag over the orifice of an external fistula.
- A urinary catheter with a vaginal tampon in vesico-vaginal fistulae.
- For all other fistulae the treatment is meticulous nursing.
- Odour may be reduced by using charcoal dressings (Denidor pads), metronidazole solution to irrigate the wound or sinus, and air fresheners (e.g. Zal-air).

Skin Problems

Fungating Tumours

The most common fungating tumour is either a primary or recurrent carcinoma of the breast. Despite the fact that it involves an important organ, is visible to the patient and is situated beneath the patient's nose, it is incredible that many patients have often delayed presentation to the doctor. They often cope with it surprisingly well. The following remedies should be considered:

- Radiotherapy or hormone manipulation.
- Infected lesions should be cleaned with half-strength eusol or hydrogen peroxide, after which the lesion is cleaned with normal saline.
- If the lesion needs to be packed, gauze soaked in half-strength eusol and liquid paraffin is applied twice daily.
- Gentian violet is a useful antiseptic, and some patients benefit from its local application. Oral metronidazole may reduce odour. Topical antibiotics are contraindicated, because sensitivity reactions are common. Regular twice-daily dressings are mandatory both for good care and also to provide padding to soak up the often profuse discharge. Temporary hospital admission may give the family or nursing staff relief from what is undoubtedly an onerous and unpleasant task for everyone.
- Occasionally, persistent capillary or small arterial bleeding occurs. Pads soaked in noradrenaline 1:1000 may be useful for capillary bleeding. Single fraction radiotherapy is most effective when the bleeding is more profuse and does not cease spontaneously. Severe bleeding is a radiotherapeutic emergency.

Insomnia

Disturbed nights or insomnia are common problems for a variety of reasons; these include unrelieved pain, anxiety, nocturnal frequency of micturition, depression and fear.

Nightsweats and rigors occasionally cause sleeplessness, and patients on steroids or those who are depressed may have a reversed diurnal rhythm. In some patients sleeping too much during the day is sufficient to produce a sleepless night. If present these symptoms must be treated, after which sleep should improve. If not, the following drugs may be used:

- Temazepam, 10–60 mg at night. This is a good, short-acting benzodiazepine that is safe and the drug of choice.
- Chlormethiazole 1 g at night is a safe hypnotic for the elderly and unlikely to cause confusion.
- Promazine, 75 mg at 7 p.m. to precede other night sedation, is beneficial in the patient who develops nocturnal confusion and restlessness. The dose may be increased if necessary.
- Chlorpromazine, 12.5–100 mg nocte, is useful in patients who cannot sleep at night because of anxiety and agitation.

- Amitriptyline, 10–20 mg nocte, is a useful antidepressant which may be given at night because it is also a hypnotic. As the depression is treated, the reversed diurnal rhythm (if present) may revert to normal.

The Last Twenty-Four Hours

Families can be left with appalling memories if the final phase in the life of a friend or relative goes wrong at the end. Obviously, the situation is helped if it occurs against a background of good pain control, bowel care and honest communication with any patient wishing to discuss his condition. If preterminal care has been poor, it may be impossible to manage the last day well, for at this stage of the illness, communication with the patient, although important, can be only superficial. The family, on the other hand, need considerable attention (see page 198).

Even when unconscious, the dying patient can hear, perceive touch and experience pain. Consequently, when talking to the family in the bedroom, the patient should be treated as if he can hear what is being said, touched to make a point, and his symptom control discussed openly, clearly explained and efficiently carried out.

Pain

Analgesics should be continued until the patient dies, or withdrawal symptoms and restlessness will occur. Oral medication may often be continued to within a few hours of death, but if parenteral drugs are necessary, the syringe driver (see page 177) provides excellent continuous medication and is easily managed in hospital or home.

Two points should be borne in mind:

- At this stage of an illness it is better to give too much than too little analgesic.
- Although restlessness may be due to pain, there are many other causes which must be considered.

Restlessness

Common causes are:

- pain
- full bladder
- faecal impaction
- mental distress
- drug-induced agitation
- hallucinations

Once recognized, the first three are easy to treat. Some drugs in suboptimal doses (e.g. pethidine, chlorpromazine) will produce confusion and hallucinations. Since the drug was presumably given to sedate, the remedy is not to reduce the dose still further, but to increase it until the restlessness and the hallucinations are controlled. A common error is to 'fiddle' with the drugs instead of making a clear decision that the patient is dying and that an adequate dosage is required to relieve his symptoms or distress.

Nursing Needs

As the patient is dying, relatives should be encouraged to participate in the nursing care if they wish, for this is the last chance they have to do anything for the patient. From time to time one sees eager nurses generously taking over all the care; although satisfying for them, this leaves the relatives feeling inadequate, useless and often guilty.

Relatives also need to be reassured that it is no longer important for the patient to eat or drink. It is also helpful to find out what horrors they anticipate as death approaches. Sensitive, but searching questions may be needed as relatives often feel that they are 'silly', or 'making a fuss' if they express their fears. Common anxieties are: a crescendo of 'agony', 'drowning' in secretions, 'bursting' abdomens, 'torrential haemorrhage' or choking to death. Cheyne-Stokes respiration—periods of regular breathing followed by apnoea—may also frighten relatives and should be explained to them. Sometimes they fear leaving the room in case the patient dies suddenly and they are absent. They need to be reassured that dying, though very sad, will be peaceful and poignant and that time given to their loved one during the final few hours or minutes of their life together is important and should not be feared.

Finally the patient should be treated with dignity and respect at this stage in their lives. They should be washed and kept clean, examined for any sign of incontinence and pressure areas cared for, provided it does not distress them. Nightsitters may be required to help an anxious elderly relative, and should be readily available in most areas of the UK. Any additional pain or restlessness should be anticipated and appropriate drugs left for the nurse to use, with clear instructions.

Care of the Family

The last twenty-four hours of the patient's life will rarely be forgotten by the family, and it is mandatory that they are involved as closely as possible if they so wish. Often one particular member of the family bears the brunt, not only of the death but of supporting other family members. They in turn should be supported by the staff. Where children are involved, it is again important that they have a chance to see their parent or grandparent. It is a common mistake to spirit them away to stay with another relative without discussing or explaining the situation to them. This causes later resentment and distress to a degree often unappreciated by the rest of the family. Children will cope better with dying than most adults. They are simple and direct: they do not hesitate to show their emotions and are often puzzled by the 'stiff upper lip' of other members of the family, who usually try not to cry in front of the children.

Sometimes old family feuds emerge at the deathbed. Occasionally these are resolved because of the death, although often they are not.

The Moment of Death

When the patient dies the doctor will not usually be in attendance. However, I believe that it is a useful part of one's education to sit with a patient who is dying. It is a surprisingly difficult thing to do, particularly for men. But in a quite unique way, it enables one to sense the importance of the event in a way quite different to that at the 'failed' cardiac massage, at which the doctor is usually present.

Witnessing such a death is also a useful reminder that whatever good doctors do, one day all their patients will be dead. Since approximately 50% of the NHS budget is spent in the last year of people's lives, this is an important and thought-provoking insight to bear in mind.

11 | Psychosocial Aspects of Cancer

J. HUGHES

The 'psycho' part of the term 'psychosocial' includes mood, attitude and cognitive function. The 'social' part includes relationships with family, workmates and friends. Having cancer causes problems in psychosocial function for between 25% and 50% of patients. Most of the others report little or no disruption in this sphere of their lives. A few claim positive improvements.

Many psychosocial problems among cancer patients are unrecognized, although such problems can often be effectively prevented or treated.

Factors Determining the Psychosocial Effects of Cancer

The impact of cancer on a patient's mental well-being and social function is influenced by many factors, some related to the illness itself and others related to the characteristics of the patient in whom that illness has developed.

Illness-Related Factors

- Physical symptoms—pain, nausea, disfigurement and limitation of activity, whether due to the cancer itself or to its treatment, are examples of common symptoms with psychological effects.
- Cerebral function—impairments, which again may be due either to the cancer or its treatment, can directly affect mood, cognition and behaviour.
- Knowledge and beliefs about illness—patients interpret what they have been told about their own case in the light of their preconceptions, often inaccurate, about cancer in general.

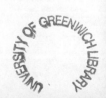

- Relationship with the medical team—is there adequate opportunity for patients to ask for information and discuss their emotional concerns?

Patient-Related Factors

- Personality—including usual pattern of response to stress, attitudes towards illness in general and cancer in particular, religious belief.
- Predisposition to psychiatric disorder—development of cancer may precipitate an episode of psychiatric illness in vulnerable people.
- Current circumstances—quality of close relationships, recent experience of life events and social difficulties, sources of satisfaction, future goals.

Mood Disorders

Mood disorders are considered first because they are the most common type of psychological problem found among cancer patients. They include anxiety state, depressive illness and, far less often, elation.

Anxious and/or depressed mood is part of the 'normal' adjustment reaction to serious illness such as cancer. Anxiety state and/or depressive illness—exaggerated forms of these mood states—should be suspected if the emotional reaction is unusually prolonged, so severe as to dominate the patient's life, or takes on a pathological quality which can no longer be logically related to the stresses of the cancer and its treatment.

The causes of mood disorder fall into three groups:

- Reactive to the stress of the illness—learning the diagnosis of cancer, experiencing side-effects from treatment.
- Cerebral dysfunction—due to brain lesions or metabolic disturbances, including side-effects of drugs.
- Independent of the cancer—history of recurrent psychiatric illness, recent adverse life events or social difficulties.

Depression

Most cancer patients feel depressed at some stage: when they learn the diagnosis; if their treatment produces gruelling side-effects; or if they know or suspect they have a poor physical prognosis. Lowering of mood and tearfulness may therefore form part of a natural 'adjustment reaction', not necessarily indicative of depressive illness.

Thoughts about suicide, feelings of guilt or worthlessness, inability to feel affection for close family or friends, and loss of interest in former sources of pleasure are *not* part of the normal adjustment reaction to having cancer, and when such symptoms develop, depressive illness should be suspected and psychiatric referral considered.

The physical accompaniments of depressive illness—early morning waking or other sleep disturbances, loss of weight and appetite, constipation, tiredness and malaise—overlap with the symptoms of cancer itself, so they are less helpful in diagnosis.

Anxiety

Anxiety is common when the physical symptoms of cancer first present. Many patients say the most stressful period of their whole illness was waiting to find out what was wrong. For this reason, although receiving confirmation of a diagnosis of cancer is not good news, patients often feel some relief of anxiety when they know exactly what they have to face up to. Anxiety is also a common reaction for patients about to start a new treatment, or those who develop symptoms which could indicate relapse.

Some patients experience more severe and persistent anxiety, which dominates their lives: such patients are suffering from an 'anxiety state'. Their pathological anxiety is usually focused on the cancer, making them continually worried about their physical health even if there is no objective sign of relapse. Sometimes they describe a 'freefloating' sense of dread or foreboding, so that all aspects of life seem inexplicably threatening. They cannot sleep at night or relax by day. There may be physical symptoms and signs indicating autonomic over-arousal: palpitations, hyperventilaton, sweating and diarrhoea. If such symptoms are spasmodic they are called 'panic attacks' and can produce a physical collapse which mimics a medical catastrophe.

Management of anxiety states and depressive illness will be discussed later.

Elation of Mood

Inappropriate elation is occasionally found in cancer patients. One cause of this is *hypomania*, a psychiatric illness also characterized by rapid copious speech, overactivity, irritability and grandiose ideas. Physical illness can precipitate hypomania in predisposed patients, many of whom have a past history or family history of affective disorder. Elation can also be a sign of organic brain disorder and corticosteroid therapy; see below.

Reactions to Diagnosis and Attitudes to Disease

The reaction patterns described below should not be labelled 'good' or 'bad', 'normal' or 'abnormal'. They represent different ways of coping with a serious disease, and all of them suit different individuals at different times. But any of them, if present to an unusually extreme degree, can lead to difficulties because they add to the patient's mental distress, damage relationships with other people or hinder compliance with anti-cancer treatment.

Stoic Acceptance. This is the most common reaction pattern. The patient acknowledges the diagnosis in a realistic fashion but shows little distress or curiosity, and seems resigned to accepting whatever outcome fate has in store.

'I just tried to do whatever the doctors told me, and carry on as normal as best I could. Sometimes I do worry about the future—but you have to accept it, you can't change what's going to happen.'

Denial.   This can be explained as an unconscious mental mechanism to prevent anxiety and depression. The patient treats the illness as a trivial matter or ignores it altogether. Extreme denial is undesirable if it prevents patients taking early action on cancer symptoms. But moderate denial can enable patients to live contentedly with their illness.

'Just one of those things; an inconvenience while it lasted. I didn't want to know too much about it. I'm quite happy—it hasn't interfered with my life at all.'

Fighting Spirit.   The patient faces the cancer as a challenge to be conquered, is keen to participate in decisions about treatment and to practise self-help strategies. Some patients are hostile and angry, others keen to build on the positive aspects of the illness experience.

'You've got to face up to it and get on with life. Calling cancer what it is—that's one of the main answers. I was very lucky I found this when I did. I've had a bone scan—after all, if there's anything to find, let's find it and meet it head-on.'

Helplessness/Hopelessness.   This involves sustained anxiety and depression, combined with a passive pessimistic attitude, guilt and low self-esteem.

'I didn't want anyone to know what was wrong with me . . . I felt ashamed, and dirty, like a leper . . . as if it was all my fault.'

Welcoming the Sick Role.   For a few patients, developing cancer is almost a relief. Patients whose lives have been spent sacrificing their own wishes out of a sense of duty, while gaining little reward in return, suddenly become the focus of concern when they develop a serious illness themselves. Without realising it, they tend to linger in the invalid role longer than is medically justified, because they are experiencing more care and attention than they have ever known before.

'I used to give, give, give all the time . . . now I make sure I leave something over for myself too.'

Effects of Anti-Cancer Treatment

Cancer surgery, radiotherapy and chemotherapy—especially the radical regimes—all have unwanted effects which can precipitate psychosocial difficulties. This does not mean the treatment is worse than the disease—most patients elect to accept whatever treatment offers the best chance of cure. Some patients are philosophical about the same kind of side-effects which would cause others to feel devastated, so it is important to take individual preferences into account when planning treatment.

Surgery

Mastectomy for breast cancer is the best-known example of a cancer operation that is often followed by psychosocial difficulties. Other procedures, like colostomy, laryngectomy or limb amputation, are just as likely to cause distress—perhaps more so, since they involve permanent loss of body function as well as disfigurement.

Surveys show that about a quarter of patients who undergo major cancer surgery develop long-term psychosocial difficulties afterwards. Many of the others seem to accept the handicap resulting from their operation with remarkable equanimity.

Psychosocial difficulties are seldom due simply to the operation alone. The anxiety, depression and sexual dysfunction observed in the months following mastectomy used to be attributed directly to the loss of a breast, and for some patients that certainly does seem to be the correct explanation. But breast cancer patients treated by local excision and radiotherapy are also prone to depression, anxiety and sexual dysfunction, suggesting that the question is more complicated and that other factors, such as the fear of cancer recurrence or the debilitating effects of radiotherapy, are just as important as disfiguring surgery in precipitating mood disturbance.

Most patients appreciate a say in choosing their treatment, in cases where a clear choice exists.

Radiotherapy and Chemotherapy

Both these forms of treatment can give rise to psychosocial problems for the following reasons:

- Physical side-effects like nausea and vomiting, hair loss, skin reactions and general tiredness tend to produce anxiety before treatment and depression afterwards.
- Direct effects on cerebral function can cause mood changes or cognitive disturbance.
- Interference with lifestyle—attending hospital for repeated treatment over several weeks or months causes prolonged disruption to patients' normal work and social routines, and serves as a continual reminder of their illness.

While the unwanted physical effects of major cancer surgery are permanent, those of radiotherapy and chemotherapy largely recover if the patient survives long term, and so do the associated psychosocial difficulties.

Organic Brain Syndromes

Cerebral function in cancer patients may be affected by brain metastases; by systemic disorders such as a severe infection, electrolyte disturbance, or organ failure; or by drugs such as steroids or certain cytotoxics.

Mental confusion is the classic presentation, but sometimes this is not obvious, and the patient develops symptoms easily mistaken for a 'functional' psychiatric disorder:

a mood change, a lack of concern about the illness, a paranoid attitude, odd behaviour, an apparent change in personality.

Simple tests of cognitive function—memory, orientation in time and place, basic mental arithmetic—often reveal quite marked deficits, even if the patient seems perfectly coherent during ordinary conversation.

A review of the medical history, physical examination and laboratory tests is indicated whenever organic impairment seems a possibility. It is surprising how many doctors fail to consider a biological basis for psychosocial disturbances among medical patients, and mismanage organic brain syndromes by giving counselling or psychotropic drugs rather than trying to identify and correct the underlying pathology.

Staff–Patient Relationships and Counselling

Communication

Good staff–patient relationships can probably do much to prevent psychosocial morbidity among cancer patients. The general principles to follow are quite simple in theory:

- *Establish a friendly trusting relationship with the patient.* This is much easier if all patients are allocated their 'own' doctor and nurse, rather than being dealt with by whoever happens to be free at the time. Hospitals and their staff systems should be designed in such a way that they care for patients and their families rather than treat diseases.

- *Give patients time to express their concerns and ask questions.* Too often, when doctors try to 'communicate', they make it a one-way process by bombarding patients with more information than they can take in at one time, asking a series of 'closed' questions without letting patients elaborate on the answers, or making assumptions about patients' feelings which may be way off the mark. Letting patients talk and listening to what they say, and being able to accept displays of emotion or periods of silence without showing criticism or disapproval, runs counter to the personality and training of many medical personnel but can be learned.

Not having sufficient time for this approach can be used as an excuse for ignoring the psychosocial aspects of patient care, but it is also a genuine problem in busy hospital settings. Fortunately, some cancer treatment units now have specialized personnel who can devote attention to counselling.

Hospital-Based Counselling

Specialized nurse-counsellors possess expertise in certain aspects of physical treatment, for example the aftercare of mastectomy or colostomy, or administration of chemotherapy. While applying their practical skills, they can also monitor patients' psychosocial welfare: listening to their concerns, answering their questions, and detecting any serious psychosocial problems which need referral to a psychiatrist, psychologist or social worker. Virtually all patients welcome the care of a skilled nurse-counsellor.

Counselling Outside the Hospital Setting

National organizations like BACUP and CANCERLINK provide telephone counselling for cancer patients who want information about their illness or support in coping with it. Local self-help groups, in which patients can discuss their condition with fellow sufferers, have grown up in many areas. 'Alternative' cancer treatment centres, such as the one in Bristol, employ a 'holistic' approach, combining counselling with the use of practical therapies such as special diets.

The demand for such facilities suggests that some NHS staff are not very good at dealing with the psychosocial aspects of cancer, or that, however sympathetic the professionals may be, some patients feel a need for something extra, independent of the hospital which is providing their physical care.

Drawbacks of Counselling

Though counselling and self-help groups can be most valuable, they are not necessarily a good thing for everybody. Many patients succeed in adapting to cancer through their own personality resources and the support of family, friends or religious faith. Formal counselling for such patients would be wasteful of time and money. Other patients, though they may seem to be in need, do not want counselling.

Counselling which is carried out by unskilled personnel, or those with a strong 'alternative medicine' philosophy, can cause harm:

- Inducing guilt by convincing patients they have caused the cancer to develop through flaws in their personality or behaviour. Some patients feel obliged to make arduous changes in lifestyle as a result.
- Encouraging undue introspection in the form of prolonged or deep-seated preoccupation with the illness.
- Fostering close contact with fellow patients who are faring particularly badly—this causes distress to patients and may give them an unduly gloomy impression of their own prognosis.
- Discrediting conventional medical treatment and encouraging patients to turn to unproven fringe remedies instead.

To sum up, all patients appreciate receiving treatment and follow-up from doctors and nurses they know and trust. Many patients feel they have not been given enough information, because they did not have sufficient chance to ask questions, or were expected to take everything in at once at the beginning when they were too bewildered to do so. Some patients value formal psychological counselling, but this is not appropriate for all, and can have adverse effects.

Family and Social Aspects

Happy families often grow even closer when one member develops cancer. Unhappy ones are sometimes dramatically reconciled, but quite often they are driven further apart. The problems can be emotional and/or practical:

- Communication barriers—when 'cancer' is a taboo word in the family, or parents feel obliged to shield children from the awareness of illness and death.
- Sexual dysfunction—when the sick partner feels unattractive following major surgery, feels contaminated by having cancer and fears infecting the healthy partner, or is worried about producing an abnormal child if pregnancy ensues.
- Practical and financial problems—these arise if patients are unable to continue their jobs or carry out household tasks, or if the illness requires extra expense such as long journeys to hospital or big home-heating bills.

Psychosocial Problems Among Relatives

Relatives themselves often become anxious and depressed when a close family member develops cancer. Nursing the patient, and taking extra responsibility for running the household, adds to their burden. They usually do their best to put on a brave face, feeling they would be failing the patient if they admitted their own distress.

These family problems can be alleviated by giving the relatives an opportunity to ventilate their concerns, and making sure they are accurately informed about the patient's illness. However, it is seldom advisable to give information to relatives unless it is also shared with the patient—this outmoded practice creates extra strain within families. Practical assistance, in the form of financial benefits or provision of aids in the home, is sometimes useful. Psychotropic drugs may be indicated for relatives who develop a formal psychiatric disorder. General practitioners, social workers, domiciliary nurses and occupational therapists can all play a useful role.

Friends and Workmates

Most patients say their relationships with people outside the family either improve or stay the same after they develop cancer. Many patients are delighted by an influx of flowers and cards, or visits from friends who had lost touch. Follow-up of patients who are able to return to work after treatment shows that the majority continue much as before. Occasionally there are problems: patients claim all their friends have deserted them, or their workmates keep out of their way. Sometimes these instances reflect genuine prejudice by ignorant insensitive people. Sometimes they reflect patients' own hypersensitivity which they have 'projected' onto others.

Recognizing and Managing Psychosocial Problems

Of the cancer patients with anxiety, depression and social difficulties identified through research studies, only a minority are receiving specific treatment. Some have not been recognized at all. In other cases, doctors have made the false assumption that because the psychosocial problems seem understandable in reaction to the physical illness, treatment will not help.

Recognizing Problems

Patients tend to be ashamed of emotional problems, so they do not complain of them spontaneously. Doctors and nurses need to be alert for signs of distress, and to ask the right questions in a sympathetic way. Depression is especially difficult to recognize because the more severe cases, far from being obviously tearful and unhappy, may be withdrawn and negative, so their suffering is easily overlooked or just put down to poor physical health.

One way to pick up psychiatric 'cases' in a busy clinic is to ask all patients to complete a brief self-rating questionnaire, such as the General Health Questionnaire or the Hospital Anxiety and Depression Scale. There is no point in doing this unless there are facilities for following up patients who obtain high scores with a personal psychiatric interview.

Though milder cases of psychosocial disturbance often improve with time and sympathetic treatment, severe ones should be referred to a psychiatrist.

Psychological Management

The principles already outlined—listening to the patients' concerns, and providing information about the illness at a level geared to individual needs—form the first stage in management, and often have considered therapeutic value in themselves.

The formal psychotherapies—including dynamic psychotherapy, cognitive therapy and behaviour therapy—are indicated for patients with more severe and complicated problems. They need to be given by trained personnel, usually drawn from the professions of psychiatry, psychology, nursing or social work.

Psychotropic Drugs

Antidepressant drugs, such as amitriptyline, imipramine, dothiepin and mianserin, work best in cases of clear-cut depressive illness, and do not relieve 'normal' unhappiness. The benefit may be delayed several weeks, whereas the side-effects such as dry mouth or drowsiness are most troublesome at the beginning of treatment. This drawback should be explained to patients so they are willing to persevere.

Anxiolytic and hypnotic drugs—most of those in current use being benzodiazepines—are more widely prescribed, often in cases where an antidepressant drug would be more effective. Benzodiazepines are best taken in the short term, as and when required, because continuous long-term administration often causes tolerance and dependence and tends to numb emotional response.

ECT

Electroconvulsive therapy (ECT) is a safe and effective treatment for severe depression. While few cancer patients develop the type of depression for which ECT is indicated, this treatment can bring great benefit in the occasional case, and it is safe unless the patient is too frail for general anaesthesia.

Do Psychosocial Factors Affect Cancer Growth?

There is some evidence for the existence of a 'cancer-prone personality'. Several studies have shown that cancer patients seldom express anger or other 'negative' emotion, and tend to be calm passive people who puts others' needs before their own.

Other studies have examined mental attitude in relation to the prognosis of cancer, and have found that patients with the 'fighting spirit' attitude tend to live longer than those with a passive or helpless response.

Another area of interest is the theory that stressful life events, such as bereavement, contribute to cancer in predisposed people. There is little evidence that this is an important effect but further studies are in progress. All this research is hampered by the difficulty of knowing whether the psychological variables are cause or effect of the cancer.

Many patients are interested in theories like this, but in the current state of knowledge it is probably unwise to set too much store by them. Patients who blame their own or their relatives' behaviour for the development of their cancer often suffer much pointless guilt and resentment.

Psychosocial Benefits of Cancer

Having cancer is not always unrelieved gloom. The positive consequences are naturally most common among long-term survivors, but even terminally ill cancer patients often report some psychological benefits. These include:

- Closer relationships with other people.
- Beliefs and priorities are revised for the better.
- Greater appreciation of life and determination to make the most of the time which remains.

Summary

Cancer may bring either problems or benefits in psychosocial functioning. The consequences depend on the personality and social circumstances of the individual patient as much as on the features of the illness and its treatment.

Good staff–patient communication, encouragement of patient participation in treatment plans and ample opportunity for open discussion about cancer all help to prevent psychosocial problems. Formal counselling is helpful for some patients; others do not want or need this.

When formal psychiatric disorders arise, psychotropic drugs and/or specialized psychotherapy are required as well as counselling, and these treatments often produce a good response even if the physical state is poor.

Further Reading

Greer, H. S. (ed.) (1987) Psychological aspects of cancer. *Cancer Surveys*, **6** (3).
Hughes, J. E. (1987) *Cancer and Emotion*. John Wiley, Chichester.

Addresses

BACUP, 122-123 Charterhouse Street, London EC1M 6AA. Tel. 01 608 1661.
CANCERLINK, 46 Pentonville Road, London N1 9HF. Tel. 01 833 2451.

Management of specific cancers

INTRODUCTION TO PART 2

The second part of the book is devoted to brief descriptions of individual tumours and an outline of their management.

These are grouped together according to system and where possible information is presented in a reproducible manner, each chapter having the same basic structure. Some information, such as detailed staging, is essentially postgraduate in nature but medical students should still know a brief outline of staging since this has therapeutic implications. Detail on different treatments has been deliberately kept to a minimum: these are essentially postgraduate topics and they (especially chemotherapy) are constantly changing.

Because of this, emphasis has been placed on epidemiology, screening (where appropriate), symptoms, investigation and symptom control rather than giving excessive detail on specific treatments.

12 | Head and Neck Cancer

C. J. WILLIAMS

This is a very heterogeneous group of tumours affecting the upper airways and digestive tract. Because the numbers of tumours seen at each of the many individual sites of primary cancer are small they tend to be grouped together for the purpose of reporting results. This is unfortunate since their causation, biology and responsiveness to therapy can vary enormously.

Incidence and Epidemiology

There is a wide variation worldwide in the incidence of head and neck cancer at the various sites (Figure 1). One of the most striking differences is in the incidence of nasopharyngeal cancer. This is relatively uncommon in Caucasians (1 per 100,000 population/year in UK) whereas the incidence is far higher in Chinese (30 per 100,000/ year in Kwangtung Province). Chinese men in Hong Kong, Singapore and San Francisco have intermediate incidence rates, as do Alaskan Eskimos.

Lip cancer also varies widely in incidence, as do cancers of the oral cavity. Oral cancers are particularly prevalent in India and Southeast Asia, with intermediate rates in westernized countries and low rates in Israel, Japan and Egypt. Laryngeal cancer is relatively uncommon in England and Wales, being most prevalent in India, Southern Europe and Thailand.

Aetiology and Pathogenesis

Although associations between risk factors and the development of different head and neck cancers have been reported, their significance is often unclear. This may be because the development of the cancer depends not on one factor but on a chain of

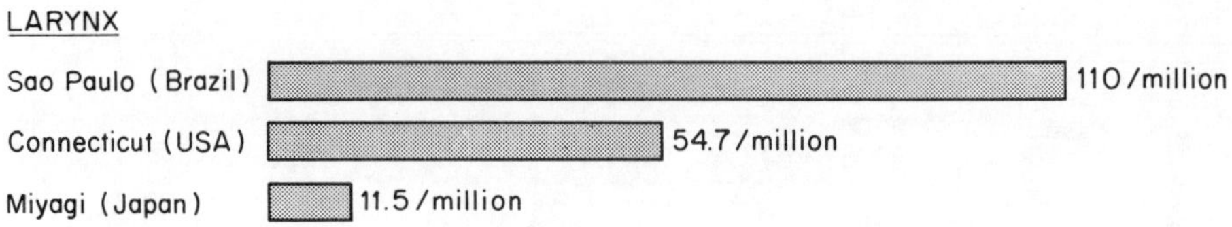

LARYNX

Sao Paulo (Brazil) [▨▨▨▨▨▨▨▨▨▨▨▨▨▨▨▨▨▨▨] 110/million

Connecticut (USA) [▨▨▨▨▨▨▨▨▨] 54.7/million

Miyagi (Japan) [▨▨] 11.5/million

Figure 1. Worldwide variation in incidence of head and neck cancer. As can be seen from the bar chart the ratio between the area of lowest incidence to that of highest incidence for laryngeal cancer is 10. The corresponding figures for other sites are: nasopharynx 40, pharynx 20, mouth 25

Table 1. Factors associated with head and neck cancers

Site	Aetiological factor
Lip	Sunlight, poor dentition, tobacco smoking or chewing
Oral cavity	Tobacco smoking or chewing, alcohol, betel nut (in lime) chewing, reverse smoking (lighted cigarette in mouth)
Oropharynx	Tobacco smoking, alcohol, wood dust
Nasal cavity/paranasal sinuses	Snuff, wood dust, industrial exposure to chemicals (nickel, chromates etc)
Nasopharnyx	Epstein-Barr virus, genetic factors
Hypopharynx	Tobacco smoking, alcohol, iron deficiency (Plummer-Vinson syndrome)
Larynx	Tobacco smoking, alcohol, nickel, wood dust

events. The major potential aetiological factors, by site, are shown in Table 1.

Some of these are particularly important since the initiating factor(s) are avoidable. Among these smoking tobacco is particularly important, though the combination of heavy usage of tobacco and alcohol is probably synergistic. Other regional factors, such as chewing betel nuts (India), use of certain uncured tobaccos ('bidi' in India and 'keego' in Thailand) and reverse smoking (parts of India and South America) are of especial importance since many cancers could be prevented if these practices were abandoned.

Of particular scientific interest is the finding of a possible causative role for Epstein-Barr virus (EBV) in nasopharyngeal cancer. There is an increased frequency of serum antibodies to EBV in patients with this tumour, though its role is not fully understood. If EBV does have a causative role it may be in conjunction with genetic factors— explaining the high incidence in Chinese from certain provinces. Two HLA haplotypes (A2-BW46 and AW19-BW17) have been associated with a high incidence and poor prognosis of nasopharyngeal cancer in Chinese.

The main preventable aetiological factors for head and neck cancers are:

- tobacco smoking or chewing
- betel nut chewing and unusual 'local' smoking habits
- poor dental hygiene
- high alcohol consumption
- wood dust and other industrial exposure

Pathology and Natural History

Most (90%) malignant head and neck tumours are squamous carcinomas. They may be:

- ulcerative
- exophytic
- endophytic or verrucous (multiple wart-like pebbly growths)

Leucoplakia is a premalignant condition usually found in the mouth of high-risk men (heavy drinkers and smokers). There are extensive thick white plaques consisting of hyperkeratosis and sarcoma *in situ*. They may progress to frank invasive carcinoma.

Squamous carcinomas of the head and neck tend to remain localized, invading local tissues remorselessly. Direct invasion of surrounding structures, including bone, is common. Spread to local lymphatics and draining lymph nodes is also frequent. Blood-borne spread to distant sites is relatively uncommon and is only usually seen in the setting of far advanced disease.

Presenting Features

These will depend on the anatomical location of the tumour and the degree of its spread. Cardinal features include:

- visible non-healing ulcer or papillary tumour
- change in speech
- oral or nasal bleeding or discharge
- halitosis
- pain in the jaw, face, eye, ear
- cranial nerve palsies
- trismus

The common symptoms and signs for the major primary sites are shown in Table 2. Their incidence varies from site to site.

Spread

Head and neck cancers are locally aggressive tumours which spread mainly via the lymphatic system. The organs involved by direct invasion and the pattern of involvement of draining lymph nodes depends on the primary site of the tumour.

Investigations and Staging

Staging System

Because the tumour is initially a locally invasive one treated mainly by surgery or radiotherapy, it is an ideal candidate for staging using a TNM system (see chapter 6). There are several staging systems dividing patients according to the extent of their primary cancer (T) and nodes (N) or metastases (M). The UICC system divides tumours into the major site and subdivides the primary tumour (T) into four groups

Table 2. Common symptoms and signs of head and neck tumours

Symptoms and signs	Sites of primary tumours
Bleeding in mouth	Whole of oral mucosa, alveolar ridges, hard palate
Halitosis	Oral cavity, tongue, hard palate, epiglottis and hypopharynx
Pain in upper teeth and maxilla, loose teeth, poorly fitting dentures	Buccal mucosa, upper alveolar ridge, nasal cavity, maxillary sinus, hard palate
Pain in lower teeth and mandible	Buccal mucosa, floor of mouth, lower alveolar ridge
Facial pain	Alveolar ridges, maxillary sinuses, nasopharynx, soft palate, salivary glands
Facial swelling	Lip, buccal mucosa, alveolar ridges, frontal and maxillary sinuses, parotid
Trismus	Buccal mucosa, maxillary sinus, soft palate, parotid
Hoarseness	Nasopharynx, epiglottic region, hypopharynx and larynx
Earache	Alveolar ridges, tongue, maxillary sinus, nasopharynx, base of tongue, epiglottic region, pharynx, hypopharynx and subglottic pharynx
Nasal obstruction, bleeding or discharge	Nasal space, paranasal sinus, nasopharynx
Headache	Nasal space, paranasal sinus, nasopharynx
Tearing	Nasal space, ethmoid and maxillary sinuses
Proptosis	Nasal space, ethmoid and maxillary sinuses, nasopharynx
Cranial nerve palsies	Paranasal sinuses, nasopharynx, parotid

Table 3. UICC classification of nodes and metastases for head and neck cancer

Classification	Description
Nodes	
N_0	No regional lymph node metastases
N_1	Metastasis in single lymph node; 3 cm diameter
N_{2a}	Metastasis in single lymph node, 3–6 cm diameter
N_{2b}	Metastasis in multiple ipsilateral lymph nodes; 6 cm diameter
N_{2c}	Metastasis in bilateral or contralateral lymph nodes; 6 cm diameter
N_3	Metastasis in one or more lymph nodes; 6 cm diameter
Metastasis	
M_0	No distant metastasis
M_1	Distant metastasis

Table 4. Stage grouping based on the TNM system

	T	N	M
Stage I	1	0	0
II	2	0	0
III	3	0	0
	or 1, 2, 3	1	0
IV	4	0,1	0
	any	2,3	0
	any	any	1

of increasingly advanced disease (details vary by site). Nodes are divided into three groups and metastases (M) are recorded as present or absent (Table 3). These data can then be used to place patients in one of four stage groups (Table 4).

Investigations

The diagnosis is made on the histopathological interpretation of a biopsy of the suspected tumour. The diagnosis is more likely to be considered if the doctor takes into account:

- a lesion in someone who smokes and drinks alcohol heavily
- symptoms such as bleeding, pain and obstruction
- development of malocclusion or ill-fitting dentures
- the presence of lymph node masses

If head and neck cancer is suspected the patient should be referred immediately to an ENT surgeon, who will undertake a careful visual inspection and palpation, and biopsies of the primary mass and palpation for lymph node involvement. Examination under anaesthesia may be required for proper assessment. If cancer is confirmed the following investigations will be considered:

- plain X-ray of skull
- chest X-ray
- routine full blood count and biochemistry
- CT imaging of the extent of the cancer and degree of invasion may be used to plan surgery or radiotherapy
- very occasionally angiography may be undertaken to assess operability
- barium swallow, especially to examine the pyriform fossa and hypopharynx

Treatment

It is impossible to discuss this in detail since there are multiple sites and stages of presentation. Choice of treatment is based on:

- primary site of the tumour
- histopathological type
- stage of the tumour (TNM)
- general physical fitness of the patient
- mental state of the patient
- the likely consequences of therapy on breathing, swallowing, speech and appearance

The advantages and disadvantages of radical therapy must be weighed carefully and discussed fully with the patient and patient's family before therapy is decided on. A multidisciplinary approach is often appropriate, including surgery, radiotherapy and chemotherapy.

If cure is the aim of therapy the following objectives should be sought:

- to eradicate the malignant tumour
- to give the best functional result possible
- to make the cosmetic result as good as possible

In order to achieve this when the patient presents with a bulky primary tumour, radiotherapy may be used to shrink the tumour prior to surgery; the scope of surgery can then be reduced. Chemotherapy has also been used in this way.

Palliative therapy aims to:

- control locally advancing cancer
- provide pain relief—especially of bone pain
- relieve obstruction and increase function
- stop bleeding

Care should be taken to ensure patients benefit from palliative care—unnecessarily toxic treatment should be avoided.

Surgery

The aim is generally gross resection of all malignant tissue: this often means dissection of draining lymph nodes as well as wide excision of the primary. Small lesions can often be removed without severely affecting the physiological functioning of the upper aerodigestive system. Larger lesions will, however, require extensive resection, which may produce a functional deficit. Such operations include:

- large laryngeal cancer—laryngectomy
- oral cavity—partial resection of mandible, palate, tongue and pharynx
- paranasal sinuses—maxillary resection or orbital exenteration

If the primary tumour is small (T_1) and there are no palpable lymph nodes, simple excision of the tumour alone is generally all that is required. Moderate-sized tumours $(T_2$ or $T_3)$ without palpable nodes are often treated by resection followed by radiotherapy to the primary site and draining lymph nodes. Patients with large primaries $(T_3$ or $T_4)$ and/or lymph node metastasis or tumours with a high risk of nodal spread, may undergo a dissection of neck lymph nodes as well as the primary tumour.

Radiotherapy

The introduction of megavoltage radiotherapy has greatly improved the care of head and neck tumours. High-energy radiation allows a radical therapy to be delivered accurately with less damage to surrounding tissues. Most normal tissues in the head and neck are not particularly radiosensitive. However, osteonecrosis, soft tissue fibrosis, radiation myelitis, salivary gland and lacrimal dysfunction, and gum disease are all potential problems.

In certain tumours, such as those of the larynx, radiotherapy may be used alone as curative treatment: the results are similar to surgery but often with less morbidity. When high doses are used 'shrinking' fields may be employed as the tumour gets smaller. Interstitial irradiation is also occasionally used to give a very high local dose.

Chemotherapy

A number of cytotoxic drugs can induce objective tumour shrinkage when used alone. The most active include:

- methotrexate
- cisplatin
- bleomycin
- cyclophosphamide
- vinblastine

Responses are seen in 30–40% of cases. When two or three of these drugs are used in combination, objective response rates rise to 50–65%. However, they do not seem to be capable of eradicating advanced or recurrent tumour. Because of their encouraging degree of activity there has been a vogue for giving chemotherapy to patients with advanced tumours before surgery and/or radiotherapy. Despite enthusiasm for this approach, large randomized trials have failed to show an improvement in long-term survival over that achieved with surgery and/or radiotherapy alone.

Currently, combination chemotherapy is toxic but yields quite high response rates though duration of remission is often short.

Outcome and Special Complications

Prognosis depends on the site of the primary tumour and its stage at presentation. Five-year survival rates for the main sites are shown in Table 5.

Tumours of the larynx and lip are especially amenable to therapy even when advanced. However, since they are detected early the overall results are excellent. In contrast, many of the other tumours are diagnosed late and cure rates are low. An additional problem is the general physical well-being of patients. Many are elderly when the cancer is found and since they are often abusers of alcohol and tobacco concomitant medical problems are common.

Special problems associated with advancing disease are generally caused by its locally infiltrative and destructive nature. These will depend upon its site but may include:

Table 5. Five-year survival by major site in head and neck cancer*

Site	Overall 5-yr survival rate (%)	(range T_1–T_4)
Mouth		
Tongue	43	(80–25)
Floor of mouth	50	(77–45)
Buccal mucosa	42	(71–25)
Lip	85	(85–75)
Oropharynx		
Tonsil	45	(89–15)
Base of tongue	26	(45–10)
Pharyngeal wall	20	(26–15)
Soft palate	50	(60–30)
Nasopharynx	43	(50–20)
Hypopharynx	25	(30–5)
Larynx		
Glottic	82	(93–36)
Supraglottic	53	(75–41)
Maxillary sinus	26	(33–19)

*Adapted from Zagars and Norante (1983) *Head and Neck Tumors in Clinical Oncology: A Multidisciplinary Approach*, pp. 241. American Cancer Society. Reproduced by permission.

- obstruction of airways or upper digestive tract
- pain, often due to bone erosion
- cranial nerve palsies
- proptosis
- rupture of major blood vessels
- the incidence of second tumours is high (25%): this may be due to tobacco acting as a carcinogen at multiple sites
- hypercalcaemia is occasionally associated with squamous head and neck cancer.

Selected Papers and Reviews

Mead, G. M. (1986) Chemotherapy in the management of head and neck cancer—a perspective. In: *Recent Advances in Clinical Oncology 2*, Williams, C. J. and Whitehouse, J. M.A. (eds.), Churchill Livingstone, Edinburgh, pp. 81–191.

Moore, C. (1980) Changing concepts in head and neck surgical oncology. *American Journal of Surgery*, **149**: 480–486.

Simons, M. J., Wee, G. B., Goh, E. W., Chan, S. H., Shanmugaratnam, K., Day, N. E. and de-Thé, G. (1976) Immunogenetic aspects of nasopharyngeal carcinoma IV. Increased risk in Chinese of nasopharyngeal carcinoma associated with a Chinese-related HLA profile (A2, Singapore 2). *Journal of the National Cancer Institute*, **57**: 977–980.

Suen, J. Y., Newman, R. K., Hannahs, K. and Fisher, J. (1980) Evaluation of the effectiveness of post-operative radiation therapy for the control of local disease. *American Journal of Surgery*, **149**: 577–579.

Wittes, R. E. (ed.) (1985) *Head and Neck Cancer*. John Wiley & Sons, Chichester.

Zut Hansen, H., Schulte-Holthausen, H., Klein, G., Henle, W., Henle, G., Clifford, P. and Santessen, L. (1970) EBV–DNA in biopsies of Burkitt tumours and anaplastic carcinomas of the nasopharynx. *Nature*, **228**: 1056–1058.

13 | Respiratory System

C. J. WILLIAMS

LUNG CANCER

Lung cancer is one of the major health problems in the western world. At the turn of the century a medical student would have been lucky to see a single case during training; now it is the commonest tumour in developed countries, with over 30,000 cases per year in England and Wales. Although anti-smoking campaigns are starting to reduce the number of smokers, there are going to be many more new cases of lung cancer in the next 30 years, and unfortunately the incidence of this tumour continues to increase in women. In fact lung cancer is poised to overtake breast cancer as the commonest tumour in American and British women.

Incidence and Epidemiology

Lung cancer is most commonly seen in the 7th and 8th decades, and in the United States one in every ten people dying in their 60s has lung cancer. In 1984, 34,000 people in Britain and 140,000 in the United States died of this tumour.

There is an extraordinarily wide geographical variation, which is partly explained by differences in tobacco consumption in various countries (Figure 1). However, Third World countries have had the greatest increase in the incidence of this tumour in recent years, and tobacco advertising and consumption are also increasing rapidly in undeveloped countries.

Aetiology and Pathogenesis

Cigarette smoking is by far the most important factor. Multiple retrospective and prospective studies have shown the following relationships between smoking and lung cancer:

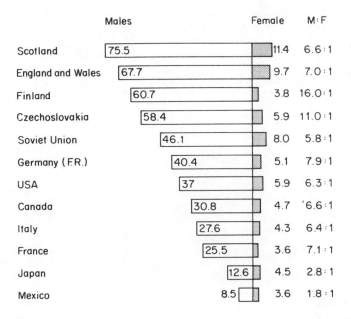

Figure 1. Incidence of lung cancer in various countries (per 100,000)

- The risk of death from lung cancer is related to the number of cigarettes smoked, the age of starting smoking, and by smoking habit (type of cigarette, length of butt, number of 'puffs'/cigarette, etc.)
- Giving up smoking reduces the risk of death from lung cancer. After about 15 years the risk falls to levels similar to that of non-smokers.

Other environmental agents, usually encountered in industry, have been identified as causal factors (Table 1).

Cancers probably result from the deposition and absorption of gaseous and particulate matter on the bronchopulmonary epithelium. The likelihood of a cancer developing depends on the integrity of the body's defence mechanism and the genetic constitution of the individual as well as the degree of exposure for the carcinogens involved. Lung cancers generally appear at the site of the most intense and prolonged exposure to inhaled carcinogens.

A latent period (often 20 or more years) elapses before cancer becomes clinically detectable. Carcinogens interact with DNA, RNA and proteins inducing changes thought to be critical to neoplastic transformation. Many biologists suspect that carcinogens affect proto-oncogenes (highly conserved genes which are probably concerned with regulation of cell development) causing them to become neoplastic by means of gene rearrangement, mutation, gene amplification or by other mechanisms. Activated oncogenes, however, can be detected in only about 25% of cases of lung cancer at the present time.

Table 1. Environmental agents associated with lung cancer

Carcinogen	Type of exposure	Associated features
Arsenic compounds	Pesticide manufacture, smelting	Keratosis on hands and face
Asbestos	Miners, pipe fitters, ship fitting	Pulmonary asbestosis
Chromate	Smelting	Dermatitis, perforated septum
Bis (chloromethyl) ether	Plastics and chemical industry	None
Radon	Mining	None
Isopropyl alcohol	Chemical industry	None
Nickel	Mining, refining, shipping	Dermatitis, nasal polyps
Tars, soot, oil	Oil refinery, asphalt, coke oven and chemical workers	Dermatitis, photosensitivity, warts
Vinyl chloride	Chemical industry	None

Pathology and Natural History

Many different tumours may arise in the lungs (Table 2). Carcinomas arising from the endobronchial epithelium account for over 90% of lung cancers. This chapter will only consider these common tumours.

Nearly all lung cancers fall into one of four common types, their incidence varying between smokers and non-smokers (Table 3). For practical purposes, small cell carcinoma is often separated from the other three common types of lung cancer, which may be collectively referred to as non-small cell lung cancer. This is because surgery is the mainstay of treatment for non-small cell tumours whilst chemotherapy has become the primary therapy for small cell lung cancers.

Both small cell and non-small cell lung cancer carry a very poor prognosis when untreated: their respective median survivals are 3 and 5 months.

Presenting Features

Over 90% of patients with lung cancer are symptomatic when they first present. Most symptoms (Figure 2) are caused by the direct effects of the tumour, though paraneoplastic effects (Chapter 8) are seen more commonly in lung cancer than in any other tumour.

On examination a variety of signs are often present. These may include:

- collapse or consolidation of the lung
- stridor
- superior vena caval obstruction
- Horner's syndrome
- recurrent laryngeal nerve palsy
- paralysis of the diaphragm (phrenic nerve)
- lymphadenopathy, usually in the supraclavicular fossae or neck
- branchial plexus involvement (pain and loss of function)

Table 2. World Health Organization classification of cancer of the lower respiratory tract (reproduced by permission)

Epidermoid (squamous) carcinoma
Small cell carcinoma
Adenocarcinoma (with or without mucin)
   Bronchogenic
   Bronchoalveolar
Large cell carcinoma
Combined epidermoid and adenocarcinoma
Carcinoid tumours
Bronchial gland tumours
Papillary tumours of the surface epithelium
Mixed tumours and carcinosarcomas
Sarcomas
Melanoma
Unclassifiable

Table 3. Common subtypes of lung cancer: percentage of cases by smoking habit

Tumour type	Men		Women	
	Smoker	Non-smoker*	Smoker	Non-smoker*
Epidermoid	39	10	23	9
Adenocarcinoma	21	56	35	68
Large cell	17	28	15	20
Small cell	23	6	27	3

*The great majority of lung cancer patients are smokers.
Data reproduced by permission from Rosenow and Carr (1979) *Cancer*, **29**:233–244.

- brain metastases
- spinal cord compression
- liver metastases
- bone metastases

Paraneoplastic syndromes, though rare, are seen relatively often in lung cancers; the principal syndromes are shown in Table 4.

Spread

Lung cancer spreads by direct extension and may cause pain by invasion of structures in the chest. Lymphatic and haematogenous spread occurs early and most patients have involvement of hilar and mediastinal nodes and distal metastases at presentation.

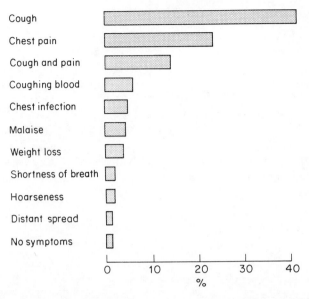

Figure 2. Incidence of symptoms of lung cancer—proportion of cases with specific symptoms

Table 4. Paraneoplastic syndromes seen in lung cancer

Osseous
  Hypertrophic pulmonary osteoarthropathy

Cutaneous
  Acanthosis nigricans
  Erythema multiforme
  Hyperkeratosis

Connective tissue
  Clubbing
  Dermatomyositis
  Scleroderma

Metabolic/endocrine
  Hypercalcaemia
  Inappropriate ADH syndrome
  Cushing's (ACTH) syndrome

Neuromuscular
  Cerebellar degeneration
  Peripheral neuropathy
  Myasthenia-like syndrome (Eaton
  Lambert)
  Polymyositis

Investigation and Staging

Staging System

Non-small cell tumours are staged using a TNM classification (Table 5), as surgery is the primary treatment. This TNM system may be used to group patients into stages according to the extent of their tumour (Table 6).

Because chemotherapy is used as the initial treatment, the staging system for small cell lung cancer is much simpler: 'limited disease' is that confined to one hemithorax with or without ipsilateral supraclavicular lymphadenopathy. Any patient with disease outside these sites is described as having 'extensive disease'. About half of patients have limited disease.

Table 5. TNM staging system for lung cancer

T—Primary Tumour

T_0 No evidence of primary
T_x Tumour proven by cytology but not visible on X-ray or bronchoscopy
T_{is} Carcinoma *in situ*
T_1 Tumour 3 cm or less, surrounded by lung or visceral pleura, no evidence of invasion proximal to lobar bronchus
T_2 Tumour more than 3 cm or tumour of any size that invades visceral pleura or has associated atelectasis or obstructive pneumonitis extending to hilum. The proximal extent of tumour must be within a lobar bronchus or at least 2 cm distant to the carina. Any atelectasis or pneumonitis must involve less than the entire lung. There must be no pleural effusion
T_3 Tumour of any size with direct extension into an adjacent structure or tumour involving the main bronchus less than 2 cm distal to the carina. Any atelectasis or pneumonitis of the entire lung or pleural effusion

N—Regional Lymph Nodes

N_0 No metastasis demonstrable in regional lymph nodes
N_1 Metastases to peribronchial and/or ipsilateral hilar nodes
N_2 Metastases to mediastinal lymph nodes

M—Distant Metastases

M_0 No distant metastases
M_1 Distant metastases

Table 6. TNM stagings grouped according to extent of tumour

Stage I	Stage II	Stage IIIA	Stage IIIB	Stage IV
$T_1 N_0 M_0$	$T_1 N_1 M_0$	$T_1 N_2 M_0$	Any T $N_3 M_0$	Any T or $N_1 M_0$
		$T_2 N_2 M_0$	T_4 any N M_0	
$T_2 N_0 M_0$		$T_3 N_{0-2} M_0$		

Investigation

Investigation is geared towards the treatment appropriate for the subtype of tumour found and the patient's general condition (Table 7). The main aim of staging in non-small cell lung cancer is to detect patients for whom surgical resection would be inappropriate.

Treatment—Non-Small Cell Lung Cancer

Surgery

Every effort should be made to select appropriate patients for surgical resection. Following physical examination, chest X-ray, bronchoscopy and, if surgery still appears feasible, CT scan and mediastinoscopy/otomy are done. A majority of patients are shown initially to be inoperable (metastatic disease, mediastinal lymphadenopathy, tumours near the carina, chest wall involvement, inadequate primary reserve). The introduction of modern staging methods has meant that a higher proportion of patients are shown to be inoperable and as an important corollary to this, fewer patients are found to be inoperable when their chest has been opened at thoracotomy. Because many patients present with obvious metastatic spread, only about 50% are assessed for suitability for surgery. Of these only 25% undergo thoracotomy and in large units about 90% will undergo surgical resection (segmentectomy, lobectomy or pneumonectomy).

Survival rates (Figure 3) are clearly related to stage at presentation; those rare patients with a T_1, N_0, M_0 tumour have an excellent chance of survival (90% alive at 3 years in recent series). For the rest of the patients with stage I disease, 5-year survival is about 50%; for those with stage II disease it is 27%; and for stage III

Table 7. Investigation of a patient with lung cancer

Non-small cell	Small cell
History	History
Physical examination	Physical examination
Chest X-ray	Chest X-ray
Full blood count and biochemistry	Full blood count and biochemistry
Bronchoscopy (biopsy)	Bronchoscopy
Mediastinoscopy/otomy (biopsy)	Bone image
CT scan mediastinum (optional)	Liver ultrasound/image
Test pulmonary function	CT scan optional
Imaging of distant sites — if clinically indicated; evaluation with multi-organ scans is NOT indicated if clinically negative	Bone marrow (optional — rarely positive when other distant sites negative)

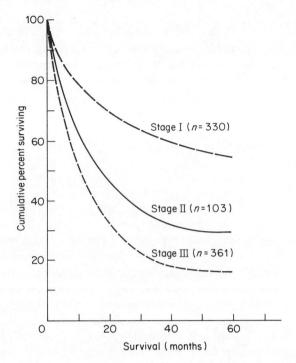

Figure 3. Survival rates for non-small cell lung cancer treated surgically

disease it is 16%. These apparently encouraging figures have, however, to be viewed in the light of the fact that most operable patients have stage II and III disease and that only 15–20% of all patients are suitable for resection.

Radiotherapy

Radiotherapy provides the best palliation for the great majority of patients who have unresectable non-small cell lung cancer. Radiation can be used to palliate the symptoms of bronchial obstruction, superior vena caval obstruction, cough, haemoptysis and pain. It is rarely used for the relief of symptoms from distant metastases apart from brain metastases. Temporary symptomatic relief is achieved in 50–80% of patients but there is little evidence that patients survive longer because of their treatment. One exception to this may be patients with a stage I cancer which is unresectable because of medical reasons precluding thoracotomy. Radical radiotherapy may, in such patients, result in long-term survival in a small proportion of patients. The disadvantages of palliative radiotherapy are frequent visits for treatment, general malaise (though this is rarely severe), and a temporary worsening of cough and dysphagia in the latter part of the treatment. There is no agreement amongst radiotherapists as to the best time to give radiotherapy—some centres treat at presentation in order to delay or prevent the onset of symptoms, whilst others wait until symptoms develop before proceeding with treatment. The median survival of patients treated with radiotherapy is about 5 months.

Chemotherapy

Although a number of drugs may cause responses in up to 20% of patients when used as a single agent, there is no evidence that combinations (causing responses in up to 40% of patients) have sufficient activity to prolong life. In recent randomized trials comparing the results of combination chemotherapy with those in patients not receiving chemotherapy, survival was identical in both groups. Since the side-effects of intensive combination chemotherapy are likely to be severe, such treatment is not good palliation and chemotherapy should not be used outside the context of clinical trials. Such trials should preferably include a 'no chemotherapy' control arm.

Treatment—Small Cell Lung Cancer

Surgery and Chemotherapy

These tumours are highly sensitive to chemotherapy, which is now the mainstay of treatment. Because this is a rapidly growing tumour which is usually widely metastatic at presentation, surgery is generally of little use: an exception to this is the rare patient presenting with a small peripheral tumour. About 30% of such patients are long-term survivors after surgery. For the rest, combination chemotherapy is used as primary treatment. Combinations usually include three or four of the following drugs: doxorubicin, cyclophosphamide, etoposide, vincristine and cisplatin. High response rates can be obtained, particularly in patients with limited disease (Table 8). However, many of these patients relapse and die within 12–18 months and despite attempts to intensify therapy most studies show a characteristic survival curve (Figure 4) with median survivals of 9–10 months for extensive disease and 14–18 months for limited disease. A small proportion (about 10–15%) of patients with limited disease survive long term.

Radiotherapy

Although early trials of radiotherapy suggested that it was superior to surgery, patients rapidly relapsed outside the radiation portal and died. Since the introduction of chemotherapy, radiation has been used as an adjuvant, in an attempt to improve the results. Radiation to the primary tumour may be given with or following chemotherapy in an attempt to prevent relapse at this site. Randomized studies have suggested that local relapse rates are reduced, but this has had little impact on survival rates. Cranial

Table 8. Response to chemotherapy in small cell lung cancer

Extent of disease	Complete response (%)	Partial response (%)	Overall response (%)
Limited	40–50	30–40	70–90
Extensive	10–20	30–40	40–50

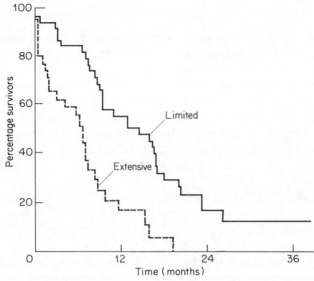

Figure 4. Characteristic survival curves for small cell lung cancer

radiotherapy is also used in an attempt to prevent relapse in the brain, which is a sanctuary site since many chemotherapy drugs do not cross the blood–brain barrier. Randomized trials have confirmed that a limited course of cranial irradiation will markedly reduce the incidence of overt brain metastases. Since the risk of clinically apparent brain metastases increases with time, radiotherapy to the brain is usually only given to those likely to survive prolonged periods (i.e. those attaining a complete remission on chemotherapy). Although such treatment can prevent this unpleasant complication it has no effect on overall survival.

Outcome and Complications

Non-Small Cell Lung Cancer

- A small proportion of patients are candidates for surgical resection, and of these about a third survive more than 5 years
- For the rest treatment is palliative, having little effect on survival, the median being about 5 months

Small Cell Lung Cancer

- Rare patients with small peripheral tumours are surgical candidates, about 30% surviving more than 5 years. These results may be improved by adjuvant chemotherapy

- The great majority will be treated with combination chemotherapy, response rates being high. Despite this, most relapse within the first 12–18 months and only a small proportion (10–15%) of patients with limited disease are long-term survivors.

Complications

The major symptomatic problems are:

- cough, haemoptysis
- dyspnoea
- anorexia
- weight loss
- nausea
- pain—usually in chest but bone pain and pain from the capsule of a grossly enlarged liver is also relatively common
- branchial plexus involvement (Pancoast tumour)
- superior vena caval obstruction
- pleural effusion
- pericardial involvement (arrhythmias, effusion)
- hypercalcaemia
- SIADH and Cushing's syndrome
- brain metastases and spinal cord compression

Selected Papers and Reviews

Arnold, A. M. and Williams, C. J. (1979) Small cell lung cancer: a curable disease? *Br. J. Dis. Chest*, **73**: 327–348.

Minna, J. D., Ihde, D. C. and Glatstein, E. T. (1986) Lung cancers: scalpels, beams, drugs and probes. *New England Journal of Medicine*, **315**: 1411–1414.

Mountain, C. F. (1977) Assessment of the role of surgery for the control of lung cancer. *Annals of Thoracic Surgery*, **24**: 365–373.

Mulshine, J. L., Glatstein, E. and Ruckdeschel, J. C. (1986) Treatment of non-small cell lung cancer. *Journal of Clinical Oncology*: **4**, 1704–1715.

Owens, A. H. and Abeloff, M. D. (1985) Neoplasms of the lung. In: *Medical Oncology: Basic Principles and Clinical Management of Cancer*, Calabresi, P., Schein, P. S. and Rosenberg, S.A. (eds.), Macmillan, New York, pp. 715–757.

MESOTHELIOMA

This is an uncommon malignancy which, because of its relationship to asbestos exposure, tends to be clustered in some population centres (Figure 5). It may affect either the pleura or peritoneum. The median age of onset is between 50 and 60 years and the male to female ratio is 2–5:1.

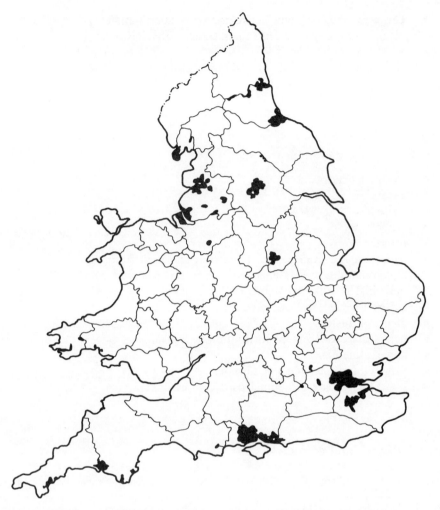

Figure 5. Malignant mesothelioma of the pleura: area of high mortality are concentrated in ports, dockyards and areas of shipbuilding and heavy engineering. (Males and females combined—adapted from Gardener, M.J. *et al.* (1984). *Atlas of Cancer Mortality in England and Wales, 1968–1978,* John Wiley & Sons, Chichester. Reprinted by permission)

Incidence and Epidemiology

The incidence of this tumour has risen sharply in the past 50 years in industrialized countries. In the United States there were about 2200 new cases of malignant mesothelioma in 1985; the mortality figure (between 1968 and 1978) for England and Wales was 1860. There is a clear relationship between development of this tumour and prior asbestos exposure, though the latent period may be as long as 40 years. Even minimal exposure can result in mesothelioma decades later. Those heavily exposed are at highest risk, the prevalence of mesothelioma being as high as 10% in such people; the risk is further increased if they are also smokers. The family of those exposed industrially also have an increased risk of developing mesothelioma—possibly due to asbestos fibres being carried into the home on clothes.

Aetiology and Pathogenesis

There is no argument over the link between asbestos and this malignancy. However, there has been much discussion on the relative importance of different types of asbestos. Asbestos is a mineral that may divide into two types of fibre:

- chrysotile: silky serpentine fibres
- amphiboles: straight rod-like fibres

These differ in their chemical composition as well as appearance. Mesothelioma risk is mainly due to the amphiboles, which are further subdivided into three major types:

- amosite
- anthophyllite
- crocidolite

Autopsy studies of the lungs of asbestos miners and unexposed controls suggest that there is preferential clearing of chrysotile fibres compared with amphiboles—this is probably determined by fibre dimension; these data also show that amosite and anthophyllite are well cleared and crocidolite is poorly cleared. The risk of mesothelioma is, therefore, greatest with crocidolite, though no type of asbestos can be considered wholly safe. Whereas it is easy to see that inhaled fibres may cause pleural mesothelioma, the mechanism by which asbestos gets to the peritoneum is unknown.

Pathology and Natural History

The major primary sites for mesothelioma are the pleura, peritoneum and pericardium, though rarely the tunica vaginalis, ovary, fallopian tube and uterus can be primarily involved. It spreads by direct invasion, chest wall and rib involvement being common in pleural tumours. Distant metastatic sites include:

- regional lymph nodes
- lungs
- adrenals
- CNS
- liver
- pericardium

Histologically, mesotheliomas appear sarcomatous, though epithelial, fibrous or biphasic forms are described. Electron microscopy and immunohistochemistry may help distinguish mesothelioma from poorly differentiated carcinoma—a not uncommon clinical problem.

Presenting Features

These will depend on the primary site of involvement:

- Pleura: chest pain
                  dyspnoea due to pleural effusion
                  weight loss
                  fever
- Peritoneum: abdominal swelling due to ascites
                  weight loss
                  abdominal pain
                  anorexia

These symptoms are often relentlessly progressive.

Investigations and Staging

Because other tumours can present with a similar picture an adequate biopsy is essential. Unfortunately needle biopsy and pleural fluid cytology are often inadequate so that an open biopsy may be necessary. Radiologically, chest films show pleural thickening, effusions, lung nodules and asbestos-related changes in the other lung. CT scan may provide further information and a more accurate estimate of the extent of the disease. Once the diagnosis has been confirmed only minimal staging tests are indicated. A simple staging system for pleural mesothelioma has been devised by Butchart and co-workers.

Stage I	Confined within the capsule of the parietal pleura.
Stage II	Involving chest wall or mediastinum or involving thoracic lymph nodes.
Stage III	Involving the diaphragm, peritoneum or opposite pleural cavity or extrathoracic lymph nodes.
Stage IV	Distant blood-borne metastases.

Treatment

Treatment has little effect on outcome and for most patients is given with palliative intent only.

Surgery

Only rarely is mesothelioma localized so that it can be excised with curative intent. Generally, it is agreed that the results of surgery for pleural mesothelioma are poor, though some centres continue to undertake radical operations. Gross resection of peritoneal disease is rarely feasible and it is usually not indicated.

Radiotherapy

This is also of little value though some patients may have temporary pain relief. Intracavitary radioisotopes have not proved to be of benefit.

Chemotherapy

Although a number of drugs have been reported to cause occasional responses they have little effect on symptoms or survival and cause toxic side-effects, hence they are not routinely indicated. Similarly, intrapleural or intraperitoneal therapy is rarely warranted.

Outcome and Special Complications

This is usually a remorselessly progressive disease whose natural history is little affected by current therapy. Survival rates are low, with less than 10% of patients living 5 years.

Major problems are:

- pain
- dyspnoea or bowel obstruction depending on the primary site
- anorexia and consequent cachexia

14 Gastrointestinal Tract

C. J. WILLIAMS

OESOPHAGEAL CANCER

There is a remarkable three hundred-fold variation in the incidence of this tumour around the world, raising the possibility that it is caused by manipulable environmental factors (Chapter 3). Its incidence in the UK has risen 30% in the past 10 years.

Incidence and Epidemiology

The areas with the highest incidence of oesophageal cancer (Figure 1) are concentrated in a belt from the Caspian Sea through Central Asia to the Chinese coast. The Southern African area of the Transkei has a similar raised incidence and there are other isolated areas where risk is high.

Male to female ratios also vary widely, being as high as 14:1 in France and as low as 2:1 in Scandinavia. In many series carcinoma of the upper oesophagus is more common in women, whereas tumours of the lower two-thirds are most common in men. The incidence of this tumour in England and Wales is 3.5 per 100,000 in men and 0.9 per 100,000 for women.

Aetiology and Pathogenesis

Fortunately, since treatment is generally poor, many tumours may be preventable. Factors known to be associated with oesophageal cancer are shown in the box.

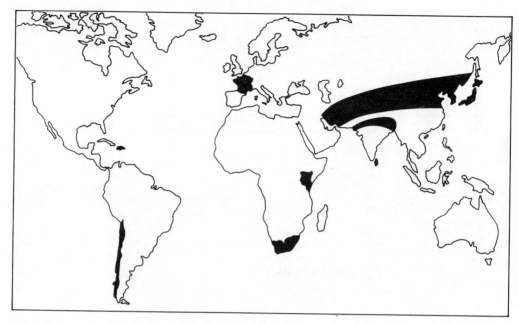

Figure 1. Outline map of the world showing areas of high incidence of oesophageal carcinoma

SOCIAL FACTORS

Tobacco — Cigarette smoking, pipe and cigar smoking and tobacco chewing.

Alcohol — The incidence rises with increasing consumption—spirits may be worse. Maize alcoholic brews may be implicated in the Transkei.

OBSTRUCTION/STASIS

Achalasia — Up to 10% incidence in long-standing achalasia.

Benign structure — Secondary to swallowing caustic foods and because of this may occur in young age group.

Barrett's oesophagus — Columnar epithelium replaces the squamous epithelium of the lower oesophagus (? chronic reflux). Adenocarcinomas occur in this situation.

DIETARY FACTORS

Sideropaenia (Plummer-Vinson syndrome)	Consists of dysphagia, hypochromic microcytic anaemia, mucosal atrophy, achlorhydria, hypoferraemia, oesophageal web. Apparently due to nutritional deficiency.
Vitamin A, B and mineral deficiency	The high incidence of this tumour in the Caspian Littoral and the Transkei has been blamed partly on nutritional deficiencies.

GENETIC

Tylosis	This is a very rare inherited disorder in which there is hyperkeratosis of the palms and soles together with a high incidence of squamous oesophageal cancer.

Avoidable factors include tobacco and alcohol (especially together) as well as vitamin deficiencies. Reduction in accidental ingestion of caustic fluids and early attention of achalasia will also prevent cases. Screening has not proven to be of any value.

Pathology and Natural History

The oesophagus is conventionally divided into three parts (Figure 2).

About 95% of oesophageal cancers are squamous carcinomas. Adenocarcinomas make up the majority of the remainder and are concentrated in the lower third in association with Barrett's oesophagus. Most squamous carcinomas in Britain are in the middle and lower thirds of the oesophagus though upper third lesions are common in the Middle East.

Tumour spread is mainly by *direct extension* and via *lymphatics*. Rapid spread and invasion within the oesophagus is the rule. There is insidious submucosal spread which has major implications for therapy. Later, mediastinal involvement occurs when the tumour has penetrated the muscular and external fibrous coats. Lymphatic drainage is initially to paratracheal and retropharyngeal nodes. Blood-borne metastasis is usually a feature of advanced disease: commonly affected sites are liver, lung, bone and brain.

Presenting Features

The most characteristic symptom of this tumour (Figure 3) is difficulty in swallowing (dysphagia). Other important and ominous features include:

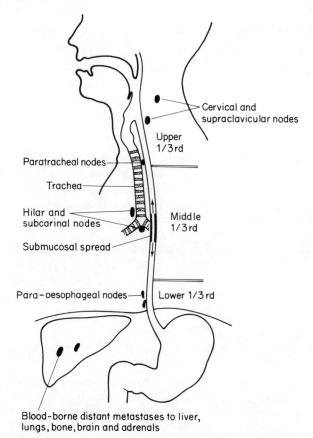

Figure 2. Diagrammatic representation of oesophageal anatomy and tumour spread. Adapted by permission from Souhami, R. L. and Tobias, J. S. (1986). *Cancer and Its Management*, Blackwell Scientific Publications, Oxford

- hoarseness (left vocal cord paralysis due to recurrent largyngeal nerve palsy)
- persistent cough (oesophageal-tracheal fistula)
- haemoptysis (communication with aorta—death imminent)

At first there are few physical findings on examination apart from evidence of recent weight loss and occasionally cervical adenopathy.

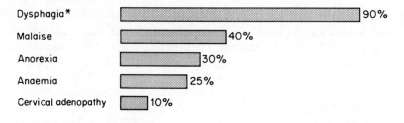

*Solids at first and then liquids

Figure 3. Presenting features of oesophageal cancer

Spread

- direct extension
- lymphatics
- haematogenous spread is generally a late feature

Investigations and Staging

All patients with dysphagia should have a barium swallow. Carcinoma is characterized by an area of *irregular narrowing*. Any potential carcinoma should subsequently be examined by oesophagoscopy and biopsied—dilatation of the strictured area may also be performed. If surgery is contemplated a chest X-ray is mandatory to look for nodal enlargement and pleural effusion. Chest X-ray also helps to exclude bronchial tumours involving the oesophagus. CT scan is useful in the search for mediastinal involvement and for assessing the thickness of the tumour prior to surgery.

Chest X-ray
Barium swallow
Oesophagoscopy—brushings and biopsy
CT scan

Staging needs to take into account:

- the site of origin of the cancer
- the depth of its invasion
- the degree of submucosal spread
- the presence of nodal or haematogenous spread

The TNM System is summarized in Figure 4.

Treatment

Before treatment is started the physician must be clear as to whether the goal is cure or, as in the majority of patients, palliation.

Surgery

Although there have been advocates for radical oesophageal surgery, the use of increasingly complicated operations has had little effect on survival—indeed in some series the operative mortality rate has been double the long-term survival rate. Such operations may require gastric mobilization into the chest or the use of colonic reconstruction of the oesophagus (Figure 5).

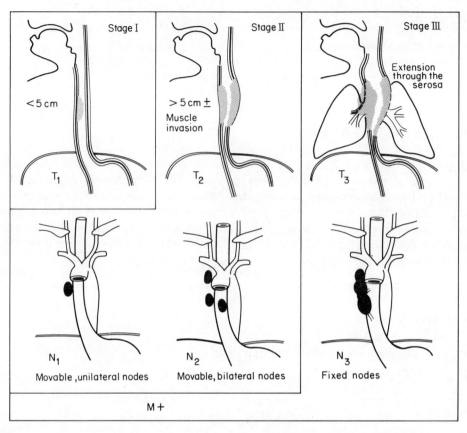

Figure 4. TNM staging of oesophageal carcinoma: there are three stage groups according to the TNM stages as shown above. Adapted by permission from the AJC and UICC staging manuals

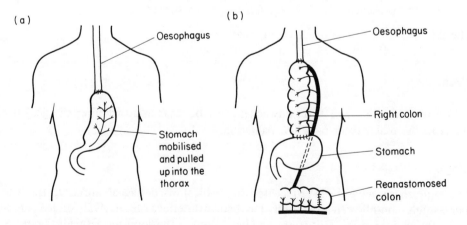

Figure 5. Radical surgery for oesophageal carcinoma. (a) Gastric mobilization and pull-through. (b) Colonic reconstruction—used for lesions too high to be treated by (a)

In the largest collected series of patients with oesophageal cancer (nearly 84,000 cases), one-third of patients died having never left hospital. The results of a policy of surgery in these series is shown in Figure 6. The very low 5-year survival rate suggests that surgery rarely prolongs survival. It may improve swallowing but at the expense of high mortality and morbidity rates. One exception to this is adenocarcinoma of the lower oesophagus. Operations at this site are technically easier with lower complication rates. In addition, these tumours are apparently less radioresponsive, so that other options are severely restricted. Only for these tumours is surgery clearly the treatment of choice.

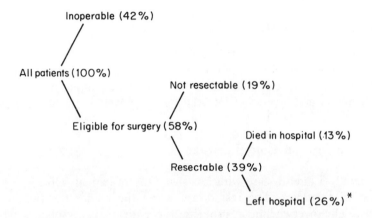

*Of those leaving hospital 18% lived 1 year, 9% lived 2 years and only 4% lived 5 years. For comparison, in these series 51% were offered palliative irradiation: 18% lived 1 year, 8% 2 years and 6% 5 years.

Figure 6. Outcome of a policy of surgery in oesophageal cancer (collected series, Earlam and Cunha-Melo, 1980, reproduced by permission)

Radiotherapy

Squamous carcinoma of the oesophagus is relatively radioresponsive and local eradication of tumour can occasionally be achieved. It is the treatment of choice for tumours of the upper third of the oesophagus, where surgery becomes increasingly hazardous the higher the site of the tumour.

Tumours of the middle third may be treated by radiation or surgery or a combination of both. Results seem little different (see Figure 6). As mentioned above, tumours of the lower third, often adenocarcinomas, are best treated surgically.

The principles of radiotherapy are:

- megavoltage irradiation
- large fields covering most of the oesophagus because of the risk of submucosal spread
- high doses

Such treatment invariably leads to oesophagitis, which may be severe. Objective responses occur in about 75% of patients and a small proportion (5–10%) treated radically survive long term. Significant palliation of dysphagia is seen in the remainder of responders.

Chemotherapy

Chemotherapy has been extensively tested, though the results have been largely disappointing. It is not indicated as a general treatment, though patients may be offered cytotoxics in trials testing new approaches. Recently chemotherapy has been used with radiotherapy in a number of trials.

Other Palliative Approaches

An alternative way of dealing with recurrent dysphagia due to cancer is to dilate the oesophagus or to pass a prosthetic tube through the cancer. The most commonly used device of this type is the celestin tube. Potential complications include gastro-oesophageal reflux and aspiration into the lungs, as well as retrosternal pain.

Outcome and Special Complications

This is generally a fatal disease with less than 10% of patients alive at 5 years despite various radical therapies. The results are worse the higher the tumour site in the oesophagus. The overwhelming problem for patients is dysphagia with resulting cachexia.

Selected Papers and Reviews

Earlam, R. and Cunha-Melo, J.R. (1980) Oesophageal squamous carcinoma I. A critical review of surgery. II. A critical review of radiotherapy. *British Journal of Surgery*, **67**: 381–391, 457–462.

Wynder, E.C. and Bross, I.J. (1961) A study of etiological factors in cancer of the oesophagus. *Cancer*, **14**: 389–413.

STOMACH CANCER

Gastric carcinoma is usually diagnosed late in its course and because of this the outlook is generally very poor. During the past half century it has become less common in most industrialized countries. Japan has, because of its unusually high incidence of stomach cancer, set up screening programmes using gastroscopy and barium contrast studies. These have had some success though their encouraging results have not been repeated in the West.

Incidence and Epidemiology

Gastric carcinoma is a tumour whose incidence varies markedly around the world (Figure 7). The highest incidence rates are found in Japan, where they are 25-fold higher than in Uganda (the area of lowest incidence). Although it remains a common tumour and one of the leading causes of death from cancer, its incidence has declined worldwide. It is twice as common in men as in women.

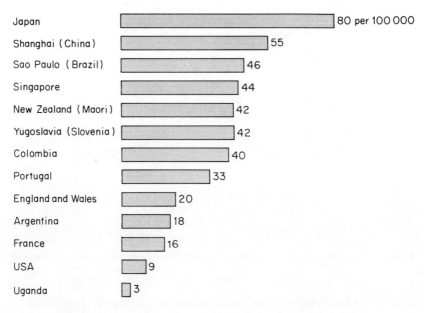

Figure 7. Incidence of stomach cancer around the world

Aetiology and Pathogenesis

The dramatic worldwide decline in incidence seen this century is a strong indicator that environmental and dietary factors play a major part in the causation of stomach cancer, since genetic changes could not be so rapid (Figure 8). Further strong evidence comes from study of Japanese who emigrated from Japan to Hawaii. In a recent study the incidence of stomach cancer in Japan was found to be 1331 per million people; comparable figures for Japanese in Hawaii were 397 and for Hawaiian Caucasians 217. Since the Japanese did not intermarry with the local inhabitants but did adopt many local habits these data favour a non-genetic cause—probably diet. One hypothesis has been that foods with a high nitrate content and those containing carcinogenic nitrosamines lead to an increased risk of stomach cancer. It has been claimed that the reduction of stomach cancer incidence in industrialized centres is a result of refrigeration of foods. This decreases bacterial reduction of nitrate and increases consumption of ascorbic acid, which inhibits nitrosamine reactions.

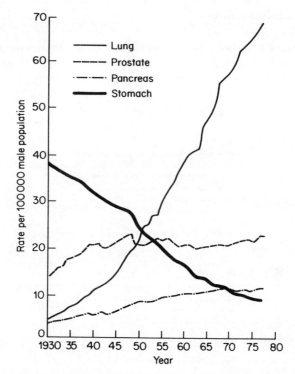

Figure 8. Changes in incidence rates of stomach and other common cancers in the United States (1930–1980). There has been a dramatic fall in the number of new cases of stomach cancer

A number of other conditions are also related to the later development of gastric cancer. These include:

- pernicious anaemia: the risk of cancer is increased 10–20 times and it may be multifocal
- chronic atrophic gastritis: independent of pernicious anaemia, has been implicated as a risk factor
- adenomas: true adenomatous lesions may be precursors of carcinoma of the stomach
- post-gastrectomy: the incidence of stomach cancer many years after gastrectomy appears to be raised 2–3-fold

A common feature of these factors is gastric mucosal injury, and it has been suggested that this acts together with carcinogens (Figure 9).

Pathology and Natural History

About 95% of stomach cancers are adenocarcinomas. Of the remaining malignant tumours, half are non-Hodgkin's lymphomas and the rest are carcinoids and sarcomas. This chapter deals only with gastric adenocarcinoma.

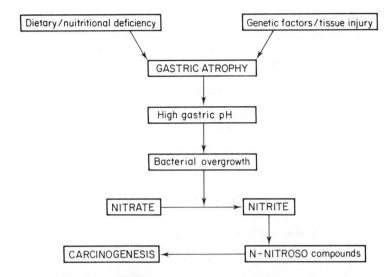

Figure 9. Possible relationship between gastric mucosal atrophy and dietary carcinogens in the causation of stomach cancer

Most tumours arise in the pyloric and antral regions (50%), with 20% arising at both the body and lesser curvature, 7% in the cardia and 3% in the greater curvature. Most tumours (75%) are ulcerating, 10% are polypoid and 10% desmoplastic (linitis plastica); the reamining 5% are characterized as superficial spreading with diffuse replacement of gastric mucosa by carcinoma cells.

The desmoplastic and diffuse spreading tumours are said to have a worse prognosis than polypoid or ulcerating carcinomas.

Presenting Features

Gastric carcinoma may cause no recognizable symptoms for long periods. Most patients complain of vague indigestion or epigastric fullness relieved by antacids. Clearly these symptoms are indistinguishable from benign peptic ulceration and oesophagitis. The discomfort gradually increases, eventually bringing the patient to the attention of their doctor. However, by this time the tumour is all too often advanced and untreatable. Other symptoms are shown in Figure 10.

Stomach cancer may occasionally be associated with various paraneoplastic syndromes (Chapter 8).

- acanthosis nigricans (p. 131)
- hyperkeratosis of soles and palms
- dermatomyositis (p. 125, 132)
- microangiopathic haemolytic anaemia (p. 129)

Signs are minimal except when the disease is far advanced. They are:

- weight loss
- anaemia

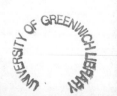

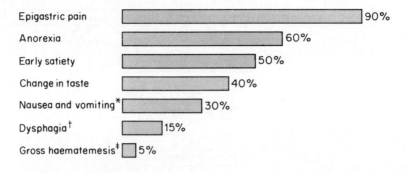

*50% of cases in which the pylorus is involved

† 60% of cases of involvement of cardio-oesophageal junction

‡ Low-grade bleeding with iron deficiency anaemia is common

Figure 10. Symptoms of stomach cancer

- supraclavicular lymphadenopathy (Virchow's node)
- epigastric mass
- hepatomegaly
- ascites
- ovarian masses (Krukenberg tumour)
- perirectal mass (Blumer's shelf)

Spread and Staging

As has already been alluded to, spread is common at presentation and is by direct extension, blood, lymph and transcoelomic implantation (Figure 11).

Investigation and Staging

Staging uses the TNM system and is shown diagrammatically in Figure 12.
  The staging can be simplified and summarized as involvement of:

T_1 Laminal propria, submucosa.
T_2 Muscularis propria, subserosa.
T_3 Penetrating serosa.
T_4 Adjacent structures.

N_1 Perigastric nodes less than 3 cm from primary.
N_2 Removable nodes more than 3 cm from primary.
N_3 Nodes which are unresectable.

M   Distant metastasis.

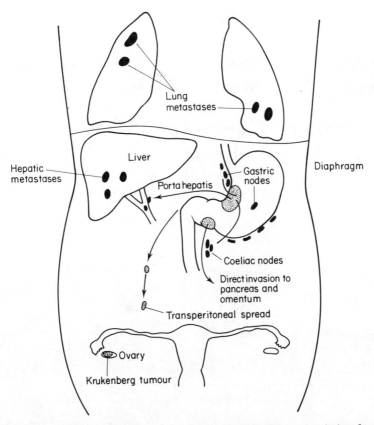

Figure 11. Modes and sites of spread of stomach cancer. Adapted by permission from Souhami, R. L. and Tobias, J. S. (1986) *Cancer and Its Management*, Blackwell Scientific Publications, Oxford

This staging system is of prognostic significance, picking out a small group of patients likely to do well compared to the rest, who have a prognosis which worsens with rising stage (Figure 13).

The diagnosis of stomach cancer is often prompted by the taking of a good history. If peripheral lymphadenopathy is found this should result in urgent investigation. Patients with symptoms of peptic ulceration should always be investigated and the possibility of carcinoma borne in mind. Early investigation offers the best chance of diagnosis of a tumour in a treatable state.

Investigation should include:

- Endoscopy—this is the most accurate investigation, with positive biopsies or cytology being obtained in more than 90% of patients with cancer. One exception is where there is diffuse infiltration of the mucosa.
- Barium meal—although this used to be the standard investigation, endoscopic studies have shown that it will fail to detect 10–30% of early cancers.

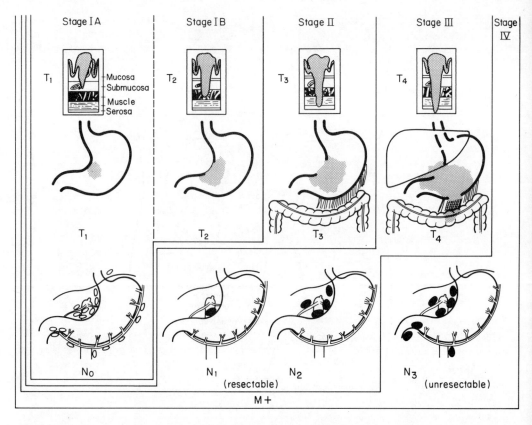

Figure 12. Diagrammatic representation of anatomical (TNM) staging of stomach cancer. See text for description of staging details, which are based on operative findings. Adapted from Rubin, P. *et al.* (1983) *Clinical Oncology: a multidisciplinary approach*, 6th edition, American Cancer Society. Reproduced by permission

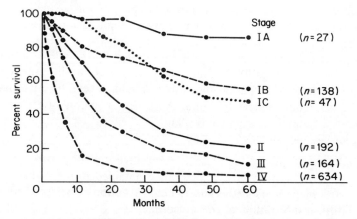

Figure 13. The relationship of TNM stage of gastric carcinoma to survival. Note that very few patients have stage IA disease whilst a great majority have stage IV disease (stage IA is T_1, N_0, M_0). Reproduced by permission

Once the diagnosis has been established the degree of spread is investigated, provided there is not obvious clinical evidence of distant metastases. Available tests include:

- liver function tests, urea and electrolytes
- full blood count
- liver ultrasound and/or CT scan
- chest X-ray

Definitive staging is only possible at laparotomy, which will be considered if these tests show no evidence of spread.

Treatment

The only curative treatment for stomach cancer is surgery—all other treatments are entirely palliative in nature.

Surgery

Selection of the type of operation to be used depends on the location and size of the primary. Patients with distant metastases or diffuse peritoneal spread of tumour are inoperable. Regional spread does not, however, mitigate against surgery—palliative resection of the primary tumour may prevent obstruction, bleeding and perforation as well as improving survival.

Even with radical surgery the overall results are not encouraging. Only about 60% of patients are suitable for surgery, and of these the majority have stage III and IV disease (see Figure 13). These poor results underline the need for early diagnosis.

Radiotherapy

Radiotherapy for stomach cancer is limited by the radiosensitivity of surrounding normal organs (small intestine, kidneys, spinal cord and liver). Doses of about 4000 cGy can be delivered in 4–5 weeks and may give useful palliation to some patients. It is generally used in patients with locally advanced unresectable cancer which has not spread to distant sites.

Chemotherapy

Gastric cancer is more sensitive to cytotoxic drugs than other gastrointestinal tract tumours, but despite this there is little evidence that such treatment prolongs survival. Combinations of drugs produce higher response rates than single agents but cause more toxicity and have no beneficial effect on survival.

Because of these data, chemotherapy has been used in patients with early stage disease undergoing potentially curative surgery. Such adjuvant chemotherapy has generally, however, failed to improve survival and cannot therefore be recommended as routine management.

Chemotherapy is not curative, but can occasionally be of palliative value.

Outcome and Special Complications

Early stomach cancer can be cured by surgery in a good proportion of cases, but unfortunately most patients present with advanced incurable disease. Median survival for these patients is usually less than 6 months.

Gastric surgery may, even if curative, result in several complications:

- dumping syndrome
- iron deficiency and B_{12} deficiency
- lactose intolerance, osteomalacia and osteoporosis

Advanced stomach cancer may cause obstruction, perforation, liver failure and ascites.

Selected Papers and Reviews

Correa, P. *et al*. (1975) A model for gastric cancer. *Lancet*, **ii**, 58–60.
Earl, H.M. *et al*. (1984) Cytotoxic chemotherapy for cancer of the stomach. *Clinics in Oncology*, **3**: 351–360.
Higgins, G.A. *et al*. (1976) Gastric cancer, factors in survival. *Surg. Gastroenterol.*, **10**: 393–400.
Lawrence, W. (1970) Surgical management of gastrointestinal cancer. *Clinical Gastroenterology*, **5**: 703–742.

PANCREATIC CANCER

Because of its position, hidden away at the back of the abdomen, diagnosis of cancer of the pancreas is often difficult. By the time it has produced symptoms and the cause for these has eventually been recognized it is usually too late for curative therapy. In view of the poor results of treatment it is particularly worrying that the incidence of this cancer continues to increase in industrialized countries.

Incidence and Epidemiology

In England and Wales, recent incidence figures for men and women are 15.2 per 100,000 and 13.2 per 100,000 respectively. Overall incidence figures for the United States are similar, though there is a greater male predominance and rates are considerably higher in black American men (25 per 100,000). Despite this, the incidence worldwide does not vary as much as many other tumours. The ratio of highest rate (New Zealand, Maori) to lowest rate (Bombay, India) is only 8. Incidence of this tumour appears to have increased gradually in the past several decades.

The median age of onset is about 60 years, incidence rising steeply with age from about 50 years (Figure 14).

Aetiology and Pathogenesis

Whilst the slow but steady increase in incidence of this cancer (Figure 15) may be partly due to improved diagnostic skills, this is unlikely to be the full explanation. In

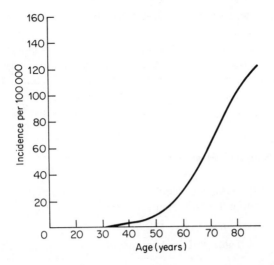

Figure 14. Incidence of cancer of the pancreas by age (England and Wales)

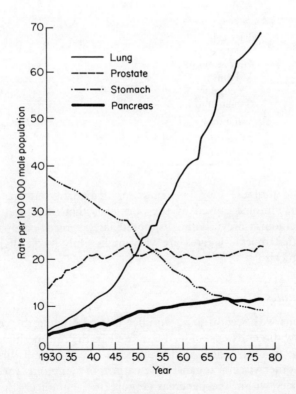

Figure 15. Incidence of pancreatic and other common cancers in the USA (1930–1980). Pancreatic cancer has become steadily more common, though not in the dramatic fashion of lung cancer

the United States the rise in incidence has been greatest in men and in blacks, suggesting an environmental cause.

Cancer of the pancreas is commonest in the lowest socioeconomic groups and in urban areas. Data suggest that chemical carcinogens are likely to play a role in its causation. However, current evidence is confusing and inconclusive. There is no clear-cut relationship to smoking, diet or occupational exposure. The role of chronic pancreatitis and diabetes mellitus is likewise controversial.

Pathology and Natural History

The great majority of pancreatic malignancies are epithelial in origin, arising in the exocrine pancreas (Table 1); this chapter refers only to this group.

Table 1. Histology of cancer of the pancreas

Tumour	Frequency (%)
Exocrine pancreatic tumours	
Adenocarcinoma of ductal origin	89
Acinar cell adenocarcinoma	1
Endocrine pancreas	5
Islet cell	
Gastrinoma	
Glucagonoma	
VIPoma	
Carcinoid	
Somatostatinoma	
Miscellaneous	5
Mixed ductal and islet cell	
Sarcoma	

The endocrine tumours may be benign or malignant but are of especial interest because of the symptoms caused by the hormones that they produce.

Exocrine carcinomas are usually diagnosed late, spread locally and via blood and lymphatics so that mortality rates are very high. Only 1–2% of patients are alive 5 years after diagnosis.

Presenting Features

Onset is insidious with weight loss, jaundice and pain being the commonest features. Pain is caused by direct extension of the tumour in the retroperitoneal space; the other features are due to obstruction of the common bile duct and direct invasion of the duodenum and other visceral organs. The pattern of symptoms varies according to the site of the primary within the pancreas (Figure 16). Jaundice is a feature of tumours of the head of the pancreas, and pain is more prominent with tumours of the body and tail.

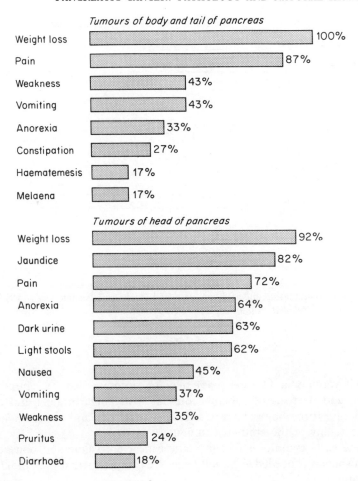

Figure 16. Symptoms of pancreatic cancer. From Howard, J.M. and Jordan, J.L. (1977), Cancer of the pancreas. *Current Problems in Cancer*, 2: 13. Copyright 1977 Year Book Medical Publishers; reproduced by permission

The pain is usually epigastric but may radiate into the lower back or be confined to the back. It gradually becomes more severe and is unremititng, often worst at night. Acute exacerbations may be due to episodes of acute pancreatitis. Left hypochondrial pain and constipation may herald direct involvement of the colon. Paroxysms of pain may be precipitated by eating. Relief may be gained by sitting or bending forwards. Such debilitating progressive pain may be accompanied by mental depression.

Jaundice is an early feature in tumours of the head of the pancreas, though it is usually preceded by epigastric pain. Pancreatic insufficiency and diabetes mellitus may result from destruction of exocrine and endocrine functions of the gland.

Signs of pancreatic malignancy are shown in Figure 17; once again they vary in frequency according to the site of the tumour. Clearly, tumours of the head of the pancreas are easier to diagnose because of their predilection for causing common bile duct obstruction and jaundice.

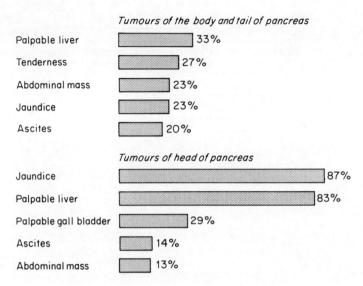

Figure 17. Signs of pancreatic cancer. From Howard, J.M. and Jordan, J.L. (1977), Cancer of the pancreas. *Current Problems in Cancer*, **2**: 13. Copyright 1977 Year Book Medical Publishers; reproduced by permission

Acinar cell carcinoma (a rare type) may be accompanied by episodes of patch inflammation and necrosis of subcutaneous fat with polyarthralgia and eosinophilia. More commonly, thrombophlebitis (classically, migratory and anticoagulant resistant) may complicate any of the epithelial tumours.

Because the early symptoms of pancreatic cancer are vague and nonspecific a high diagnostic suspicion is needed. The following are symptoms that may indicate the need for investigation:

- recent upper abdominal or back pain, or both, consistent with a retroperitoneal origin
- vague upper abdominal pain with investigations negative for a gastrointestinal origin
- unexplained weight loss
- pancreatitis in the absence of gallstones or a history of excessive alcohol intake
- maturity onset diabetes and epigastric or back pain

Obstructive jaundice is always an indication for assessment of the pancreas.

Spread

The head of the pancreas is involved in about two-thirds of cases and the body and tail in about one-third. Tumours in the head spread to involve the duodenum and obstruct the common bile duct (Figure 18). They will also spread backwards into the retroperitoneal space and forwards to the lesser sac. Tumours of the body also spread to the retroperitoneal and forwards to the peritoneal cavity. Occasionally the portal

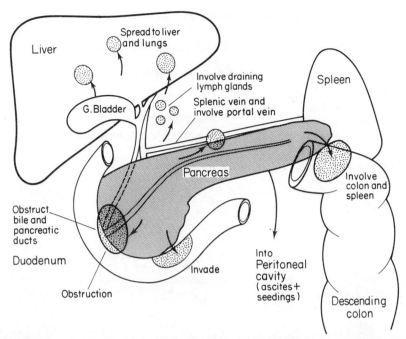

Figure 18. Nature and sites of spread of adenocarcinoma of the pancreas. Adapted by permission from Souhami, R. L. and Tobias, J. S. (1986) *Cancer and Its Management*, Blackwell Scientific Publications, Oxford

and splenic veins may be involved. Distant spread to the liver, lungs and peritoneal surfaces is common.

The main sites of spread in a large series of more than 7000 cases are shown in Table 2.

Investigations and Staging

Despite new and improved diagnostic tests, over 90% of pancreatic carcinomas have spread beyond the gland at the time of diagnosis. Unfortunately, increasingly sensitive

Table 2. Main sites of spread with pancreatic adenocarcinoma

Site of spread	Site of primary	
	Head ($n=5233$)	Body and tail ($n=1912$)
Regional nodes	75%	76%
Liver	65%	71%
Lungs	30%	14%
Peritoneum	22%	38%
Duodenum	19%	5%
Adrenals	13%	24%
Stomach	11%	5%
Spleen	6%	14%

tests are unlikely to improve the situation since most patients remain asymptomatic until the tumour is advanced.

Some or all of the following tests are indicated if the malignancy is suspected.

- biochemical and haematological screening tests
- barium meal
- ultrasonography
- CT scan
- endoscopy with retrograde cholangiopancreatogram (ERCP)
- needle biopsy or laparotomy
- liver biopsy if there is clinical malignant infiltration

These tests will usually confirm the nature of the tumour and the degree of spread. A simple TNM staging system is used (Table 3 and Figure 19).

Table 3. TNM staging system for pancreatic cancer

Stage	Description
T_1	Limited to pancreas (<2 cm)
T_2	Limited to pancreas (2–6 cm)
T_3	>6 cm
T_4	Extrapancreatic spread
N_0	No regional nodes involved
N_1	One regional group involved
N_2	Two or more regional groups involved
N_3	Clinical evidence of regional nodal involvement
N_4	Juxta-regional nodes involved
M_0	No distant metastases
M_1	Distant metastases

Treatment

The outlook is nearly always bad and the toxicity of treatment must always be balanced against the potential gains for the patient.

Surgery

Since over 90% of tumours have spread beyond the confines of the pancreas at diagnosis, curative surgery plays little role. In general only small tumours of the body

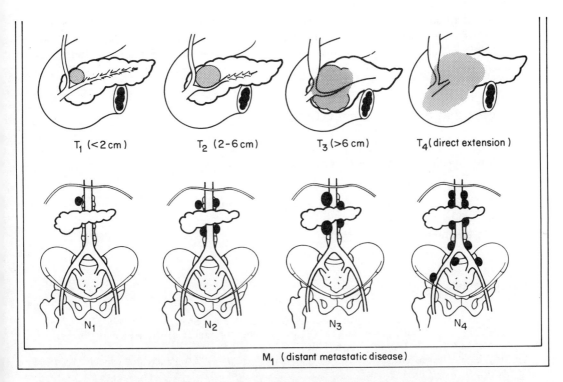

T_1 (<2 cm) T_2 (2-6 cm) T_3 (>6 cm) T_4(direct extension)

N_1 N_2 N_3 N_4

M_1 (distant metastatic disease)

Figure 19. Diagrammatic representation of anatomical TNM staging of pancreatic cancer (see Table 3) modified from Rubin, *et al.* (1983) *Clinical Oncology: a multidisciplinary approach*, 6th edition, American Cancer Society. Reproduced by permission

and tail of the pancreas are curable by resection. In these rare cases total pancreatectomy may be justified. However, the operation is formidable and postoperative mortality (15%) often exceeds the reported 5-year survival figures.

Palliative operations may be useful in patients who have unresectable tumours. Biliary and/or gastrointestinal obstruction can often be bypassed by cholecystojejunostomy and gastrojejunostomy.

Radiotherapy

Such treatment is essentially palliative, though occasional long-term survival has been reported after radical irradiation. Pain can be reduced by doses of up to 5000–6500 cGy in 7–8 weeks, and in some institutions iodine-123 implants have been used intraoperatively.

Chemotherapy

Objective responses are seen in about 20% of patients with a number of drugs when they are used singly. However, responses are usually partial and of short duration. Improved response rates (40%) can be achieved with drug combinations but, disappointingly, randomized trials comparing such therapy with single agent treatment have failed to show that multiple drugs improve survival. The chances of temporary palliation in less than half the patients must be weighed against the toxicity of combination chemotherapy. For many sick and symptomatic patients such therapy is unlikely to be helpful.

Outcome and Special Complications

This cancer is almost universally fatal—the median survival is less than 6 months from diagnosis. Special problems are numerous and include:

- biliary obstruction
- gastrointestinal obstruction and malabsorption
- diabetes mellitus
- thrombophlebitis migrans

Selected Papers and Reviews

Holyoke, E.D. (1981) New surgical approaches to pancreatic cancer. *Cancer*, **47**: 1719–1723.
Wynder, E.L., Mabuchi, K. *et al.* (1973) Epidemiology of cancer of the pancreas. *Journal of the National Cancer Institute*, **50**: 645–667.
Yarbro, Y.W., Bornstein, R.S., Mastragelo, M.J., *et al.* (1979) Pancreatic cancer. *Seminar Oncol.*, **6**: 273–394.

HEPATOCELLULAR CARCINOMA (HEPATOMA)

Incidence and Epidemiology

Though malignancy of the liver and biliary tract is relatively uncommon in the western world, liver cancer is one of the commonest malignancies in some Third World countries. The incidence of hepatocellular carcinoma in England and Wales, 2.0 per 100,000 in men and 0.7 for women, is similar to that in the United States and many other industrialized countries. There are, however, dramatic variations around the world (Figure 20); for instance, the rate in Bantu males in Mozambique is about 500 fold that in Britain. In some Third World countries hepatocellular cancer is the leading cause of cancer death.

The average age of onset in men in western countries is between 65 and 75 years. For women incidence rates continue to increase beyond 80 years of age.

Aetiology and Pathogenesis

The development of hepatocellular carcinoma is closely related to pre-existing cirrhosis. Between 60 and 80% of patients with this tumour have evidence of cirrhotic changes in their liver, and it has been estimated that 5% of patients with cirrhosis will go on to develop hepatocellular carcinoma, a figure which increases with time. The risk is

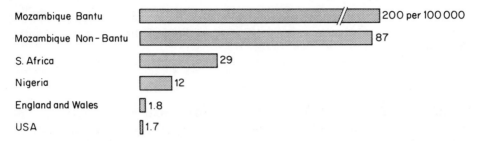

Figure 20. Incidence of hepatocellular carcinoma around the world

highest for those with post-necrotic cirrhosis secondary to hepatitis B infection and haemochromatosis. The correlation with alcoholic cirrhosis is less strong but is important in western countries. Coexisting alcoholic cirrhosis and hepatitis B infection result in a particularly high risk of hepatocellular cancer.

Fungal infection of food with aflatoxins has also been implicated, though much of the data refer to animal models. These fungi produce highly potent carcinogens, and contamination of peanuts and other foodstuffs has been linked to a high incidence of hepatoma. Despite this, the very high incidence seen in some parts of the world is more likely to be linked to the hepatitis B virus, where there may be perinatal transmission of the virus from mother to child. Up to 80% of patients with hepatocellular carcinoma in some parts of the world are HBsAg positive. Hepatitis A does not seem to predispose to hepatoma.

The worldwide variations are explained by differences in risk factors:

- hepatitis B infection—prevalent in parts of Africa and Asia
- haemochromatosis—sporadic
- alcoholic cirrhosis—important in industrialized countries
- aflatoxin contamination of food—tropical areas
- parasitic infections of the intestine (especially schistosomiasis) have been blamed in some tropical areas

Pathology and Natural History

The great majority of primary liver cancers are hepatocellular carcinomas, though other rare tumours are seen (see box).

HISTOLOGICAL CLASSIFICATION OF LIVER CANCER

Hepatocellular carcinoma
Cholangiocarcinoma (intrahepatic)
Combined hepatocellular and cholangiocarcinoma
Hepatoblastoma (childhood)

In a majority of cases there are multiple nodules of hepatoma throughout the liver, though in about a quarter of cases there is a single large tumour with or without satellite nodules.

Presenting Features

In patients with pre-existing cirrhosis there is often rapid decompensation of their condition with development of liver failure. However, less than half are jaundiced at the onset, and right upper quadrant pain and mass together with weight loss and ascites are the commonest symptoms (Figure 21). Ascites may be due to cirrhosis or to the sudden onset of the Budd-Chiari syndrome caused by hepatic vein occlusion. Figure 22 summarizes the incidence of typical signs with hepatocellular carcinoma.

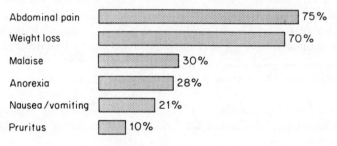

Figure 21. Symptoms of hepatocellular cancer

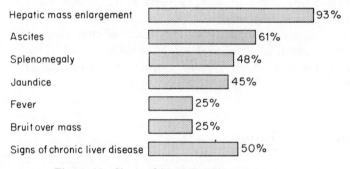

Figure 22. Signs of hepatocellular carcinoma

The condition may, additionally, produce a variety of paraneoplastic syndromes. These include:

- fever, cachexia
- leucocytosis and eosinophilia
- hypertrophic osteoarthropathy
- migratory thrombophlebitis
- gynaecomastia
- hypoglycaemia
- hypercalcaemia

- dysfibrinogenaemia
- porphyria

Spread

Hepatoma spreads by direct invasion within the liver: by parasinusoidal extension, by retrograde venous extension and by lymphatic invasion. Distant metastasis is seen in about half of patients; sites include regional lymph nodes, lungs and brain. There is no specific staging system.

Investigations

In parts of the world where hepatocellular carcinoma is common, the diagnosis is generally relatively straightforward. However, in western countries where the disease is sporadic an antemortem diagnosis is only made in about two-thirds of cases. Diagnosis is an especial problem if the patient has a cirrhotic liver to which the patient's symptoms can be ascribed.

Routine liver function tests are of relatively little value in sorting out the differential diagnosis. Fortunately, most hepatomas produce a protein (alpha-fetoprotein: AFP) which is a useful marker of the tumour. Up to 90% of patients with hepatoma have levels of AFP in excess of 40 ng/ml; frequently levels are greater than 1000 ng/ml. High levels, while not diagnostic, are strongly suggestive of hepatoma. Other tests include:

- liver ultrasound, CT or radioisotope image
- liver biopsy (may be unsafe if prothrombin time is prolonged or if the tumour is highly vascular)
- arteriography (usually only done if surgery is contemplated)

Treatment

The underlying condition of the patient with cirrhosis will often affect what therapy is possible.

Surgery

This offers the only chance of cure, but most patients are unsuitable for resection because of extensive cirrhosis and liver failure. Candidates for surgery should:

- have tumour confined to one lobe of the liver, ideally a single mass
- preferably not be cirrhotic
- have no evidence of distant spread

These selection criteria mean that less than 10% of patients are candidates for resection. Operative mortality rates are falling but may still be as high as 10–15%. Despite extensive surgery, long-term survival rates are relatively poor in patients who have undergone resection: 15–25% at 5 years.

Selective hepatic artery embolization or ligation has also been used but often causes severe temporary worsening of liver function. It may be of palliative value in some cases.

Radiotherapy

This has no curative value since hepatoma cells are not radiosensitive and the tolerance of normal hepatocytes is only about 3000 cGy. Some patients may have temporary pain relief at this dose.

Chemotherapy

Chemotherapy has been extensively tested without much success. Doxorubicin, an anthracycline, is the most active drug but only produces objective responses in about 20% of patients. It may be of occasional palliative benefit but does not prolong life. Drug combinations are not recommended.

Outcome and Special Complications

In most patients, i.e. where the tumour is unresectable, there is a rapidly progressive course, most patients dying within 6 months. Where resection is possible, many patients rapidly relapse, though up to 20% will survive long term. In view of the endemic nature of this tumour in some parts of the world and its relationship to hepatitis B, prevention by vaccination programmes for hepatitis B virus is very important. The complications of hepatoma are legion and are outlined in the section on presenting features.

Selected Papers and Reviews

Beasley, R.P., Hwang, L-Y., Lin, C-C, and Chein, C-S. (1981) Hepatocellular carcinoma and hepatitis B virus. A prospective study of 22,707 men in Taiwan. *Lancet*, **ii**, 1129.
Lee, F.I. (1966) Cirrhosis and hepatoma in alcoholics. *Gut*, **7**: 77–85.
Trichopoulos, D., Sizaret, P., Tabor, E., *et al.* (1980) Alphafetoprotein levels in liver cancer patients and controls in a European population. *Cancer*, **46**: 736–740.

BILIARY TRACT CANCERS

Incidence and Epidemiology

Cancers of the gall bladder and cholangiocarcinomas (i.e. cancers of the biliary ducts) are relatively uncommon. Most cases are seen after the age of 65 years, gall bladder tumours being more common in women, whereas cholangiocarcinoma is more often seen in men. There are about 2000 new cases per year in the UK, accounting for around 5% of gastrointestinal malignancy.

Aetiology and Pathogenesis

Numerous factors have been linked to biliary cancer. The higher incidence of gall bladder cancer in women may be related to the higher rate of gallstones in the female population. Calculi have been reported to be present in 70–90% of operations for gall bladder cancer. The association of cancer and gallstones appears to be independent of age and sex and has been used as a reason for undertaking prophylactic cholecystectomy. However, recent data have suggested that the link is not strong. The rate of elective cholecystectomy has markedly fallen in Denmark without any effect on the rate of gall bladder cancer. Any link between gallstones and cholangiocarcinoma is even more tentative.

In some areas of the world there is a strong link between liver infestation with liver flukes and cholangiocarcinoma. An excess of biliary cancers is also seen in patients with ulcerative colitis.

Pathology and Natural History

Cancer of the gall bladder is more common than cholangiocarcinoma and usually arises in the body of the organ. Histologically, biliary malignancy comprises:

- adenocarcinoma (90%)
- anaplastic or small cell tumour (6%)
- squamous carcinoma (3%)

These tumours frequently spread locally and to the liver before diagnosis so that the results of treatment are generally very poor.

Presenting Features

The main signs and symptoms of these types of cancer are similar (Figure 23) though jaundice is, not unexpectedly, very much more common with cholangiocarcinoma.

Many of these features are similar to those of benign gall bladder disease, and it is hardly surprising that many biliary carcinomas are not recognized until surgery is performed for supposedly benign disease.

Spread

These tumours spread in a variety of ways:

- via lymphatics
- bloodstream
- intraductally
- intraperitoneally
- by perineural invasion

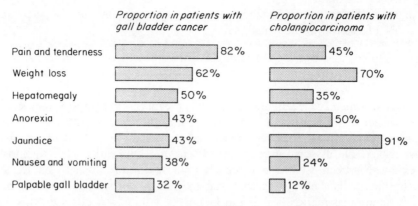

Figure 23. Symptoms and signs of biliary cancer

As a result of this, involvement of the following structures is common:

- lymph nodes in the porta hepatis
- liver
- stomach
- duodenum
- colon
- omentum
- abdominal wall

Investigations and Staging

Unfortunately most diagnostic tests are unable to differentiate between benign and malignant disease. Because of this, less than 20% of gall bladder cancer is diagnosed pre-operatively. Tests include.

- cholecystogram (usually unhelpful as the gall bladder is nonfunctioning)
- ultrasound and CT (may show a mass)
- percutaneous transhepatic cholangiogram (shows dilated bile ducts and may allow relief of jaundice)
- endoscopic retrograde cholangiopancreatography (ERCP)

There is no widely accepted staging system.

Treatment

Resection of the malignancy is the only chance of cure, but most tumours are already too advanced at the time of surgery.

Surgery

Presurgical and intraoperative assessment is crucial since the surgeon must decide whether complete excision is technically feasible. Where possible the gall bladder should be removed completely. If there is evidence of invasion a margin of normal liver tissue should be excised as well. Where there is extensive local invasion or distant spread bypass surgery can be used for relief of jaundice, though non-surgical procedures may be preferred.

Only about 15% of patients have gall bladder cancer that is resectable. Morbidity and mortality (10%) of such surgery remains high. Cholangiocarcinoma is treated in much the same fashion.

Radiotherapy

Temporary relief of pain and obstructive jaundice can be achieved in the great majority of patients using a dose of 4000–5000 cGy.

Chemotherapy

Chemotherapy has not been systematically studied. Responses have been reported to a variety of single agents and combinations but none has been shown to prolong life.

Outcome and Special Complications

The majority of patients with these tumours are dead within months. Only a small proportion are suitable for definitive surgery. In this group median survival is about 30 months.

Because of its invasion of nearby structures a wide variety of complications are common. Obstructive jaundice is a particularly common problem—it may be relieved by percutaneous transhepatic biliary drainage.

Selected Papers and Reviews

Bismuth, H. and Malt, R.A. (1979) Carcinoma of the biliary tract. *New England Journal of Medicine*, **301**: 704–706.

Broden, G. and Bengtsson, L. (1980) Carcinoma of the gall bladder. Its relationship to cholelithiasis and to the concept of prophylactic cholecystectomy. *Acta. Chir. Scand.*, [Suppl] **500**: 15–18.

Kopelson, G., Harisiadis, L., Tretter, P., *et al.* (1977) The role of radiation therapy in cancer of the extrahepatic biliary system. *Int. J. Rad. Oncol. Biol. Phy.* 2: 883–894.

Tanga, M.R. and Ewing, J.B. (1970) Primary malignant tumours of the gall bladder. *Surgery*, **67**: 418–426.

SMALL BOWEL CANCER (CARCINOID)

The small bowel is one of the largest epithelial organs in the human body, but despite this and its potential exposure to carcinogens it is rarely the primary site of cancer. Adenocarcinoma is the commonest tumour and is managed in a fashion similar to large bowel tumours. It may arise in the presence of regional enteritis (Crohn's disease), Peutz-Jeghers syndrome (polyps in bowel and oral pigmentation), familial polyposis coli (autosomal dominant—mainly large bowel cancer) and Gardener's syndrome (adenoma of bowel, epidermoid cysts and bony osteomas). Although carcinoid tumours are second in frequency to adenocarcinoma they have attracted much more attention because of the characteristic hormonal syndrome that they cause. This section concentrates on these unusual cancers.

Incidence and Epidemiology

The incidence of small bowel tumours of all types is low in western countries—around 1 per 100,000. There is a slight excess in men, but the real point of interest is the very low cancer rate in a large organ, constantly exposed to carcinogens, whose mucosa is constantly undergoing cell division. Various explanations for this have been advanced; they include:

- liquid content of the bowel dilutes carcinogens and transit time is short, reducing exposure
- bacterial population (capable of converting fat and bile salts to carcinogens) is much lower than in the colon
- enzymes present in high concentrations in the small intestine may metabolize ingested carcinogens
- the local immune system may have an effect
- it has been suggested that the rapid cell turnover has a protective effect

Aetiology and Pathogenesis

There is little information on the aetiology of these tumours.

Pathology and Natural History

Macroscopically carcinoid tumours are usually yellow or orange in colour. They are mainly seen in the ileum, in contradistinction to other tumours of the small bowel (Table 4).

Carcinoid tumours are derived from enterochromaffin cells of the APUD (amine precursor uptake decarboxylation) system. Microscopically they consist of densely packed epithelial cells which stain with silver nitrate (argentaffinomas). They may occasionally occur outside the bowel.

Table 4. Distribution of cancers of the small bowel

Cancer	Proportion (%) involving		
	Duodenum	Jejunum	Ileum
Adenocarcinoma	40	40	20
Carcinoid	5	10	85*
Lymphoma	15	50	35
Leiomyosarcoma	10	35	55

*Includes appendix

They are often relatively slow growing and usually produce the characteristic carcinoid syndrome only when metastatic to the liver.

Presenting Features

Carcinoid tumours are occasionally an unexpected finding at routine surgery. However, most patients present with the characteristic syndrome. Occasional patients may come to surgery because of intussusception.

Carcinoid syndrome is caused by the release of a variety of vasoactive peptides (Figure 24). The commonest symptom is flushing. This is intermittent at first, often precipitated by alcohol, but gradually becomes more frequent so that in the end the patient is almost permanently flushed. Telangiectases occur on the face together with thickened violaceous skin. Diarrhoea is a common problem. It is watery in character and sometimes patients are labelled as having 'irritable bowel syndrome'. The diarrhoea is not related to flushing attacks and appears to be caused by increased gut motility. Diagnosis is an especial problem when diarrhoea is the sole presenting symptom. Late-onset asthma may also pose diganostic difficulties when it occurs as an isolated symptom prior to development of the full-blown syndrome.

Less common complications include pellagra (niacin deficiency) and tricuspid incompetence and pulmonary stenosis due to deposition of fibrous material in the heart valves. The frequencies of the different manifestations of carcinoid syndrome are shown in Figure 25.

Local symptoms due to metastases may also occur. Pain in the left hypochondrium, caused by liver involvement, is common as is weight loss, malaise and anorexia when the disease is advanced. Other hormones, such as ACTH, may be released by carcinoid tumours though this is more common when the tumour develops at sites outside the small bowel.

Spread

Carcinoid of the small bowel spreads by blood to involve the liver. Involvement of draining lymph nodes is often seen; less commonly, bone and lung may be sites of metastases.

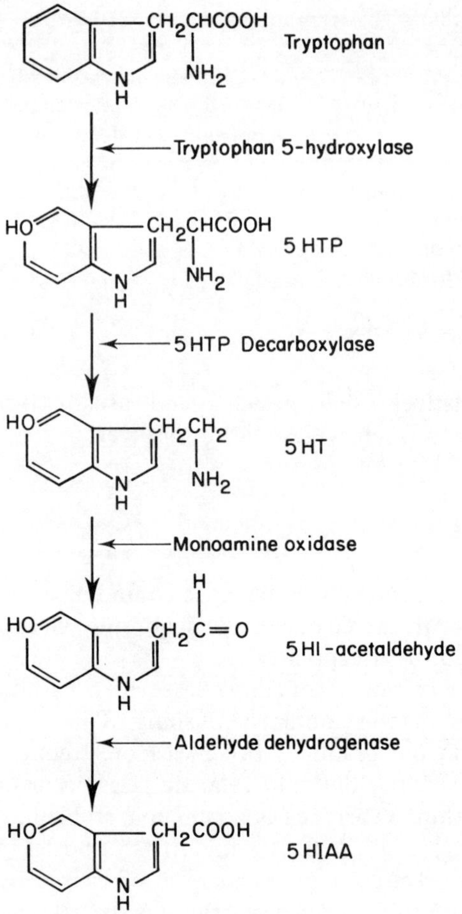

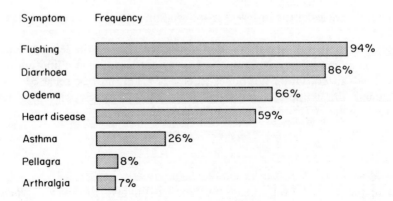

Figure 24. Synthesis and metabolism of serotonin (5 HT)

Symptom	Frequency	
Flushing		94%
Diarrhoea		86%
Oedema		66%
Heart disease		59%
Asthma		26%
Pellagra		8%
Arthralgia		7%

Figure 25. Frequency of symptoms in patients with carcinoid syndrome

Investigations and Staging

The diagnosis may occasionally be made at surgery, for instance appendicectomy for right lower quadrant pain. However, in most instances patients present with symptoms of liver involvement with or without carcinoid syndrome.

Investigations include:

- liver biopsy
- measurement of urinary 5-HIAA (variable and not a good marker of tumour response)
- liver function tests
- ultrasound or CT imaging

There is no formal staging system.

Treatment

Surgery, the only curative mode of treatment, is rarely possible since most patients with small bowel carcinoid only present when they have liver metastases.

Surgery

Whenever small bowel carcinoid is found localized to the bowel it should be completely excised. The results are best when there is no lymph node involvement (Figure 26). When metastatic carcinoid is found to be localized to one lobe of the liver this may be excised since it may provide good palliation for a long time. Temporary relief of symptoms may be gained by embolization of the liver.

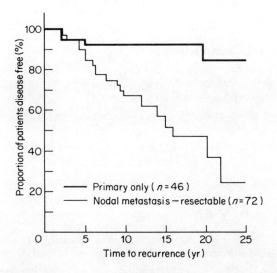

Figure 26. Survival free of disease recurrence after surgery for carcinoid tumour

Radiotherapy

This has no role in the management of this tumour.

Chemotherapy

This is usually ineffective. Objective tumour responses are very unusual though symptom relief may occur in up to 30% of patients. Such symptom control may be better achieved with drugs chosen for their antihormone effects.

Antihormone Treatment

Drugs may be selected according to the symptom being palliated.
- Diarrhoea:
  Codeine phosphate or diphenoxylate
  Methysergide (5HT antagonist)—may cause abdominal cramps and nausea
      and risk of retroperitoneal fibrosis
  Cyproheptadine (5HT and H_1 antagonist)
  Parachlorophenylalanine (PCPA)—causes headache, mental changes,
      lethargy, necessitating stopping treatment in 50% of patients
  Corticosteroids may sometimes be helpful
- Flushing:
  Indomethacin to antagonize prostaglandin effects
  Phenothiazine—block bradykinin
  Phentolamine—alpha-adrenergic blockade since catecholamines can
      precipitate bradykinin release
- Bronchospasm
  Results are generally disappointing, though cyproheptadine and
      phenothiazines may occasionally be helpful

Outcome and Special Complications

Since most patients with small bowel carcinoid have metastatic disease at presentation, cure is rarely possible. Although symptoms can be partially controlled there is no treatment to arrest the disease, which progresses remorselessly, albeit often slowly over many years.

There are many complications of this tumour as outlined in the section on presenting features.

Selected Papers and Reviews

Grahaeme-Smith, D.C. (1972) *The Carcinoid Syndrome.* Heinemann, London.
Hill, G.J. (1971) Carcinoid tumours: pharmacological therapy. *Oncology*, 25: 329–343.
Moertel, C.G. (1987) An odyssey in the land of small tumours. *Journal of Clinical Oncology*, 5: 1503–1522.

Moertel, C.G. *et al.* (1961) Life history of the carcinoid tumour of the small intestine. *Cancer*, **14**: 901–902.

LARGE BOWEL CANCER

This is the second commonest cancer, after carcinoma of the lung, in western countries. The incidence varies markedly in different geographical locations, suggesting the importance of an environment factor, possibly diet.

Incidence and Epidemiology

The incidence rates for colon and rectal cancer in England and Wales are 24 per 100,000 and 16 per 100,000 respectively. These figures are similar to other industrialized countries but are much higher than African, Asian and South American countries (Figure 27). The variation from areas of lowest incidence to highest is 28-fold.

The average age of onset is 60 years though the incidence of the disease continues to increase well past 80 years. The sex ratio is roughly unity. Epidemiological studies, especially among migrants, suggest a dietary aetiology for this tumour. The incidence of large bowel cancer in Hawaiian Japanese is four times that seen in native Japanese. Similarly the incidence is much higher in Puerto Ricans living in the USA compared with those in their home country. Bowel cancer has increased dramatically in the American black population—in marked contrast to the very low levels seen in Africa. Dietary factors may also be important in Seventh-Day Adventists, who have a very low incidence of this malignancy—they consume low levels of meat and animal fats.

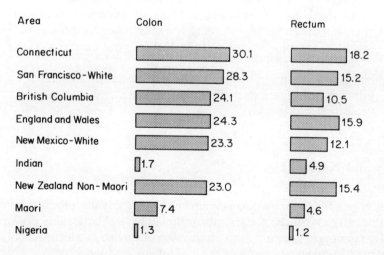

Figure 27. Incidence of colorectal cancer (males) around the world (per 100,000)

Aetiology and Pathogenesis

Animal models show that colorectal tumours may be induced by chemical carcinogens. A number of foodstuffs and factors have been implicated, though clear-cut evidence for a role in human cancer is awaited. Among these putative factors are:

- a high meat and animal fat diet producing a bacterial flora whose enzymes convert steroids into carcinogens
- bile acids may act as cocarcinogens
- low dietary fibre leading to a long transit time

Dietary fibre is largely indigestible and the increased bulk leads to rapid transit time. It has been claimed that this reduces the time high concentrations of carcinogens are in contact with the bowel mucosa. Some population-based studies have shown a correlation between bowel transit time and colorectal cancer risk, though others have not. Overall, the evidence is suggestive of a link between fibre and colon cancer but it is not conclusive.

Other conditions predisposing to colorectal cancer include:

- Familial polyposis coli (a dominant genetic condition in which the bowel mucosa contains hundreds of polyps—there is a marked tendency for malignant change. Prophylactic sub-total or total colectomy is indicated)
- Chronic ulcerative colitis (the risk increases with duration of active colitis and with the extent of bowel involvement. Sub-total colectomy is indicated in selected cases)
- Colorectal adenomatous polyps may become malignant. Conclusive data are awaited. Villous adenomas are considered to be definitely premalignant
- Cancer family syndrome (autosomal dominant predispositon to cancers of colon, breast and endometrium as well as other sites. Early age of onset and multiple primary sites common)
- Other inherited conditions predisposing to colorectal tumours include Turcot syndrome, Peutz-Jeghers syndrome and Gardener's syndrome
- Other predisposing inflammatory bowel diseases are: Crohn's disease, schistosomiasis, lymphogranuloma inguinale and radiation proctocolitis

Pathology and Natural History

Most large bowel tumours are adenocarcinomas—they usually produce mucin; some which produce large volumes of extracellular mucin have a particularly poor prognosis. Occasionally tumours present as a scirrhous carcinoma, which usually has an undifferentiated histology and poor outlook. Tumour grading correlates with survival, and histological findings are used to stage the cancer (see below).

The gross features are variable, often changing with location in the bowel. Right-sided tumours are more likely to be polypoid, while left-sided carcinomas are more often infiltrating and constricting. Most tumours are found in the left side of the large bowel (Figure 28), a finding which has been attributed to stasis of carcinogenic bowel contents at this site.

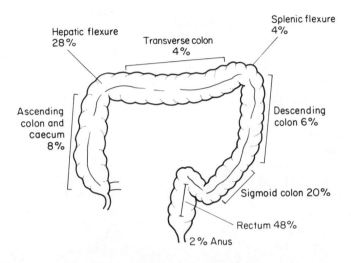

Figure 28. Anatomical sites of large bowel cancer

Presenting Features

These vary greatly according to the site of the tumour in the large bowel. Right-sided cancers often present with insidious symptoms such as anaemia due to unrecognized chronic blood loss and non-specific pain, whereas rectal tumours often cause changes in bowel habit and frank rectal bleeding at an early stage. The common symptoms, by site, are shown in Figure 29.

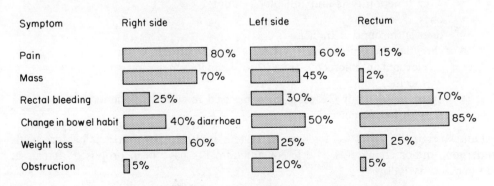

Figure 29. Common symptoms of large bowel cancer

The key part of physical examination, if a carcinoma of the colon is suspected, is a rectal examination. Up to half of all large bowel tumours can be detected by digital examination. Proctosigmoidoscopy will detect two-thirds of all colorectal cancers. Abdominal masses may be palpable if the tumour is of right- or left-sided origin.

Spread

Colorectal cancers spread by all the classical routes:
- Local:
  - Circularly within the bowel wall
  - Up and down the bowel wall
  - Perpendicularly out from the bowel
  - Perineurally to adjacent structures
- Lymphatic
- Haematogenous:
  - Colon → liver → lungs
  - Rectum → liver → lungs
  - Rectum → Batson's venous plexus → vertebral column
- Implantation:
  - Incisional
  - Anastomotic
  - Intraperitoneal

Local spread is common and the liver is by far the most common site of distant spread.

Investigation and Staging

The diagnosis is usually reached without great difficulty, though final staging can usually only be made at a laparotomy. Tests include:

- proctosigmoidoscopy
- barium enema
- colonoscopy
- liver function tests and full blood count
- chest X-ray
- liver ultrasound if indicated
- carcinoembryonic antigen (CEA—a marker protein often elevated in colorectal cancer: unfortunately it is not very specific)
- cystoscopy and/or CT scans may be used in selected patients with low lesions

Dukes originally proposed his staging system in 1930. Since then it has gradually undergone minor changes as a series of amendments have been proposed. It can be summarized as follows:

A. Tumour confined to mucosa and submucosa.
B. Invasion through submucosa without nodal involvement.
C. Lymph node involvement:
  C_1. Involved lymph nodes limited to paracolic region.
  C_2. Involved lymph nodes to point of vascular pedicle.
D. Metastatic involvement.

Subtle variations of this 1935 classification produce groups with differing prognoses; there is confusion because of the number of versions suggested. The UICC and AJC groups have produced TNM classifications which are complicated and are generally not used.

Treatment

In common with most solid tumours the patients' only real chance of long-term survival is surgical resection of all disease.

Surgery

Carcinoma of the large bowel is removed by wide segmental resection of the involved bowel and mesentery with intestinal anastomosis or abdominoperineal resection and permanent colostomy, depending upon the level of the tumour. The exact procedure depends on the anatomy of the vascular supply and lymphatic drainage of the portion of the bowel affected. With the introduction of new techniques for forming an anastomosis, quite low rectal cancers can be resected and permanent colostomy avoided. Cancers in the distal 5 cm of the rectum require an abdominoperineal resection. Using this radical approach good results are achieved in patients with early stage disease.

5-YEAR SURVIVAL AFTER RESECTION BY STAGE

Dukes A_____95%
     B_____70%
     C_1_____65%
     C_2_____50%
     D 4%

However, many patients present with advanced disease. Surgery may be indicated in such patients since it may prevent unpleasant complications, such as obstruction or fistulae. Bypass procedures or formation of a colostomy may be undertaken if an unresectable tumour is formed.

Radiotherapy

Because local relapse is still relatively common after radical resection of bowel cancer, perioperative radiotherapy has been used as an adjuvant treatment, especially for rectal cancer. The results of a series of randomized trials, though often conflicting, do not often show an obvious improvement in survival. Similar studies, often involving combined chemotherapy, continue.

If radiation is not used as an adjuvant its only role is as a palliative treatment for painful or bleeding local recurrence.

Chemotherapy

Cytotoxic drugs have been tested in this malignancy for several decades, without great success. There are several drugs which induce responses in a moderate proportion of patients. Fluorouracil (5-Fu) is the standard single agent used to treat selected patients with advanced disease. Its role is entirely palliative since it does not prolong survival. Combinations of cytotoxic drugs have been compared to 5-Fu but none seems much more active.

Drugs have also been used as an adjuvant soon after surgery. Until recently all randomized studies have been negative. A large cooperative group in the USA has reported that a combination of drugs can improve survival in a selected subgroup of patients (young men). A British group has also reported that a short course of intraportal 5-Fu improves survival of patients with colonic cancer by reducing deaths from liver metastases. Both these trials need to be confirmed by other groups but hold a hope for the future.

Outcome and Special Complications

Survival of this tumour is closely linked to stage at presentation. Unfortunately, many patients still present with advanced disease. Screening has so far been cumbersome and expensive and is not routinely used in the United Kingdom. Metastatic disease at presentation or relapse is incurable with present therapy and most effort is directed to improving initial treatment. Studies of new surgical techniques and intra-arterial or portal chemotherapy for hepatic metastases continue.

The problems of uncontrolled disease are:

- bowel obstruction
- liver metastases
- local failure leading to pain and bleeding

Selected Papers and Reviews

DeCosse, J.J. (1984) Are we doing better with large-bowel cancer? *New England Journal of Medicine*, **310**: 782–783.

Klugerman, M.M. (1976) Radiation therapy for rectal carcinoma. *Seminars in Oncology*, **3**: 407–413.

Moertel, C.G. (1978) Chemotherapy of gastrointestinal cancer. *New England Journal of Medicine*, **299**: 1049–1057.

Muto, T., Bussey, H.J.R. and Morson, B.C. (1975) The evolution of cancer of the colon and rectum. *Cancer*, **26**: 2251–2260.

Sherlock, P., Lipkim, M. and Winawer, S.J. (1975) Predisposing factors in carcinoma of the colon. *Adv. Intern. Med.*, **20**: 121–150.

Wooley, P.V. (1976) Clinical manifestations of cancer of the colon and rectum. *Seminars in Oncology*, **3**: 373–376.

15 | Gynaecological Cancers

C. J. WILLIAMS

BREAST CANCER

This is the leading malignant cause of death in women in western countries: its incidence has risen steadily in the past 30 years. Whilst there have not been major improvements in survival rates, methods of managing breast cancer have changed radically in the last 10 years and there is hope that more women will be cured in future and that treatment will be more acceptable.

There are about 21,000 new cases registered each year in England and Wales, the incidence increasing with age (Figure 1). Male breast cancer is rare, only accounting for 1% of cases. There is a only a modest variation in incidence around the world, rates being six times higher in western countries compared with Asia and Africa. Rates tend to be highest in industrialized regions (Figure 2).

Aetiology and Pathogenesis

A number of factors have been related to the risk of developing breast cancer, most through possible hormonal effects.

- Age at menarche and menopause. Women who start menstruating before 12 years have nearly double the risk of breast cancer compared to those whose menarche was after 13 years. Women who reach menopause after 55 years of age have twice the risk of those whose menopause is before 45 years.
- Age at first *full term* pregnancy. The earlier the first baby is born the greater the protective effect. Multiparity itself has

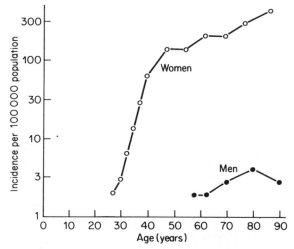

Figure 1. Age-specific incidence of breast cancer for England and Wales (1974)

no protective effect, operating simply through age at first
pregnancy.
- Weight and diet. There is a strong correlation between
  increasing body weight and risk of subsequent breast cancer.
  High-fat diets may be an additional factor.
- Recent data suggest that the risk of breast cancer increases with
  increasing alcohol consumption.
- Benign breast disease. There is a small increase in the chances
  of developing breast cancer in women with benign breast
  disease.
- Family history. Studies have shown that women with first-degree
  relatives with breast cancer have a higher risk themselves. If
  mother and sisters are involved, this risk may be very high.
- Oral contraceptives. The multiple studies published show
  contradictory results. The risks, if they exist, are unlikely to
  be large and are probably confined to young women using a
  high-oestrogen pill for a prolonged period.
- Postmenopausal hormone therapy. The results of studies are
  contradictory and further long-term observation is needed.

Pathology and Natural History

Although several classifications have been proposed, the most commonly used one is
that of the World Health Organization (Table 1). The majority (65%) of invasive
carcinomas are ductal tumours which, unfortunately, have a less good prognosis (38%
10-year survival). Histological grade also appears to correlate with survival (Figure 3).

Breast cancer incidence rates in different countries

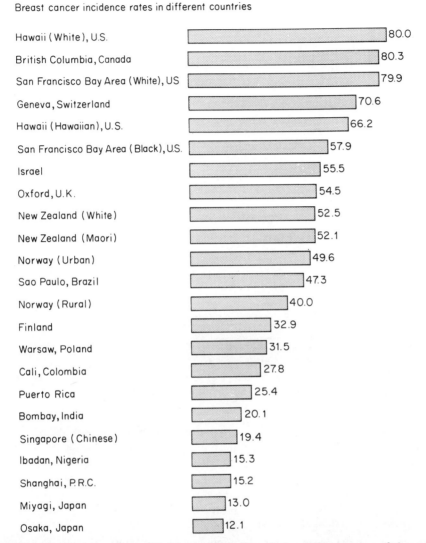

Hawaii (White), U.S.	80.0
British Columbia, Canada	80.3
San Francisco Bay Area (White), US	79.9
Geneva, Switzerland	70.6
Hawaii (Hawaiian), U.S.	66.2
San Francisco Bay Area (Black), U.S.	57.9
Israel	55.5
Oxford, U.K.	54.5
New Zealand (White)	52.5
New Zealand (Maori)	52.1
Norway (Urban)	49.6
Sao Paulo, Brazil	47.3
Norway (Rural)	40.0
Finland	32.9
Warsaw, Poland	31.5
Cali, Colombia	27.8
Puerto Rica	25.4
Bombay, India	20.1
Singapore (Chinese)	19.4
Ibadan, Nigeria	15.3
Shanghai, P.R.C.	15.2
Miyagi, Japan	13.0
Osaka, Japan	12.1

Figure 2. Female breast cancer incidence, age adjusted, for different parts of the world

As can be seen from these data, a high proportion of patients will have recurrent or metastatic disease. It used to be thought that breast cancer spread in a logical sequence:

- by direct extension within the breast
- by intramammary lymph vessels
- to draining lymph nodes
- and then via the bloodstream to distant sites

This hypothesis was the reason that radical mastectomy was developed as the 'definitive' cancer operation. However, its failure to have a major impact on survival should have

Table 1. Simplified histopathological classification for breast cancer (WHO, reproduced by permission)

CARCINOMA

1. Intraduct and intralobular non-invasive carcinoma
2. Invasive carcinoma
3. Common histological variants of carcinoma:

    Medullary carcinoma
    Ductal carcinoma
    Mucous carcinoma
    Lobular carcinoma

4. Paget's disease of breast

SARCOMA

CARCINOSARCOMA

UNCLASSIFIED TUMOURS

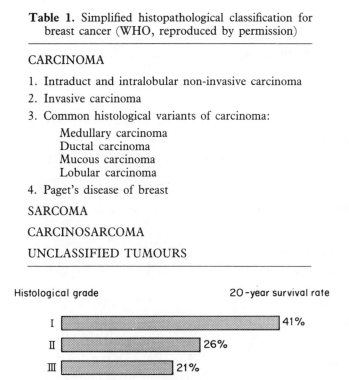

Figure 3. 20-year survival rates by histological grade for epithelial breast cancer (Reproduced by permission from Bloom and Richardson, 1957)

led to an early re-examination of the hypothesis on which it was based. It was not until recently that the operation and underlying hypothesis were successfully challenged. Current opinion holds that spread via the bloodstream occurs at an early stage in many if not all women. Tumour cells are distributed widely, being arrested in capillaries in various organs. Here they may perish, lie dormant or grow to form a metastasis—the fate of malignant cells depending upon their own biological properties and the environment in which they find themselves.

This theory explains the later development of metastatic disease in women who apparently have small tumours which should be eminently curable by mastectomy if they have not spread. Such relapse may occur quickly or in some cases as late as 20 or more years after initial surgery: presumably cancer cells lie dormant until triggered into action in such patients. Recently, monoclonal antibodies have been used to demonstrate the presence of epithelial cells (presumably metastatic breast cancer) in the bone marrow of women undergoing surgery, providing additional support for this hypothesis of micrometastatic disease.

Presenting Features

The great majority of women present with a lump in the breast (*generally* painless), but with the introduction of mammographic screening an increasing proportion of cancers will be detected before the patient is aware that anything is wrong. Presentation with gross local disease or metastatic disease is still all too common—usually in older women. Occasionally patients present with nipple discharge or bleeding, a painful breast or axillary adenopathy.

Several randomized and case-control studies of mammographic screening have shown that the screened population have smaller tumours, less involvement of axillary nodes and better survival than unscreened controls (Figure 4). Because of this the National Health Service is introducing breast screening for women aged 50–74 years in the UK. The lower age was chosen since significant improvement in survival has been seen only after this age (see page 67).

On examination of a woman with a breast lump the clinician needs to look for:

- mass in the breast; record size in centimetres
- nipple inversion or discharge/bleeding
- fixation to skin or chest wall
- peau d'orange
- erythema and skin infiltration
- presence and state of draining lymph nodes
- signs of distant metastases (bone, lung, pleura, liver, CNS)

Spread

This has already been alluded to. There is undoubtedly progressive spread within the breast and to draining lymph nodes, but haematogenous dissemination also occurs early. The sites of spread are illustrated in Figure 5.

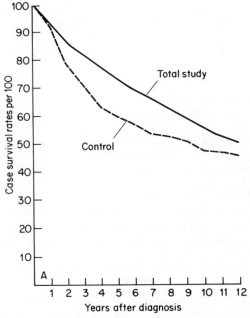

Figure 4. Case survival rates in the HIP randomized study comparing a screened group with an unscreened control population

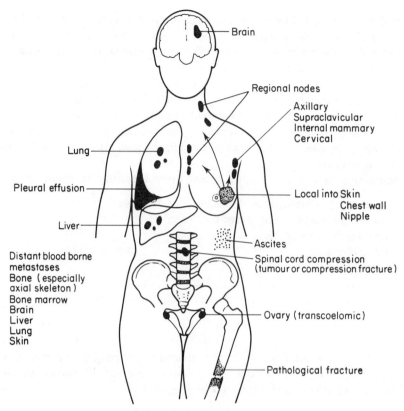

Figure 5. Mode and sites of spread of breast cancer. Adapted by permission from Souhami, R. L. and Tobias, J. S. (1986) *Cancer and Its Management*, Blackwell Scientific Publications, Oxford

Investigations and Staging

Techniques to make preoperative diagnosis of invasive cancer have improved markedly in the last decade, so that the diagnosis is clear in 80% or more of patients prior to surgery. Patients should ideally be assessed by:

- clinical examination by an experienced breast specialist
- mammography and/or ultrasonography
- fine-needle aspirate for cytology

If all these tests clearly show malignancy or a benign tumour then management can be planned on the basis of their findings. Only in the intermediate case where the findings are unclear or unsatisfactory is an excision biopsy needed before definitive therapy. Other tests that are justified when cancer is found clinically include:

- examination for draining lymph nodes and skin deposits
- examination of the contralateral breast
- chest X-ray

Additional tests, such as bone scan and CT or ultrasonic liver imaging, are rarely helpful and are expensive.

Staging is based on the TNM system. The UICC system is shown in simplified form in the box and diagrammatically in Figure 6.

T T_1 tumour less than 2 cm
T_2 tumour 2–5 cm
T_3 tumour more than 5 cm
T_4 tumour of any size fixed to skin or chest wall

N N_0 no palpable axillary lymph nodes
N_1 mobile ipsilateral nodes
N_2 fixed ipsilateral nodes
N_3 supraclavicular or infraclavicular nodes

M M_0 no distant metastases
M_1 distant metastases

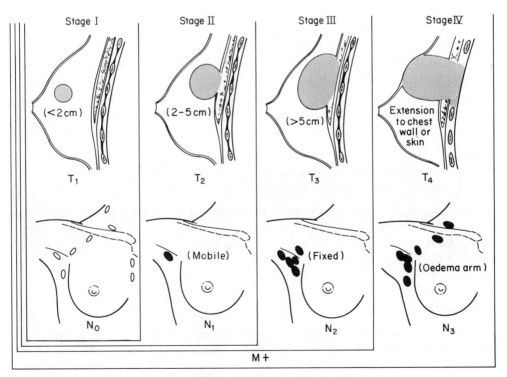

Figure 6. UICC anatomical (TNM) staging for breast cancer

Treatment

A number of modalities are available and their use has changed dramatically in the past 20 years. Surgery is still the mainstay of curative therapy but is now often used with adjuvant treatments.

Surgery

There has been a major swing away from radical surgery. Although there have long been proponents for limited surgery and/or radiation it was not until major trials showed that there was no survival benefit for radical operations that the pattern of surgery changed. These studies, led by the National Surgical Adjuvant Breast Project (NSABP) in the United States and the National Cancer Institute in Milan, have successively shown that:

- Supra-radical surgery (radical mastectomy plus excision of supra- and infraclavicular and internal mammary nodes) is no better than radical mastectomy (complete mastectomy, axillary clearance, thick flaps and excision of the pectoralis major muscle).
- Radical mastectomy is no better than simple mastectomy (mastectomy with thin flaps and axillary node dissection) with or without radiation.
- Radical mastectomy is no better than segmental resection and irradiation.
- Simple mastectomy is no better than wide local excision with or without irradiation (higher local relapse without irradiation).

Currently many patients appear to have disease which is appropriate for breast-conserving surgery. Since these data have been collected from randomized clinical trials, most clinicians feel that patients should be selected and treated according to the methods used in these trials. Those treated with breast conservation include patients who have:

- tumour up to 4 cm in diameter
- mobile axillary lymph nodes

Women excluded are those with more advanced disease and those in whom a good cosmetic result cannot be obtained because the breast is small, or in whom there is an increased risk of residual disease because the tumour is directly beneath the nipple and may involve the ducts.

Radiotherapy

Postoperative irradiation has been extensively tested and the consensus is that it does not improve survival. It can, however, reduce the risk of local relapse and for this reason it is usually used after wide local excision and for selected high-risk patients after mastectomy.

Radiation is a very useful palliative treatment, particularly for local recurrence and painful bone metastases. It is also used in women presenting with advanced unresectable breast cancer and in inflammatory breast cancer (mass in breast with erythema and skin infiltration).

Hormone Therapy

Beatson, as long ago as 1896, noted that advanced breast cancer would regress in some women undergoing oophorectomy. More recently, hormonal receptors for oestrogen and progesterone have been identified in cancer cells. Up to 50% of tumours contain such receptors and nearly all women destined to respond to hormonal treatment have tumours with these receptors.

Assays are available for clinical use and the chances of response to hormonal treatment are directly related to the level of the receptor. Oestrogen interacts with the receptor to form a complex which is transported to the nucleus where it initiates or modifies RNA synthesis (Figure 7). Such assays are useful in choosing treatment as only 5% of receptor negative patients will respond to hormone treatment compared with 60% of positive patients.

Although hormones were originally only used for advanced or metastatic disease, they are now being used as an adjuvant treatment—this is considered in the section on adjuvant therapy. For patients with advanced disease hormone therapy may provide the simplest non-toxic way of controlling disease. For this reason it has often been used as a first line therapy in such patients in the UK. It should generally be avoided, however, in women with rapidly advancing visceral breast cancer or those who are hormone receptor negative since their chances of response are very low.

Originally hormonal therapy consisted solely of surgical ablation but over the last 20 years a number of pharmaceutical preparations have become available. These include:

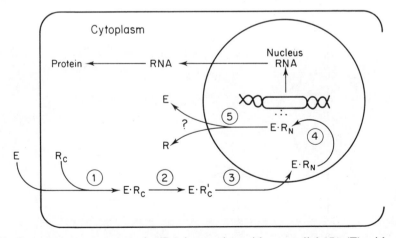

Figure 7. Oestrogen receptor protein (R_c) interaction with oestradiol-17β (E) with subsequent translocation to the cell nucleus as a complex (ER_N) where it influences RNA synthesis. ER^1_c = Transformed complex

- tamoxifen—an anti-oestrogen which is very well tolerated
- progestogens (megestrol acetate or methoxyprogesterone
  acetate)—relatively well tolerated drugs generally used as a
  second line to tamoxifen
- aminoglutethimide—an adrenal and aromatase blocker which
  prevents adrenal and peripheral production of oestrogen.
  Used as a second or third line therapy
- traditional drugs, such as oestrogen and androgens, are less
  commonly used these days as they are more toxic than the
  newer agents

If a patient responds to one hormonal treatment it is usually worth trying a second, different, hormonal therapy as the chances of a subsequent response are still good. Although claims have been made that certain hormonal treatments are more effective in patients with particular patterns of metastases (bone, for example), these are poorly documented and hormonal therapy should be chosen on the basis of least side-effects. Combinations of hormones are probably not beneficial.

Chemotherapy

Breast cancer is quite sensitive to the effects of cytotoxic drugs, with objective response rates of more than 25% being reported for eight different drugs. These can be used in combination, when response rates as high as 60–80% have been claimed in advanced disease. Unfortunately, most responses are partial and even when there is apparent complete resolution of disease the effect is temporary—the median duration of response is only 9 months. Chemotherapy is, therefore, never curative (Figure 8); most patients only survive 1–2 years after starting cytotoxic therapy. Because of this, it is important that the therapeutic balance is seen to favour the patient—toxic, ineffective therapy is never worthwhile. However, if chemotherapy is to be given, a combination of known efficiency should be used in full dose in an attempt to get maximum tumour regression.

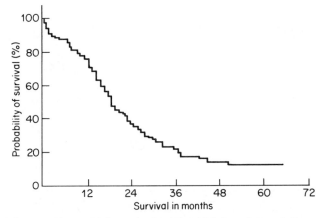

Figure 8. Chemotherapy (doxorubicin-cyclophosphamide) for advanced disease: survival (COSA ANZ study)

Chemotherapy has also been used as an adjuvant treatment, as discussed in the next section.

Adjuvant Therapy

Because up to 70% of patients are destined to have recurrent disease at local or distant sites, attempts have been made to test the value of systemic treatments at the time of surgery, when patients have the least tumour burden. Patients at higher risk of relapse have been chosen for such studies—usually those with axillary node involvement. Originally, such clinical trials tested the value of hormonal treatments. Oophorectomy, at the time of mastectomy, was tested in a series of trials. It was found to delay relapse but did not improve survival and was largely abandoned in the late 1960s. In retrospect, none of the studies reported was adequate in terms of size or design. More recently, a series of trials have tested the value of tamoxifen as an adjuvant treatment. These seem to show not only a delay in time to relapse, but also a modest improvement in survival (Figure 9). Surprisingly, this benefit does not seem to be restricted to patients whose tumour contains hormone receptors. This suggests that tamoxifen may also have a non-hormonal action. Trials are now testing for how long the drug should be used— so far it seems necessary to continue for at least 5 years for the best result. Benefit is most marked in postmenopausal patients but may also be seen in younger women.

Chemotherapy has been extensively tested in the past 20 years. Studies have concentrated on women with axillary node involvement and recommendations can only be made in this group. Overall there seems to be an improvement in survival of about 15%, which is *confined* to premenopausal women.

Consensus conferences on adjuvant therapy recommend:

- Adjuvant chemotherapy significantly increases disease-free survival and overall survival in premenopausal women with less than 10 axillary nodes involved with cancer. Combination chemotherapy is preferred.
- Adjuvant tamoxifen improves the disease-free survival and overall survival of postmenopausal women. Tamoxifen should

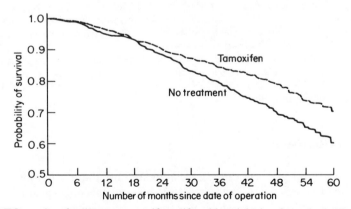

Figure 9. NATO study of adjuvant tamoxifen: life table analysis of survival. Note the vertical axis omits probability of survival below 50% (Reproduced by permission of Professor M. Baum)

be continued for at least 5 years. It may be beneficial in premenopausal women though further trials are necessary.

Outlook and Special Complications

There are, at last, hopes that the outlook for women with breast cancer will be improved. Hopefully, screening and the use of adjuvant therapy will result in more women being cured, while less radical operations will make treatment more acceptable. Despite this many patients still present with advanced incurable disease or relapse after initial therapy. Breast cancer may recur in different patterns:

- primarily local—very extensive and unpleasant tumour may occur (sometimes called 'en cuirasse')
- mainly bone involvement
- visceral metastatic disease

Complications such as pleural/pericardial effusion, hypercalcaemia, CNS involvement and bone fracture are common and require specific symptomatic care (see Chapters 9 and 10).

The psychological consequences of mastectomy and chemotherapy for breast cancer have received a lot of attention (Chapter 11). Depression and anxiety are very common, and the earlier problems are recognized and treated the better.

Selected Papers and Reviews

Baum, M., Brinckley, D.M., *et al.* (1985) Controlled trial of tamoxifen as single adjuvant agent in management of early breast cancer: analysis of six years by Nolvadex Adjuvant Trial Organisation. *Lancet*, i: 836–840.

Bonadonna, G. and Rossi, A. (1985) Adjuvant CMF chemotherapy in operable breast cancer: ten years later. *Lancet*, i: 976–977.

Fisher, B., Bauer, M., *et al.* (1985) Five-year results of a randomized clinical trial comparing total mastectomy and segmental mastectomy with or without irradiation in the treatment of breast cancer. *New England Journal of Medicine*, 312: 665–673.

Fisher, B., Redmond, C., *et al.* (1985) Ten-year results of a randomized clinical trial comparing radical mastectomy and total mastectomy with or without irradiation in the treatment of breast cancer. *New England Journal of Medicine*, 312: 674–681.

Shapiro, S., Venet, W., *et al.* (1982) Ten to fourteen year effect of screening on breast cancer mortality. *Journal of the National Cancer Institute*, 69: 349–355.

Williams, C.J. and Buchanan, R.B. (1987) *Medical Management of Breast Cancer*. Castle House Publications, Tunbridge Wells.

OVARIAN CARCINOMA

Although both cervical and endometrial carcinoma are more common than ovarian cancer, the latter is the leading cause of death from gynaecological malignancy. This is because, unlike other gynaecological cancers, it does not cause characteristic symptoms until, usually, it is far advanced. Early diagnosis is usually by chance and screening has so far been unsuccessful. Recently ultrasound screening has shown that it is possible to detect early disease, but whether this will improve survival is unclear and the cost will be high. Measurement of a marker antigen (ca-125) may be helpful.

Incidence and Epidemiology

There are about 5000 new cases of ovarian cancer each year in England and Wales (14 per 100,000); the incidence in the USA is similar with 18,000 cases per year. About 70% of these women are destined to die of their disease; cancer of the ovary is the fourth leading cause of cancer death in the United States. The incidence of the common epithelial types of ovarian cancer increases with age; the median age at diagnosis is 56 years.

Incidence rates vary quite widely around the world: rates are highest in industrialized countries (Figure 10) and are increasing (Figure 11). Japan is something of an exception to this since incidence rates are rather low. However, the incidence increases in Japanese who move to the USA, suggesting the influence of environmental factors.

Aetiology and Pathogenesis

Little is known about aetiology, but the ovary is indirectly exposed to environmental factors via the bloodstream and to the external environment through the Fallopian

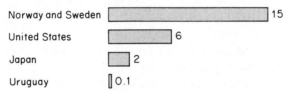

Figure 10. Incidence of malignant ovarian neoplasia in various countries (per 100,000)

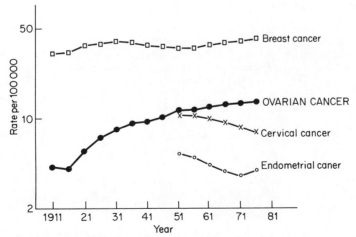

Figure 11. Death rates from gynaecological cancer in England and Wales from 1911 to 1981

tubes, uterus and vagina. Although it has been shown that talc rapidly gains access to the peritoneal cavity, there are no data to support the theory that the asbestos in talc causes ovarian cancer.

There is, however, evidence which suggests that the contraceptive pill quite markedly *reduces* the risk of women developing this tumour. This is the first piece of evidence to show that hormonal factors may play a part in the aetiology of cancer of the ovary. It has also been reported that multiparity has a protective effect.

A few families with a very high risk of cancer of the ovary have been reported, but the genetic implications of this are unclear. It is interesting to note, however, that women with breast cancer (in which there is a clear genetic component) have a higher risk of developing an ovarian malignancy.

Pathology and Natural History

The pathology of ovarian neoplasms is very complicated, though this section is only concerned with the common epithelial tumours (Table 2). Although the WHO classification lists 27 histological subtypes of ovarian malignancy, over 90% are epithelial tumours which originate from the epithelial surface of the ovary.

Malignant epithelial tumours are further described according to their appearance as serous cystadenocarcinoma, mucinous, endometrioid, clear cell and undifferentiated adenocarcinomas. Tumour grading is important in this cancer and in some series has been found to be a better predictor of outcome than histological subtype. The presence of psammoma bodies (small aggregations of calcium, also known as calco-sphereites) is helpful in making the diagnosis when there is doubt over the origin of the tumour.

The natural history of these tumours is very variable, the patient's chances of survival being dictated by the biology of the tumour. Some, such as borderline tumours, are exceedingly indolent, slow-growing neoplasms which have a good outlook, even when metastatic. Others, whilst clearly malignant, are of good histological grade and are less likely to metastasize so that the chances of cure are fairly good. The remainder are undifferentiated tumours which have a propensity to invasion and early spread, hence the chances of cure are poor.

Table 2. Simplified classification
of ovarian tumours

I.   Epithelial tumours:
      A. Benign
      B. Borderline malignant
      C. Malignant

II.   Germ cell tumours

III. Stromal tumours

IV. Sarcomas

V.   Unclassified

Presenting Features

Nearly all ovarian tumours are large before they cause symptoms. Even early stage tumours (see below) tend to be of considerable size by the time they are detected— stage 1 disease is more a function of favourable biology than early diagnosis. Although in retrospect many patients will give a history of vague upper abdominal discomfort for some time prior to diagnosis, this is too non-specific or mild to precipitate investigation likely to reveal the cause. Since ovarian tumours do not invade nearby structures, symptoms are usually caused by the pressure caused by a large tumour, ascites or torsion of an ovarian mass (Figure 12).

Nearly all patients will have a palpable mass on examination. This may only be demonstrable on bimanual pelvic examination, but often a mass may be felt, on abdominal palpation, arising out of the pelvis. Ascites is commonly found whilst pleural effusions are much less frequent (Figure 13).

Occasionally, women will present without an obvious mass, even when there is advanced disease. This is because of the plaque-like nature of this malignancy. The presence of an adnexal mass in a postmenopausal woman is always a cause for investigation, whilst masses greater than 5 cm deserve attention in younger women.

Spread

This is primarily by direct extension, intraperitoneal seeding and lymphatic spread to pelvic and para-aortic nodes. Blood-borne spread is rare in this type of cancer. Within the abdomen, negative pressures caused by respiration result in fluid in the peritoneal cavity being sucked up the right paracolic gutter to the diaphragmatic surface of the liver. Because of this, the upper surface of the liver is a common hidden site of metastases. Figure 14 shows the common modes of spread diagrammatically.

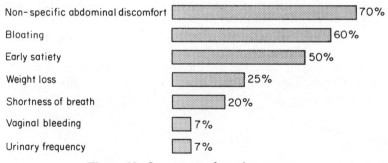

Figure 12. Symptoms of ovarian cancer

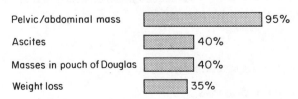

Figure 13. Signs of ovarian cancer

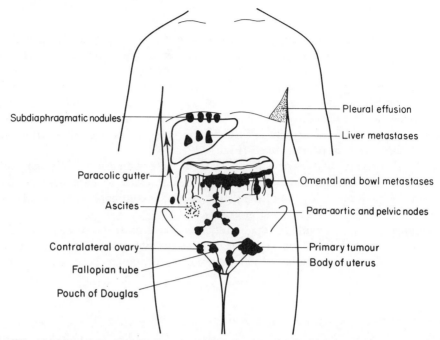

Figure 14. Modes and sites of spread of ovarian cancer. Peritoneal fluid and malignant cells are carried up the right paracolic gutter to the diaphragm. Spread by the lymphatics is also common. Adapted by permission from Souhami, R. L. and Tobias, J. S. (1986) *Cancer and Its Management*, Blackwell Scientific Publications, Oxford

Investigations and Staging

Physical examination is usually indicative of the diagnosis. This can be confirmed by ultrasound or computed tomographic imaging. If ascites or a pleural effusion is present, diagnostic paracentesis may confirm the presence of malignant cells but will not detect the primary site. Other investigations prior to surgery may include chest X-ray, barium enema and intravenous pyelography.

Several similar staging systems are in use. However, that of the International Federation of Gynaecology and Obstetrics (FIGO) is most often used (Table 3 and Figure 15).

Treatment

Surgery is still the key to treatment, though both chemotherapy and radiotherapy have become increasingly important. Management will be planned according to the findings at surgery (stage) and the tumour grade.

Surgery

The aims of surgery for ovarian cancer are:

- to make the diagnosis
- to stage the extent of tumour involvement

Table 3. FIGO staging system in carcinoma of the ovary

Stage	Description
Stage I	Growth limited to ovary (26%)*
Ia	One ovary involved
Ib	Both ovaries involved
Ic	Ascites present, or positive peritoneal washings
Stage II	Growth limited to pelvis (21%)
IIa	Extension to gynaecological adnexae
IIb	Extension to other pelvic tissues
IIc	Ascites or positive washings
Stage III†	Growth extending to abdominal cavity — including peritoneal surface seedlings, omentum, etc. (37%)
Stage IV	Metastases to distant sites (including hepatic parenchymal disease) (16%)

*Proportion of total cases presenting with each particular stage.
†May be subdivided (a or b) by bulk of intra-abdominal disease.

- to excise all or as much of the tumour as possible (bilateral salpingo-oophorectomy and hysterectomy (BSOH) and omentectomy)

The requirements of an exploratory operation for ovarian cancer are shown in Table 4.

Although the concept of surgical debulking has fallen out of favour for most primary tumours, it remains standard therapy in ovarian cancer (Figure 16). Because ovarian cancer is rarely deeply invasive, tissue planes are often intact so that widespread cancer is often resectable.

Radiotherapy

Because the whole of the peritoneal cavity is at risk radiotherapy confined to the pelvis is unlikely to be effective. This has proved to be the case in trials of postoperative pelvic irradiation. More recently, trials have tested the utility of radiotherapy to the whole abdomen and pelvis (Figure 17). These have shown improved survival, but only in patients who have had an abdominal hysterectomy and bilateral salpingo-oophorectomy. The tolerance of the abdominal contents to irradiation is low, so that a relatively small dose is used (2250 cGy), the pelvis being treated to a total of about 4500 cGy. Treatment is given over 6–7 weeks. Toxicity is quite high, with nausea prominent in the middle of treatment and diarrhoea during the latter part. In the long term, the incidence of recurrent bowel obstruction is increased by the use of this

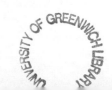

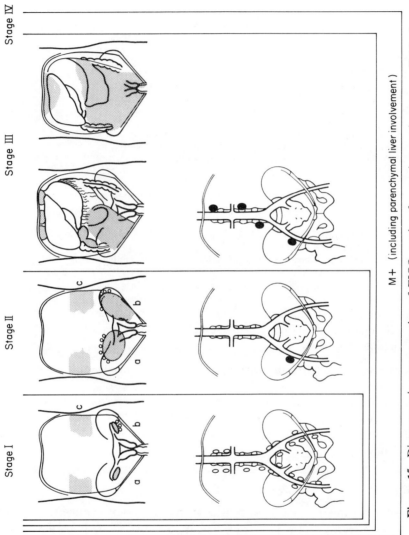

Figure 15. Diagrammatic representation of FIGO staging for ovarian carcinoma: see Table 2 for details

Stage I   Stage II   Stage III   Stage IV

M+ (including parenchymal liver involvement)

Table 4. Surgery for epithelial ovarian carcinomas

Inspection: exploratory laparotomy

Free fluid

Parietal peritoneum:	Anterior abdominal wall, paracolic gutters, sub-diaphragmatic areas, posterior abdominal wall
Upper abdominal contents:	Liver, gall bladder, spleen, stomach, large and small bowel, appendix, mesentery and meso-colon, omentum
Retroperitoneal structures:	Kidneys, para-aortic lymph nodes, pelvic lymph nodes
Pelvic organs:	Uterus, ovaries and Fallopian tubes, bladder and rectum with sigmoid colon

Surgical resection and biopsy

Aspiration of ascites/peritoneal washings for cytology
Sub-diaphragmatic biopsy and scraping

Radical oophorectomy:	Extended total abdominal hysterectomy, bilateral salpingo-oophorectomy
	Omentectomy (total)
	Appendicectomy
Debulking of further tumour masses as indicated:	
	Pelvic peritoneum
	Bowel resection
	Dome of bladder

Pelvic and para-aortic lymphadenectomy as indicated

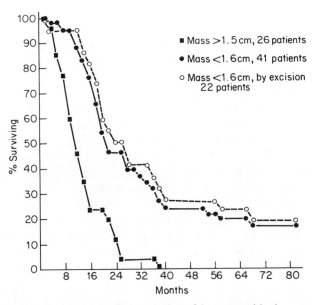

Figure 16. Relationship between survival and size of largest residual metastasis after primary operation for stage III ovarian carcinoma. The survival curve of patients whose tumour size was reduced to ≤ 1.5 cm by excision of larger metastases was identical to that of all patients with a residual tumour size below this limit. From Griffiths *et al.* (1978). *Surg. Clin. North America,* **58:** 131–142. Reproduced by permission

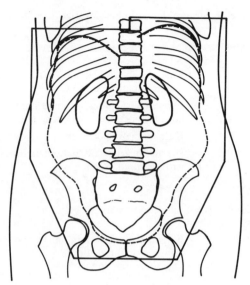

Figure 17. Line drawing from a simulator X-ray showing the treatment volume for abdomino-pelvic radiotherapy

type of irradiation after surgery. The use of abdomino-pelvic radiotherapy remains controversial.

Chemotherapy

Chemotherapy, which has long been used in the management of advanced disease, is now being used in patients with earlier stage disease. There is a wide selection of drugs which are able to produce objective responses in more than 20% of cases; most of these drugs are alkylating agents.

Traditionally oral alkylating agents have been used alone—they can induce clinical response in 25–50% of patients. The introduction of a new drug, cisplatin, coincided with the development of combination chemotherapy. This resulted in an increase in response rates to 60–80% and survival seemed to be improved. However, a number of randomized clinical trials have failed to confirm better survival (Figure 18), though all have shown higher response rates and disease-free survival. Currently, cisplatin is the most active single drug though there is still controversy as to whether it should be used alone or with other drugs. Unfortunately, cisplatin is a toxic drug so that the therapeutic ratio should be assessed for each individual patient. Recently a new analogue of cisplatin, carboplatin, has been introduced. This causes less subjective toxicity though increased bone marrow suppression is a potential problem when used with other drugs.

Results of Different Management Policies

Debate about the most effective treatments for the various stages and grades of ovarian cancer abound. The following are commonly used policies:

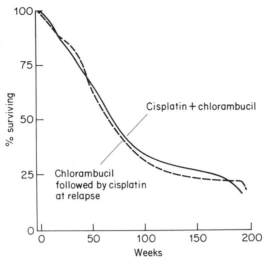

Figure 18. COSA study of combination chemotherapy versus sequential therapy—overall survival

- Borderline tumour regardless of stage—surgery (BSOH) only, followed by observation.
- Stage Ia, good grade tumour—complete surgery (BSOH) followed by observation.
- Stage Ia, poor grade tumour—complete surgery (BSOH) followed by abdomino-pelvic irradiation, or complete surgery followed by chemotherapy.
- Stage Ib–IIc, regardless of grade—complete surgery (BSOH) followed by abdomino-pelvic irradiation, or complete surgery followed by chemotherapy. Where surgery is incomplete (less than BSOH) chemotherapy should be used and not irradiation.
- Stage III–IV, maximum surgery possible followed by chemotherapy.

Surgery should, where possible, be complete excision (including bilateral salpingo-oophorectomy and hysterectomy) or maximal tumour debulking.

Irradiation should ideally include the whole abdomen and pelvis. Chemotherapy is contentious, varying from simple treatment with an oral alkylating agent to cisplatin-based combination chemotherapy, with single agent cisplatin as the middle road.

Outcome and Special Complications

The chances of cure are closely related, as stated, to the amount of residual disease after surgery, stage and grade (Figure 19). Complications of ovarian cancer include:

- recurrent ascites
- recurrent subacute bowel obstruction

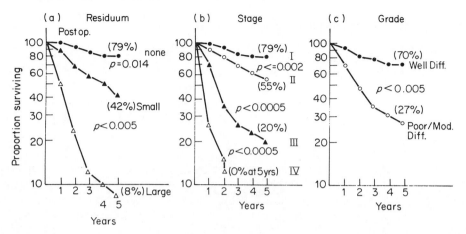

Figure 19. Survival data for patients with ovarian carcinoma according to (a) bulk of residual disease after surgery; (b) stage and (c) grade. (R. Bush, Princess Margaret Hospital, Toronto.) Reproduced by permission

- pleural effusion
- cachexia

Selected Papers and Reviews

COSA (1986) Chemotherapy of advanced ovarian adenocarcinoma: a randomized comparison of combination versus sequential therapy using chlorambucil and cisplatin. *Gynecologic Oncology*, **23**: 1–13.

Dembo, A.J., Bush, R.S., *et al.* (1980) Ovarian carcinoma: improved survival following abdominopelvic irradiation in patients with completed pelvic operation. *American Journal of Obstetrics and Gynecology*, **134**: 793–800.

Ozols, R.F. (1983) The case for combination chemotherapy in the treatment of advanced ovarian cancer. *Journal of Clinical Oncology*, **3**: 1445–1447.

Richardson, G.S., Scully, R.E., *et al.* (1985) Common epithelial cancer of the ovary. *New England Journal of Medicine*, **312**: 415–424, 474–483.

Williams, C.J., Mead, G.M., *et al.* (1985) Cisplatin combination chemotherapy versus chlorambucil in advanced ovarian carcinoma: mature results of a randomized trial. *Journal of Clinical Oncology*, **3**, 1455–1462.

Williams, C.J. and Whitehouse, J.M.A. (eds.) (1985) *Cancer of the Female Reproductive System.* John Wiley & Sons, Chichester.

CANCER OF THE BODY OF THE UTERUS (ENDOMETRIAL CANCER)

The survival rates for this tumour are among the highest of the common solid tumours. This reflects relatively early diagnosis—because of easily recognizable symptoms—late penetration through a large muscular organ and the underlying tumour biology. This is fortunate, since there seems to have been an increase in its incidence in the last 30 years.

Incidence and Epidemiology

The incidence rate in England and Wales (13 per 100,000) is rather lower than in the United States. UK figures show higher incidence rates for cervical cancer; endometrial carcinoma rates are similar to those for ovarian cancer, whereas in the USA uterine cancer leads the gynaecological cancer incidence rates with 39,000 cases each year.

The median age of onset is about 63 years, the incidence reaching a plateau after 60 years (Figure 20). Around 20% of patients are premenopausal, and only 4% are younger than 40 years.

There is a fairly wide variation in incidence worldwide, highest rates being in the USA and lowest in Japan (Figure 21). Interestingly, the rates for Japanese emigrating to Hawaii (41 per 100,000) are much higher than in Japan and approach those of Caucasian Hawaiians (70 per 100,000), strongly suggesting environmental effects.

Aetiology and Pathogenesis

The cause of this malignancy is unknown though it seems likely that both endogenous and exogenous oestrogens have a role to play. Retrospective and case-control studies have revealed a number of associations with this cancer:

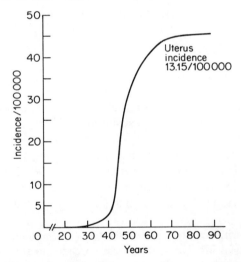

Figure 20. Incidence of cancer of the uterus by age in England and Wales

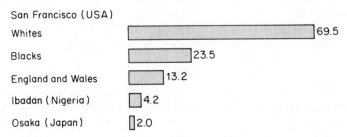

Figure 21. Incidence rates per 100,000 for uterine cancer around the world

- use of oestrogens
- obesity
- late menopause (> 52 years)
- diabetes
- infertility and anovulatory cycles

Support for an underlying derangement in oestrogen metabolism comes from a number of sources:

- Endometrial cancer is uncommon in women who have undergone an oophorectomy.
- Adenomatous hyperplasia (a precursor of malignancy) is common in granulosa tumours of the ovary which produce oestrogen.
- There are defects in sex hormone-binding globulin in obese women which result in raised levels of free oestrogens.
- During anovulatory cycles there is failure to produce a corpus luteum so that there is no progesterone to oppose the effects of oestrogen.
- Chronic exogenous oestrogen administration leads to hyperplasia and an excess of endometrial carcinomas. This risk falls when oestrogens are stopped or if they are given with a progestogen.

Pathology and Natural History

Nearly 90% of cancers of the body of the uterus are adenocarcinomas. Squamous elements are occasionally present (adenoacanthoma). Sarcomas, carcinosarcomas and pure squamous carcinomas are all rare. Only the common adenocarcinoma will be dealt with here. Diagnostic problems may occur in biopsies showing adenomatous hyperplasia, where differentiation from carcinoma may be difficult.

Tumour grade is important, correlating with survival, and is used in the staging system (see below). Fortunately, most patients have well-differentiated tumours (grade 1).

The size of the uterine cavity also correlates with outcome, probably because it partly reflects myometrial involvement. Direct spread into the vagina, Fallopian tubes and ovaries is relatively common, as is spread to draining lymph nodes. Contamination of the peritoneal cavity by penetration through the uterine wall or via the Fallopian tubes is a relatively late event. Visceral metastases (lung, liver, bone) are usually seen in the setting of advanced disease though not invariably. Tumour recurrence is usually seen within 36 months of primary treatment, late recurrences being uncommon.

Presenting Features

The cardinal symptom of endometrial cancer is abnormal vaginal bleeding. This is postmenopausal in most patients, though about 20% are premenopausal, when intermenstrual bleeding, irregular periods and/or excessive bleeding may occur.

Coexisting symptoms may include pelvic or back pain. Abnormal vaginal bleeding is always a reason for investigation by an experienced gynaecologist.

On examination, there are often no abnormal findings or simple uterine enlargement; infiltration with or without thickening of the cervix and of associated pelvic structures may sometimes be found. Occasionally signs of extensive disease are present from the outset.

Spread

In most cases spread is confined to local invasion. However, with increasing myometrial invasion and worsening grade, lymphatic involvement becomes more common. As discussed above, spread into the peritoneum and bloodstream are less common, normally later events (Figure 22).

Investigations and Staging

Peri- or postmenopausal vaginal bleeding should be considered to be a symptom of endometrial cancer until proved otherwise. Investigation includes:

- history for risk factors
- pelvic examination

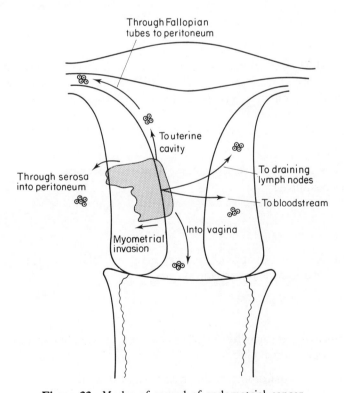

Figure 22. Modes of spread of endometrial cancer

- cervical cytology (positive in about half of cases but a negative smear never excludes the diagnosis)
- curettage (D & C) of the endometrium for histological examination or aspiration cytology of the endometrium is mandatory in all cases of abnormal vaginal bleeding. Curettage is the favoured procedure, though aspiration cytology is also used in the United States since it can be done on an outpatient basis

Staging is according to the International Federation of Gynaecologists (FIGO) system shown below.

Stage I   Confined to the corpus.*
           Ia Uterine length 8 cm or less.
           Ib Uterine length more than 8 cm
Stage II   Extension to the cervix.
Stage III Extension beyond uterus, within true pelvis.
Stage IV   Involvement of bladder or rectum or extension outside pelvis.

---

* Subclassified grade 1, 2 or 3.

There is a TNM system which is similar to the FIGO system but includes nodal disease and metastatic disease in stages III and IV respectively (Figure 23). The depth of invasion into the myometrium is also an important prognostic factor used in selecting therapy for early stage disesae.

If an endometrial cancer is diagnosed, additional investigations may include:

- cystoscopy
- CT scan   in selected cases of advanced disease
- lymphography

Treatment

In general, the results of treatment are very good, the choice of therapy being made on the basis of well-known prognostic factors.

Surgery

This is the principal treatment; radiation is used as an adjuvant in high-risk patients. An appropriate operation includes:

- exploratory laparotomy with careful surgical staging
- peritoneal washings for cytology

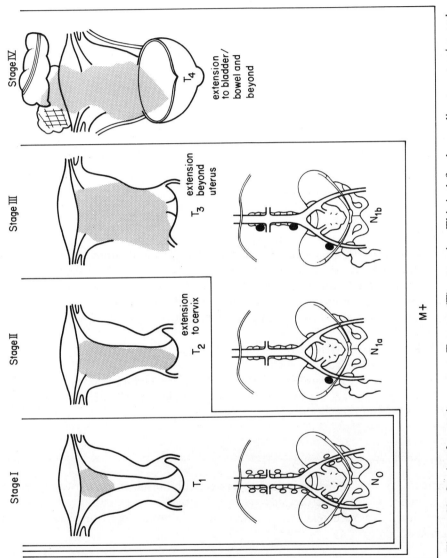

Figure 23. Staging for uterine cancer. Tumour (T) categories: This is defined according to extension and depth of invasion. T_1 is confined to the uterine fundus; extension to cervix signifies T_2; parametrial invasion signifies T_3 and invasion into bladder and/or rectum denotes T_4. Node (N) categories: $N_{1a} =$ pelvic node; $N_{1b} =$ para-aortic nodes. *Stage grouping*: This is identical to T categories. However, N_1 is grouped with T_3

- total abdominal hysterectomy
- bilateral salpingo-oophorectomy

Some American surgeons have recommended lymphadenectomy, though there is little evidence that this improves survival. Radical hysterectomy may be undertaken in some patients with stage II tumours.

Radiotherapy

Radiation may be used preoperatively with the intention of preventing spread before surgery. The theoretical advantages of this approach are:

- reduce tumour spill and implantation metastasis
- reduce uterine size to improve operability

Postoperative irradiation is used by some centres; the advantage of this approach is that treatment is planned on the basis of full surgical staging.

Treatment by Stage

Since surgery may be used alone or in combination with radiotherapy, treatment is best outlined by stage:

- *Stage IA or IB, Grade I or II*: surgery alone is the treatment of choice
- *Stage IA or IB, Grade III*: surgery with or without postoperative irradiation. Irradiation is generally used when myometrial invasion is greater than one-third of the thickness of the uterine wall
- *Stage II*: preoperative irradiation (intra-cavity ± external beam) followed by radical surgery
- *Stage III or IV*: treatment is individualized, depending upon the circumstances, but will probably include irradiation, with or without surgery

Chemotherapy/Hormonal Therapy

Disseminated or recurrent disease is usually treated with hormones, progestogens being the drug of choice. Cytotoxic drugs are largely ineffective and are not indicated because of their toxicity. Local recurrence may be treated by radiotherapy if this has not been used previously.

Outcome and Special Complications

Over two-thirds of patients survive long term, the chances of cure being closely related to stage at presentation (Table 5). Recurrence in the pelvis can pose problems that are difficult to palliate.

Table 5. 5-year survival by FIGO
stage for endometrial carcinoma from
eight collected studies

Stage	Surviving patients at 5 years		
	No.	%	% range in studies
I	2785*	84	76–96
II	309	57	32–79
III	282	36	4–61
IV	203	7	0–13
TOTAL	3579	78	–

*Note the great majority (82.5%) of
patients have stage I disease.

Selected Papers and Reviews

Gusberg, S.B. (1980) Current concepts in cancer: the changing nature of endometrial carcinoma. *New England Journal of Medicine*, **302**: 729–731.

McMahon, B. (1974) Risk factors for endometrial cancer. *Gynecologic Oncology* 2: 122–128.

Morrow, C.P. and Townsend, D.E. (1981) *Synopsis of Gynecologic Oncology*. John Wiley & Sons, Chichester, pp. 133–185.

Piver, M.S. and Malfetano, J.H. (1985) Management of carcinoma of the endometrium. In: *Cancer of the Female Reproductive System*, Williams, C.J. and Whitehouse, J.M.A. (eds.), John Wiley & Sons, Chichester, pp. 217–228.

Williams, C.J. (1986) Cervical, endometrial and vulval cancer. In: *Randomized Trials in Cancer: a Critical Review by Sites*, Slevin, M.L. and Staquet, M.J. (eds.), Raven Press, New York, pp. 417–446.

CERVICAL CANCER

Although cancer of the cervix is the commonest gynaecological cancer in Britain, only about 2000 women per annum in England and Wales die of this tumour. Although survival rates are relatively high, it is an important tumour since effective screening is available and we are learning more about its causes and hence about how it can be avoided.

Incidence and Epidemiology

There have been major changes in the incidence and mortality from cervical cancer in industrialized countries. These are shown clearly in Figure 24, which records the changes in mortality and incidence of invasive cancer and *in situ* cancer in the United

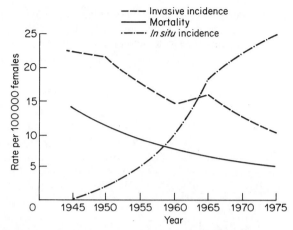

Figure 24. Incidence and mortality in cervical cancer in the United States. Taken from DiSaia, P.J. and Creasman, W.T. (1984), *Clinical Gynaecologic Oncology*, Second Edition. C.V. Mosby Missouri; reproduced by permission

States between 1945 and 1975. As can be seen, whilst there has been a progressive decline in both mortality and incidence of invasive tumours, there has, at the same time, been a dramatic increase in the incidence of *in situ* cervical cancer. The increase in cases of *in situ* cancer is undoubtedly due in part to the introduction of cervical screening. The fall in invasive tumours and mortality is probably due to this, though a number of other factors are clearly involved (see below).

Rates for cervical carcinoma vary widely around the world (Figure 25), low levels being found in Jewish women, whilst high levels are found in Third World countries.

Aetiology and Pathogenesis

Cancer of the cervix has many of the characteristics of a venereal disease. It is associated with:

- poor socioeconomic status
- early sexual activity
- multiple partners
- frequent pregnancy

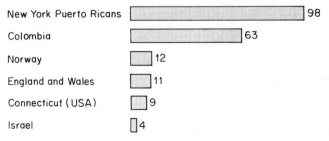

Figure 25. Incidence rates per 100,000 for cervical cancer around the world

Because of these findings infectious agents that could cause this cancer have been sought. Most of this research has centred on the herpesvirus HSV2 and more recently, and perhaps significantly, on the human papillomavirus (HPV).

Age at first intercourse may be important since it is thought that the drift of squamous epithelium, by a process of metaplasia, into the mucus-secreting columnar epithelium of the endocervix leaves an area of epithelial 'unrest'. This area may be susceptible to carcinogenic factors in young women soon after puberty. A second period of similar cellular activity may be associated with first pregnancy.

Currently there exist persuasive data that a virus (possibly human papillomavirus) may be involved in the development of this cancer, though multiple other steps may be necessary (see Chapter 3). An example of this is the recent finding that smoking may increase the risk of cervical cancer by reducing the number of Langerhan's cells in the cervix.

Pathology and Natural History

In situ lesions are now more common than invasive cancer. They are usually treated by ablation since it was thought that such areas automatically progressed to frank invasion. There is some evidence that this is not always the case. In several studies only one-third of untreated patients with *in situ* lesions developed invasive cancer during a follow-up period of up to 14 years. These data suggest that reduced mortality rates worldwide in industrialized countries are not simply a result of screening, though this has undoubtedly played an important part.

The precancerous lesions of the cervix are known collectively as cervical intraepithelial neoplasia (CIN). Carcinoma *in situ* is CIN3, there being a continuum from mild dysplasia (CIN1) through to frankly invasive cervical cancer.

Over 90% of cervical cancers are squamous cell carcinomas, other malignant tumours being adenocarcinoma, adenoacanthomas or sarcomas. Only squamous carcinomas are considered here.

Relatively early in its natural history cervical carcinoma invades lymphatics, metastasizing to pelvic wall and parametrial lymph nodes. As the tumour grows local invasion becomes more extensive, involving the bladder and eventually the rectum. There is with time diffuse involvement of pelvic and parametrial tissues. Spread to distant metastatic sites, primarily lung, is usually a late event.

Presenting Features

Where possible the diagnosis should be made at screening (see page 65) when the patient is asymptomatic. Recommendations for screening vary around the world. Many gynaecologists would accept that:

- screening should be started when a woman becomes sexually active
- screening should continue to age 65 years
- if negative, the test should be repeated every 3 years

The symptoms of invasive cervical cancer are shown in Figure 26. Overall, between 80 and 90% of patients will present with some form of abnormal vaginal bleeding.

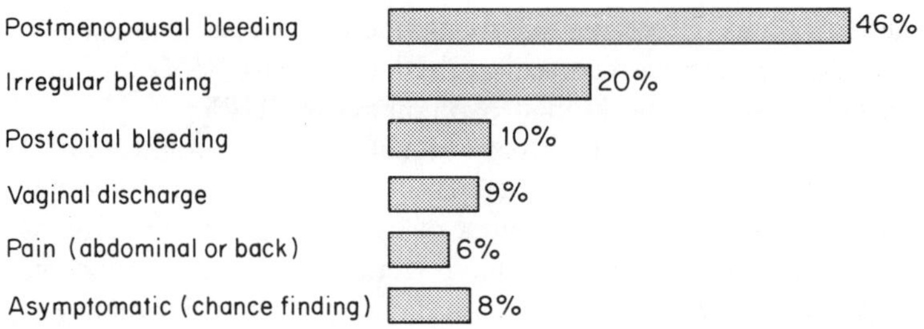

Postmenopausal bleeding ▏46%

Irregular bleeding ▏20%

Postcoital bleeding ▏10%

Vaginal discharge ▏9%

Pain (abdominal or back) ▏6%

Asymptomatic (chance finding) ▏8%

Urinary or rectal symptoms are uncommon but suggest locally extensive disease.

Figure 26. Incidence of symptoms of invasive cervical carcinoma

The great majority of patients have no abnormal findings on general physical examination. Gynaecological examination is of paramount importance. Vulvar and vaginal metastasis are uncommon but should be looked for. The cervix should be examined though it may look normal if there is a very small tumour or if it is endocervical in location. If tumour is identified the extent of invasion should be assessed.

Investigations and Staging

Any patient with a possible cervical carcinoma should be investigated by a gynaecologist. Work-up should, ideally, include colposcopy (direct microscopic examination of the cervix). If an invasive carcinoma is found additional investigations are:

- chest X-ray
- blood count and biochemistry
- intravenous pyelogram
- barium enema, lymphangiogram (Figure 27) in selected patients
- examination under anaesthetic

Staging is complicated (Table 6 and Figure 28) with multiple subgroups of increasing disease extent.

Treatment

The two keys to cure in these malignancies are early diagnosis and adequate local therapy to eradicate the tumour. Since there is a wide variety of different approaches according to stage, treatment will be discussed for each major stage rather than under the usual heading of surgery, radiotherapy, etc.

Staged-CIN

A variety of approaches are available for these premalignant lesions:

- conization (excision of the lesion with a cone of normal tissue)
- cryotherapy

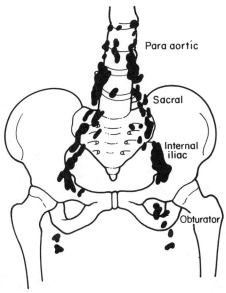

Figure 27. Lymphatic drainage of the cervix. Lymphatic involvement in carcinoma of the cervix generally occurs in an orderly progression from obturator up to para-aortic

Table 6. UICC staging of cervical cancer

Stage	Description
T_{IS}	Carcinoma *in situ*
T_1	Confined to cervix
T_{1a}	Microinvasive
T_{1b}	Invasive
T_2	Extension to vagina (not lower third)/parametrium/not pelvic wall
T_{2a}	Vagina (not lower third)
T_{2b}	Parametrium
T_3	Extension to lower third vagina/parametrium/pelvic wall
T_{3a}	Vagina/lower third
T_{3b}	Parametrium/pelvic wall
T_4	Extension to bladder/rectum/beyond true pelvis
M_1	Distant organs

- laser therapy
- hysterectomy

Their use depends on the detailed colposcopy finding, local custom and availability of equipment.

318

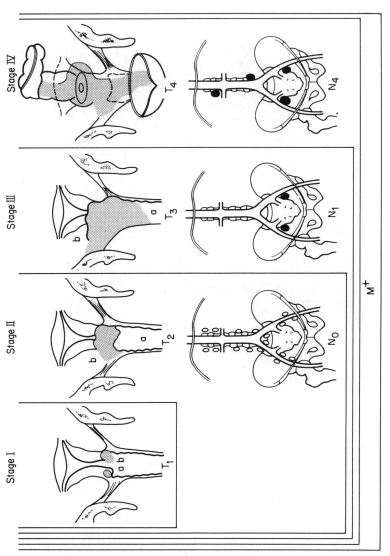

Figure 28. Staging for cervix cancer. Tumour (T) categories: The extent and depth of invasion are the critical factors. Node (N) categories: Only location is considered. There are no N_2 or N_3 categories. Stage grouping: Each T category determines stage; evidence of involved nodes or metastases also indicates stage. Modified from Rubin, P. *et al.* (1983) *Clinical Oncology: a multidisciplinary approach*, 6th edition, American Cancer Society. Reproduced by permission

Stage IA (Microinvasive Cancer)

If, after careful assessment, the cancer is truly microinvasive, simple hysterectomy is all that is required. If there is doubt treat as IB.

Stages IB and IIA

Surgery and radiotherapy are equally effective. Radiotherapy is given by intra-cavity insertion (Figure 29) and external beam. Surgery is radical—a Wertheim's hysterectomy.

Stages IIB–IIIB

Radiotherapy is the treatment of choice. Surgery may also be used in conjunction with irradiation.

Stage IV

Cure is rarely possible—radiotherapy is the mainstay of treatment.

Recurrent or Disseminated Disease

Selected patients with local recurrence may be cured with irradiation if initially treated surgically.

Chemotherapy produces responses in 30–60% of cases, but so far there is little evidence that patients live longer. Because of encouraging responses, trials of new chemotherapy approaches continue, though their place in routine management is so far doubtful.

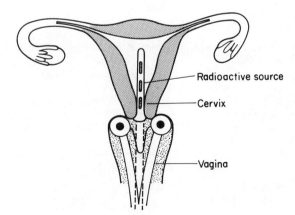

Figure 29. Typical disposable after-loading system of intra-cavitary irradiation in carcinoma of the cervix

Outcome and Special Complications

Outcome is closely related to stage (Figure 30). Complications are common and relate to the tumour itself and also result from surgery and radiotherapy. They include:

- fistulae
- haemorrhage and discharge
- bowel damage from irradiation
- pelvic pain (bone and nerves)
- fibrous cystitis (irradiation)
- bowel obstruction
- bladder involvement
- pulmonary and bone metastasis
- oedema of leg(s)

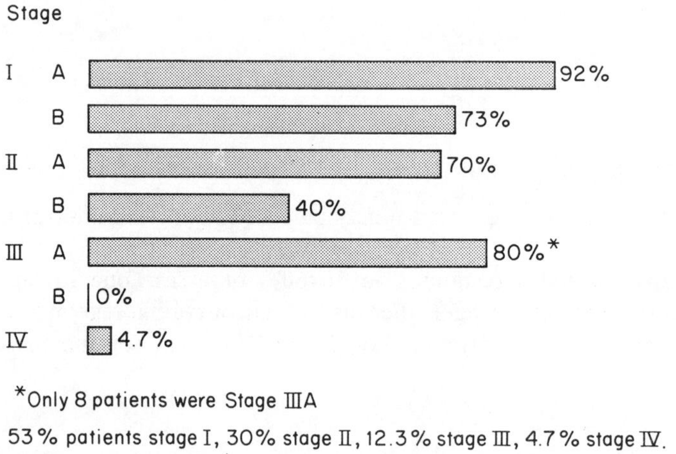

Stage

```
I    A  [================================] 92%
     B  [=========================] 73%
II   A  [========================] 70%
     B  [============] 40%
III  A  [=============================] 80%*
     B  |0%
IV      [] 4.7%
```

*Only 8 patients were Stage IIIA

53% patients stage I, 30% stage II, 12.3% stage III, 4.7% stage IV.

Figure 30. Five-year survival for cervical cancer: a series involving 869 patients (reproduced by permission from Shingleton *et al.*, 1979 University of Alabama)

Selected Papers and Reviews

Anderson, M. (1976) The aetiology and pathology of carcinoma of the cervix. *Clinical Obstetrics and Gynecology*, 3: 317–337.

Chamberlaine, G. (1981) Aetiology of gynaecological cancer. *Journal of the Royal Society of Medicine*, **74**: 246–261.

Guzick, D.S. (1978) Efficacy of screening for cervical cancer: a review. *American Journal of Public Health*, **68**: 125–134.

Morrow, C.P. and Townsend, D.E. (1981) *Synopsis of Gynecologic Oncology.* John Wiley & Sons, New York, pp. 61–132.

Williams, C.J. (1986) Cervical, endometrial and vulvar cancer. In: *Randomized Trials in Cancer: a Critical Review by Site*, Slevin, M.L. and Staquet, M.J. (eds.), Raven Press, New York, pp. 417–446.

16 Urogenital Cancers

C. J. WILLIAMS

BLADDER CANCER

The incidence of bladder cancer in men is three-fold that in women, probably reflecting work exposure to carcinogens. Mortality has remained unchanged in the past 40 years, though incidence has increased.

Incidence and Epidemiology

The incidence rate rises with age in both men and women (Figure 1). The rates are modestly variable with a six-fold difference between areas of lowest and highest incidence (Figure 2).

Aetiology and Pathogenesis

At the end of the last century it became clear that workers in the aniline dye industry were at much higher risk of this tumour than workers in other industries—one of the earliest demonstrations of a carcinogen, later identified as β-naphthylamine. In western countries exposure to carcinogens remains important, the main aetiological factors being:

- aniline dye—used in rubber and cable industry; there is a long latent interval (10–20 years)
- β-naphthylamine, 4-amino diphenyl and tobacco tar cause bladder cancer in animals. There is strong evidence that cigarette smoking may at least potentiate the risk (smokers have twice the incidence rate of non-smokers)

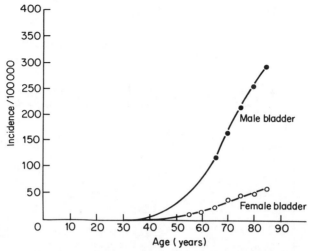

Figure 1. Incidence of bladder cancer by age in England and Wales

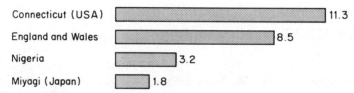

Figure 2. Age standardized incidence rates (per 100,000) for male bladder cancer around the world

- chronic bladder infections or calculi may lead to squamous cancer of the bladder. *Schistosoma haematobium* is the commonest infectious cause.

Pathology and Natural History

In western countries about 90% of tumours are derived from transitional epithelium (Figure 3). Where schistosomal infections are common, such as Egypt, squamous carcinoma is much more common. The discussion of management in this section is directed towards the common transitional tumours.

The natural history of bladder cancer is very variable; some tumours are of low grade and locally recurrent whilst others are anaplastic and invade locally in an aggressive fashion as well as spreading to distant sites.

Presenting Features

Haematuria is the cardinal symptom of bladder cancer; it is usually painless (Figure 4). Routine testing for microscopic haematuria may be used as a screening procedure in industries where workers are at potential risk of bladder cancer.

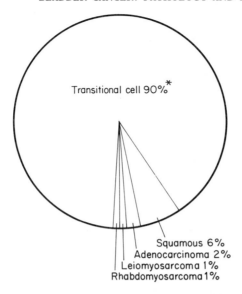

Transitional cell 90%*

Squamous 6%
Adenocarcinoma 2%
Leiomyosarcoma 1%
Rhabdomyosarcoma 1%

* About 20% of transitional tumours contain foci
of squamous cell carcinoma or adenomatous features

Figure 3. Pathology of bladder cancer in western countries

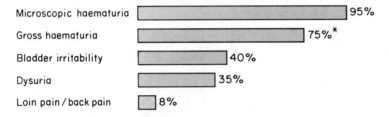

Microscopic haematuria   95%

Gross haematuria   75%*

Bladder irritability   40%

Dysuria   35%

Loin pain / back pain   8%

*Haematuria is usually intermittent.

Figure 4. Common symptoms of bladder cancer

There are generally no abnormal findings on clinical examination. Despite this lack
of signs, haematuria, even one episode, should be fully investigated.

Spread

This depends very much on the biological characteristics of the tumour, histologically
demonstrated by grade and depth of penetration of tumour (see staging system below).
Sites of distant spread are draining lymph nodes, lung, liver and bone.

Investigations and Staging

When bladder cancer is suspected or if unexplained haematuria occurs, some or all of
the following investigations should be undertaken:

- cystoscopy with biopsy
- rectal and bimanual palpation (EUA)
- urinary cytology
- intravenous pyelogram
- biochemical assessment of renal function
- full blood count

If cancer is found, some centres will also perform CT imaging and lymphography.

There are, unfortunately, several staging systems though they all take the same general approach—assessing the tumour by the TNM system with a special emphasis on depth of tumour penetration. Since clinical staging is rather imprecise, greater emphasis should be laid on surgical staging (Figure 5). Patients may be grouped into various stages (A–D) according to their TNM characteristics (Figure 6). The most important distinction to be made is that between T_2 and T_3 tumour, since the prognosis worsens dramatically as the depth of penetration increases.

Treatment

A variety of therapies are available. Choice of appropriate treatment depends on:

- stage and grade of tumour
- location of the lesion

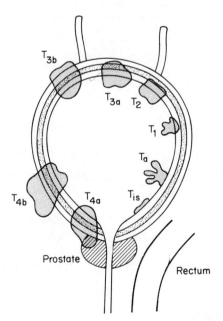

Figure 5. T staging of bladder cancer. T_{is}: *in situ* carcinoma; T_a: non-invasive papillary carcinoma; T_1: limited to lamina propria; T_2: superficial muscle involvement; T_{3a}: deep muscle involvement; T_{3b}: full thickness of bladder wall; T_{4a}: invading neighbouring structures (prostate, vagina); T_{4b}: involvement of rectum, fixed to pelvic wall

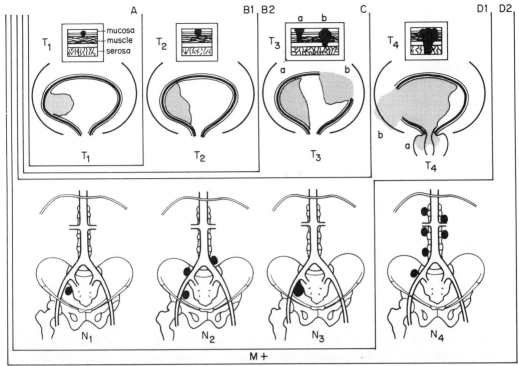

Figure 6. Anatomical staging for bladder carcinoma. Tumour (T) categories: The depth of invasion is the important criterion and follows that of hollow viscera. Size and location, though important, are not critical factors. Progression is to muscle and then serosa, then to pelvis or abdominal wall for T_1, T_2, T_3 and T_4, respectively. Node (N) categories: The regional nodes are defined by single vs. multiple, ipsilateral vs. bilateral for N_1 vs. N_2. Fixed nodes are N_3 and para-aortic nodes are juxtaregional. Stage grouping is used in some systems (A–D). Adapted from P. Rubin *et al.* (1983). *Clinical Oncology: a multidisciplinary approach*, 6th edition. American Cancer Society

- general health of patient
- other genito-urinary problems.

Surgery

The type of operation to be used depends on the particular situation (especially stage and grade). Options are:

- Endoscopic resection and fulguration—used for diagnosis and treatment of superficial or multiple tumours and control of bleeding.
- Segmental bladder resection—for large single lesions on the dome of the bladder or lateral wall.
- Total cystectomy with urinary diversion—used for large tumours or those which are invasive, anaplastic or involve the trigone and when there is no evidence of metastatic disease.

Radiotherapy

Radiation is often used in conjunction with surgery. Although there have not been randomized trials which have demonstrated benefit for this approach, many centres use combined modality treatment for selected patients. Some hospitals have tested radical radiotherapy (6000 cGy in 6 weeks) alone against a lower dose of radiation and cystectomy. Survival in the Royal Marsden Hospital and other studies suggests an advantage for the combined modality group, though the difference does not achieve statistical significance.

Complications of irradiation to the bladder include:

- immediate bladder irritation—depends on degree of bladder involvement, infection and prostatic hypertrophy
- persistent cystitis
- fibrotic contracted bladder
- haemorrhage of bladder
- ileitis and colitis

Chemotherapy

Several drugs, used individually, induce responses in 20–30% of patients, and recently much improved results have been claimed for combinations. These are now being tested in phase III trials, not only for metastatic disease but also as an adjuvant in high-risk patients. Until definitive evidence is available from these trials, chemotherapy cannot be considered to be a routine treatment. Drugs may also be given directly into the bladder (intravesical therapy) to treat extensive superficial disease within the bladder.

Outcome and Special Complications

The choice of optimal therapy is still controversial. Discussions about the relative merits of surgery, radical radiotherapy or combined modality therapy for patients with aggressive tumours continue. Attitudes may need to be adjusted if current trials of adjuvant chemotherapy demonstrate improved survival.

Survival rates are closely correlated with stage (Figure 7).

In common with other pelvic tumours, uncontrolled disease may lead to unpleasant complications, which include:

- haematuria
- pelvic pain
- fistulae
- renal failure

Selected Papers and Reviews

Bloom, H. J. G., Hendry, W. F., *et al.* (1982) Treatment of T$_3$ bladder cancer; controlled trial of pre-operative radiotherapy and radical cystectomy versus radical radiotherapy. *British*

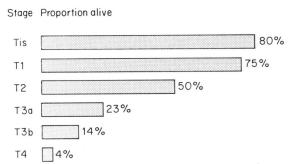

Stage   Proportion alive

Tis   80%
T1   75%
T2   50%
T3a   23%
T3b   14%
T4   4%

Figure 7. Survival at 5 years by T stage at diagnosis (Memorial Sloan-Kettering Cancer Centre, New York)

Journal of Urology, **54**: 136–151.
Denis, L., Dalesio, D. and Van Dosterom, A. T. (1986) Bladder carcinoma. In: *Randomized Trials in Cancer: A Critical Review by Sites*, Slevin, M. L. and Staquet, P. (ed.s), Raven Press, New York, pp. 645–660.
Rubin, P. (1968) Cancer of the urogenital tract: bladder cancer—incidence, frequency, aetiological factors. *Journal of the American Medical Association*, **206**: 1761–1776.
Soloway, M. S. (1980) The management of superficial bladder cancer. *Cancer*, **45**: 1856–1865.
Whitmore, F. Jr. (1979) Management of bladder cancer. *Cur Probl. Cancer* **4**: 3–48.
Wynder, E. L. and Goldsmith, R. (1977) The epidemiology of bladder cancer—a second look. *Cancer*, **40**: 1246–1268.

CANCER OF THE KIDNEY

Malignant tumours of the kidney account for about 3.0% of all cancers. The behaviour and management of renal tumours in children (Wilms' tumour or nephroblastoma) are very different from adults and are considered in Chapter 10. Tumours of the ureter and renal pelvis are usually transitional cell tumours and behave more like bladder cancer, though their prognosis is poor as early spread from such a small organ is common.

Incidence and Epidemiology

There are about 450 new renal cancers in adults in the UK each year; the figure for the United States is 2000 per annum. This gives an incidence rate of about 4 per 100,000 in both countries.

Renal cancers are more common in men than women (2.5:1), and incidence increases with age, though most patients are aged between 50 and 70. There is only a modest variation in incidence in different countries (Figure 8). About 1% of renal cancers are bilateral.

Aetiology and Pathogenesis

The aetiology of most cases remains obscure. The predominance in men suggests an environmental factor, and there is evidence that renal cancer is more common in

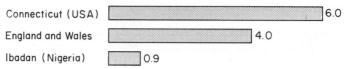

Connecticut (USA)	6.0
England and Wales	4.0
Ibadan (Nigeria)	0.9

Figure 8. Variation in incidence of kidney cancer around the world (males per 100,000)

smokers. Heavy cigarette smokers have a risk which is five-fold that of non-smokers. Interestingly, unlike lung cancer, the risk is also increased in cigar smokers and in men who chew tobacco. There is a clear-cut association between renal cell cancer and von Hippel-Lindau syndrome (cerebellar and retinal haemangioblastomas with phaeochromocytoma). About one in three patients with this syndrome develop renal carcinoma. A higher incidence is also seen in obese women.

Recently a family with a high incidence of bilateral renal cancer in three generations has been shown to have a chromosomal abnormality (reciprocal translocation of chromosomes 3 and 8). In summary, the causative factors in renal cell cancer are unknown in most cases; however, the following are important in some cases:

- smoking
- obesity in women (? hormonal effect)
- von Hippel-Lindau syndrome
- chromosomal abnormalities (t[3;8][14;q24])

Pathology and Natural History

Nearly all adult tumours of the parenchyma are renal cell adenocarcinomas. The old term hypernephroma is now inappropriate since there is no evidence that these tumours arise from adrenal rests.

Most tumours are diagnosed relatively late. Median survival is about 18 months, though late relapse may occur.

Presenting Features

Patients may present with a wide variety of symptoms and signs (Figure 9). Haematuria may be microscopic or minimal but is common. Loin pain usually indicates local spread or pelvic obstruction. The classic triad of haematuria, mass and pain only occurs in 10% of cases. Symptoms may sometimes be present for a long period before diagnosis. Non-specific symptoms such as fever, weight loss and anaemia are relatively common, whilst specific paraneoplastic phenomena, such as polycythaemia (caused by erythropoietin production), are rare. Liver function tests may be abnormal when there are no hepatic metastases; these may return to normal when the primary cancer is removed.

In addition, patients may present with symptoms and signs of metastatic disease:

- lung—cough and/or haemoptysis
- bone—fracture or pain

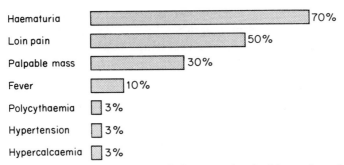

Haematuria	70%
Loin pain	50%
Palpable mass	30%
Fever	10%
Polycythaemia	3%
Hypertension	3%
Hypercalcaemia	3%

Figure 9. Incidence of symptoms and signs associated with renal carcinoma

- spinal cord or brain
- liver

Spread

The disease spreads by local invasion to adjacent structures and to distant sites via the bloodstream and lymphatics (Figure 10). In up to half of cases there is involvement

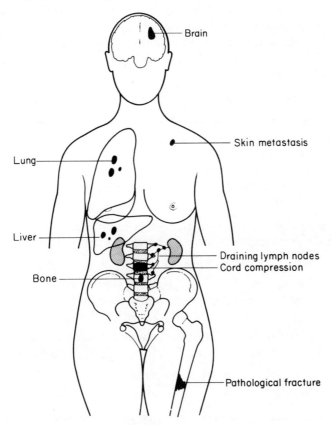

Figure 10. Sites of spread of cancer of the kidney

of the perinephric fat. Local extension into adjacent viscera and the adrenal occur in 10% of cases. Renal vein invasion is seen in 30% of cases and extension of thrombosis into the inferior vena cava in 10%. Regional lymph node involvement is seen in about 20% of patients undergoing nephrectomy.

Investigations and Staging

Three-quarters of patients present with urological symptoms, though in up to 10% of cases the tumour is found incidentally. Investigations used to make the diagnosis include:

- Urinalysis—microscopic haematuria.
- Intravenous pyelogram—may reveal pelvocalyceal displacement suggestive of a mass in the kidney. Renal calcification is present in 5% of tumours.
- Ultrasonography—particularly helpful in differentiating solid from cystic lesions.
- CT scan—useful in delineating the mass and looking for nodal spread and involvement of the veins.
- Renal arteriogram—less often required with the introduction of the non-invasive techniques described above.
- Biopsy of the lesion under ultrasound or CT guidance. These are vascular tumours and some surgeons prefer to go straight to laparotomy.

If cancer is confirmed the following additional tests may be needed:

- chest X-ray—though thoracic CT is a much more sensitive method of detecting lung metastases
- isotopic bone scan
- Full blood count and biochemistry
- Liver ultrasound may be used if biochemistry suggests involvement

Staging is based on the TNM system, though there is no internationally accepted standard (Table 1). A simplified system is shown in Figure 11.

Treatment

Surgical excision is the optimum treatment, though difficulties may be encountered when there is a horseshoe kidney or in the case of bilateral renal cancer.

Surgery

Radical nephrectomy with lymph node dissection is the treatment of choice for patients with stage II–III disease. For more advanced disease, a palliative nephrectomy may

Table 1. Tumour (T) node (N) classification of kidney cancer

Classification	Description
T_1	Small tumour (<2.5 cm) no enlargement of kidney
T_2	Large tumour (>2.5 cm) cortex not broken
T_3	Perinephric or hilar extension. Venous involvement
T_4	Extension to neighbouring organs
N_1	Single homolateral regional (<2 cm)
N_2	Contra- or bilateral/multiple regional
N_3	Fixed regional
N_4	Juxtaregional

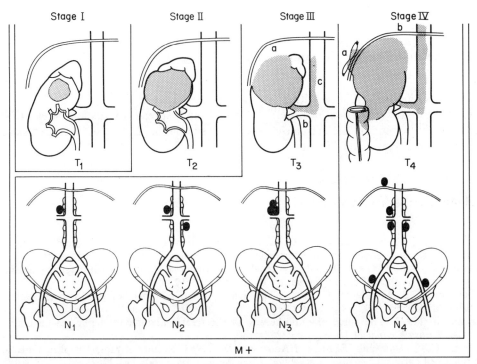

Figure 11. Staging for renal carcinoma. Tumour (T) categories: Extension through the renal capsule and renal vein is the major type of advancement. Node (N) categories: Advancement of nodal disease in the regional nodes (para-aortic) is: single homolateral (N_1), multiple and bilateral (N_2), fixed nodes (N_3) and juxtaregional (N_4)

be indicated for control of bleeding and pain. Long-term survival has occasionally been reported following nephrectomy and resection of a solitary metastasis. There is no good evidence that metastases regress when the primary is removed, despite extensive anecdotal data.

Radiotherapy

Radiation has a limited role in treatment of this tumour. Routine use pre- or post-operatively is controversial, studies in general not showing improved survival or lower local relapse rates. Palliative treatment for metastatic disease to bone, spine and brain can be helpful for selected patients.

Chemotherapy

This is one of the most chemoresistant of all tumours. There is no role for routine cytotoxic therapy. Hormones (progestogens) were reported to be useful in the early 1970s; but since then large trials have shown responses in less than 5% of patients. Immunotherapy and more recently interleukins have been used with some success but remain entirely experimental.

Outcome and Special Complications

Survival is closely correlated with stage at diagnosis (Figure 12).

Complications are those of local recurrence and spread to distant sites. CNS involvement is common and can cause devastating symptoms. Lung and bone metastases are frequent in advanced disease.

Selected Papers and Reviews

Bennington, J. R. and Laubscher, F. A. (1978) Epidemiologic studies on carcinoma of the kidney. I. Association of renal adenocarcinoma with smoking. *Cancer*, **21**: 1069–1071.

Cohen, A. J. *et al.* (1979) Hereditary renal cell carcinoma associated with a chromosomal translocation. *New England Journal of Medicine*, **301**: 592–595.

Dekernion, J. B. and Berry, D. (1980) The diagnosis and treatment of renal cancer. *Cancer*, **45**: 1947–1956.

Finney, R. (1973) The value of radiotherapy in the treatment of hypernephroma—a clinical trial. *British Journal of Urology*, **45**: 258–269.

Robson, C. C., Churchill, B. M. and Anderson, W. (1968) Results of radical nephrectomy for renal cell carcinoma. *Trans. Am. Assoc. Genitourinary Surg.*, **60**: 112–126.

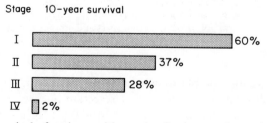

Figure 12. Survival of patients with renal cell adenocarcinoma by stage

CANCER OF THE PROSTATE

The incidence of malignant tumours of the prostate is second only to that of lung cancer in men. The reported clinical incidence of this tumour, however, underestimates the number of cases; autopsy studies have shown cancer is present in the prostate of 14–46% of men over 50 years of age.

Incidence and Epidemiology

Prostatic cancer is the third leading cause of malignant death in England and Wales, the incidence rising rapidly with age above 50 years (Figure 13). There is a wide variation around the world, highest rates being seen in US blacks and lowest among the Japanese (Figure 14). Data concerning Japanese emigrating to Hawaii suggest that the variation is due to environmental factors, as their rate rises to approach that of Caucasians. Data from the United States show a much higher incidence in blacks than in whites.

Aetiology and Pathogenesis

Prostatic cancer is uncommon before 50 years of age, but rapidly increases in incidence in successive decades, doubling in incidence with each 5-year increment in age. The discrepancy between incidence rates and autopsy findings suggests a quiescent period

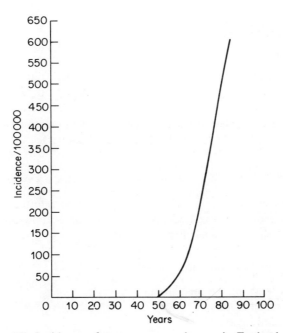

Figure 13. Incidence of prostate cancer by age in England and Wales

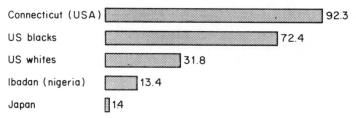

Figure 14. Incidence of prostatic cancer around the world (per 100,000)

of several decades between malignant transformation and the clinical detection of cancer.

The aetiology of this disease is obscure. A hormonal basis has been suggested by experimental and clinical data but much remains to be learned. Factors that may be relevant include:

- Prostatic cancer does not occur in castrated men and is uncommon in hepatic cirrhosis where oestrogen metabolism may be abnormal.
- It has been suggested that the incidence is higher in men who are sexually more active.

Studies have failed to demonstrate any variation in incidence by socio-economic status, educational achievement, alcohol consumption or cigarette smoking. Any relationship between benign prostatic hypertrophy and prostatic cancer remains speculative.

Pathology and Natural History

Nearly all cases are adenocarcinomas, though occasionally transitional cell tumours are seen. Three-quarters of tumours arise in the posterior or peripheral part of the prostate gland. Histological grade is important, though the majority of tumours are well or moderately differentiated. Five-year survival for poorly differentiated tumours is only 5% compared with 60% for well-differentiated cancers.

Presenting Features

This tumour is often asymptomatic when diagnosed, being found on routine rectal examination. One half of prostatic nodules felt on rectal examination turn out to be malignant. Classically the gland feels firm, indurated or craggy with obliteration of the median sulcus.

Symptoms of early presentation are:

- difficulty in starting urinary stream
- urinary tract infections
- terminal dribbling
- bladder retention

Advanced presentation includes these symptoms:

- bladder outlet obstruction with retention
- ureteral obstruction with anuria
- renal failure
- anaemia
- weight loss and anorexia
- bone pain

Spread

This tumour infiltrates locally as well as spreading by draining lymphatics and the bloodstream. The prime site for distant metastatic disease is the skeleton. The pelvis, lumbar vertebrae, ribs and skull are the bones most often affected. Typically the metastases are osteosclerotic, though lytic lesions are also seen.

Investigations and Staging

Tissue from the lesion is needed to make the diagnosis; this can be done by transrectal needle biopsy. If tumour is found some or all of these tests may be used:

- full blood count and biochemistry
- isotopic bone scan
- X-rays of bone
- intravenous pyelogram
- ultrasound or CT scan to assess local extent of tumour
- blood for prostatic acid phosphatase
- creatinine phosphokinase

There is no universally accepted staging system, though the available ones are similar in concept. A simplified system is shown in Table 2 and Figure 15.

Treatment

There are no commonly accepted approaches to the treatment of the various stages of prostatic cancer; indeed, controversy has raged for many years. Although radical treatment is used for clinically localized disease, much of the debate surrounds the extent of surgery needed for patients with early stage disease (T1).

Surgery

For relatively young men with well-circumscribed tumours and without bone metastases, radical prostatectomy may be used. This has been the treatment of choice for such patients in some centres in the United States. The operation may be done by several routes (transpubic, retropubic or perineal). Some surgeons have carried out a pelvic

Table 2. Tumour (T), node (N) classification for prostate cancer

Classification	Description
T_0	Incidental carcinoma
T_1	Intracapsular/normal gland
T_2	Intracapsular/deformed gland
T_3	Extension beyond capsule
T_4	Extension fixed to neighbouring organs
N_1	Single homolateral regional
N_2	Contra- or bilateral/multiple regional
N_3	Fixed regional
N_4	Juxtaregional
M_0	No metastatic disease
M_1	Metastatic disease

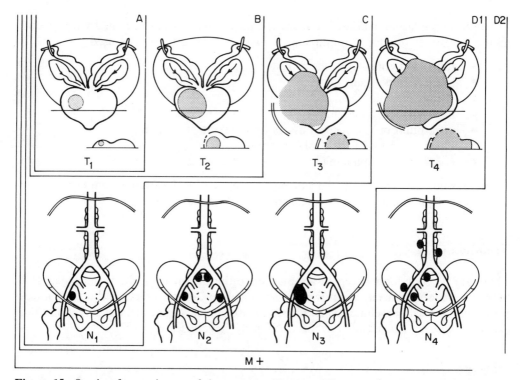

Figure 15. Staging for carcinoma of the prostate. Tumour (T) categories: The extension of the cancer beyond the capsule (not size), and to surrounding structures determines the T category. Node (N) categories: The regional nodes are pelvic nodes and advancement is measured from single homolateral (N_1) to multiple homolateral (N_2) to fixed nodules (N_3), and juxtaregional or para-aortic (N_4). Stage groupings: This follows the T categories

lymphadenectomy, though there are no data to suggest that this improves survival rates.

These surgical procedures will cause impotence in all patients and incontinence in about 10% of patients. However, only relatively few patients (8%) are suitable for radical surgery.

Radiotherapy

The normal prostate tolerates high doses of radiation well, though surrounding tissues are radiosensitive. Although interstitial implants of radium have been used, external beam treatment is generally preferred. High doses (6000 cGy over 6 weeks) are delivered to the prostatic bed, with a lower dose to the rest of the pelvis. Recently, the use of radio-iodine (I-125) has renewed interest in interstitial therapy. Side-effects of irradiation include long-term bladder fibrosis and urethral stricture as well as the acute effects of treatment. Impotence is usually avoided.

Hormonal Therapy

Patients who are not candidates for surgery or irradiation may be treated by hormonal means. The options (Figure 16) include:

- orchidectomy
- oestrogens (low doses reduce the cardiovascular side-effects)
- anti-androgens
- LHRH agonists
- aminoglutethimide (peripheral aromatase inhibitor)

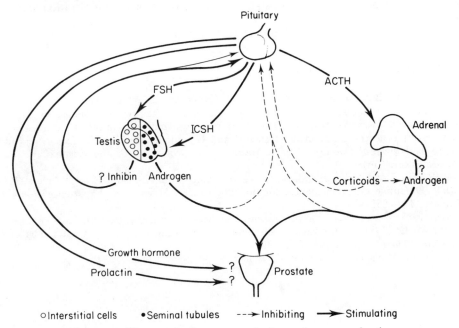

Figure 16. Hormonal effects on testicular androgen production

Orchidectomy is probably the treatment of choice since it is simple, cheap and free of side-effects apart from impotence (a feature of the other hormonal treatments). About three-quarters of patients respond to such treatment, bone pain being particularly helped. When a patient relapses from one hormonal manoeuvre, another may be tried though the success rate will be lower.

Chemotherapy

There is no standard cytotoxic treatment available. Few patients respond usefully and such treatment cannot be recommended. Recently, radioactive strontium (which is taken up by bone) has been used to treat generalized bone metastasis with some success.

Outcome and Special Complications

Prognosis depends very much on stage at presentation. Five-year survival rates of 60% have been claimed for selected patients with early disease treated surgically or with irradiation. However, late relapse is common. Median survival of patients with advanced disease is about 2 years. It is difficult to know how much treatment of early disease influences survival. In a review of patients with clinically recognized stage I disease treated by placebo, radical prostatectomy, or oestrogen and prostatectomy, Byar found a minimal difference in time to disease progression but no difference in survival. Moreover, survival for patients found to have focal cancer in a resection specimen of prostate (removed for hypertrophy) is similar to an age-matched group.

The problems of uncontrolled prostate cancer are those of local infiltration and bone metastases.

Selected Papers and Reviews

Bagshaw, M. A., Ray, G. R., Pistenma, D. A., Castellino, R. A. and Meares, E. M. (1975) External beam radiation therapy of primary carcinoma of the prostate. *Cancer*, 36: 723–728.

Byar, D. P. (1980) Review of the Veterans Administration studies of cancer of the prostate and new results concerning treatment of stage I and II tumours. In: *Bladder Tumors and Other Topics in Urological Oncology*, Parone-Macaluso, M., Smith, J. P. and Edsmyo, F. (eds.), Plenum, New York.

Cupps, R. E., Utz, D. L., Flemings, T. R., Carson, C. C., Zinckle, H. and Myers, R. A. (1980) Definitive radiation therapy for prostatic cancer; Mayo Clinic Experience. *Journal of Urology*, 124: 855–859.

Editorial (1985) Dilemmas in the management of prostatic cancer. *Lancet* ii: 1219.

Resnick, M. E. (1981) Non-invasive techniques in evaluating patients with carcinoma of the prostate. *Journal of Urology*, 17: 25–30.

Various (1980) Management of prostatic cancer. Supplement to *Cancer*, 45.

CANCER OF THE TESTIS

Although relatively rare, testicular cancer is of particular importance as it is the commonest cancer in young men (15–35 years), is increasing in incidence and is highly curable even when there is metastatic spread.

Incidence and Epidemiology

Cancer of the testis accounts for 1% of all male malignancies. The average age of onset is 27 years, there being a bimodal pattern of incidence by age (Figure 17). Teratomas are seen in younger men (peak incidence 18–30 years), whilst seminomas are seen in a slightly older group (peak incidence 30–45 years). The small second peak (50–60 years) is mainly seminomas, though occasionally lymphoma is found in this age group.

The incidence of testicular tumours has been rising for the past 40 years in western countries (Figure 18). Incidence figures in England and Wales (3.8 per 100,000) are very similar to those in the United States. North American figures show that testicular tumours are less common in blacks and orientals than in Caucasians. Worldwide variation in incidence is relatively small in western countries though markedly lower rates are seen in some less prosperous nations. Highest rates are seen in Denmark and lowest in Nigeria and Jamaica (Figure 19). This type of cancer is more common in men of higher socio-economic groups.

Aetiology and Pathogenesis

Little is known about the aetiology of this tumour apart from an association with maldescent of the testis:

- Men with a maldescended testis have a ten-fold increase in risk of testis cancer.

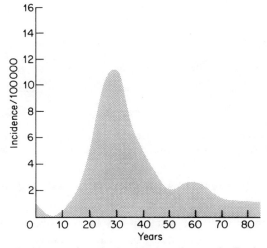

Figure 17. Incidence of testicular tumours by age in England and Wales

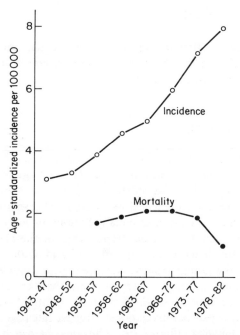

Figure 18. Age-standardized average annual incidence rates (○) and mortality rates (●) of testicular cancer in Denmark, 1943–1982 (Reproduced by permission from A. Østerlind (1986). *Br. J. Cancer*, **53**, 501–505). Despite a rising incidence of testicular cancer, mortality is falling because treatment has improved so much

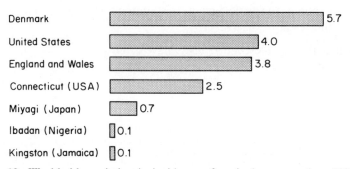

Figure 19. Worldwide variation in incidence of testicular cancer (per 100,000)

- This risk also applies to the contralateral testis in men with unilateral maldescent.
- 24% of men with bilateral cryptorchidism and a testicular cancer go on to develop a second tumour in the contralateral testis.

This suggests that cancer may not just develop because the maldescended testis is affected in such a way as to induce cancer, but that the cancer-causing events can lead to both maldescent and cancer.

So far, epidemiological studies have failed to explain the increasing incidence. One possible explanation of the link between maldescent, testicular cancer and its increasing incidence, is that it is related to increasing maternal weight during pregnancy. There is a correlation between maternal weight at birth and maldescent of the testis (which is increasing in incidence)—possibly due to altered oestrogen metabolism during pregnancy. Such altered steroid metabolism might also cause a germinal defect which could result in cancer in later life. This theory is unproven but illustrates how a subtle change in way of life might induce cancer in an indirect fashion.

Pathology and Natural History

Ninety-four percent of testicular malignancies are of germ cell origin (just the opposite to the situation in ovarian cancer). Non-germinal tumours (lymphoma, sarcoma, Sertoli and Leydig cell tumours) are all exceedingly rare and will not be considered further. There are several different histopathological classifications: the two most commonly used in Britain and the United States are shown in Table 3. Carcinoma *in situ* is found in the contralateral testis of some patients with a malignant germ cell tumour.

Rarely, germ cell tumours develop in extragonadal sites; these include the retroperitoneum, mediastinum and pineal gland; they will not be discussed further. The natural history of gonadal seminoma is very different to that of testicular teratoma—see 'Spread' and 'Treatment' below.

Presenting Features

The great majority of patients present with a simple testicular swelling. This is often painless, though pain by no means rules out the diagnosis. Unfortunately, all too often this mass is diagnosed as epididymitis and is treated with antibiotics, thereby wasting valuable time. The finding of a mass in a testis is always reason for referral to a urologist rather than a therapeutic trial of an antibiotic. Sometimes the testicular swelling may be masked by a concomitant hydrocoel.

Other important symptoms include:

- breast enlargement and tenderness—suggests raised β-human chorionic gonadotrophin levels (β-HCG)
- back pain—a sign of extensive retroperitoneal spread

Table 3. Histopathological classification of testicular germ cell malignancies and their frequencies

Classification		Frequency
British testicular tumour panel	Dixon and Moore (USA)	
Seminoma	Pure seminoma	40%
Malignant teratoma undifferentiated	Embryonal carcinoma	25%
Malignant teratoma intermediate	Teratoma with malignant areas	25%
Malignant teratoma trophoblastic	Choriocarcinoma	2%
Teratoma differentiated	Teratoma	6%

Other symptoms due to distant spread (CNS involvement and extensive lung metastases) are uncommon.

On examination there is usually a firm scrotal mass that cannot be separated from the testis and which does not transilluminate. If disease is advanced an abdominal mass of retroperitoneal lymph nodes may be found as well as supraclavicular adenopathy. Signs of distant metastatic disease at other sites are uncommon.

Spread

This tumour spreads by two main routes:

- lymphatic
- blood-borne

Local invasion is less important and scrotal involvement is rare, unless transcrotal biopsy has been done erroneously. Sites of metastases are shown in Figure 20.

Seminomas spread by the lymphatic route; bloodstream spread is really very uncommon. This means that metastases are much more regional in nature—an important factor in planning treatment.

Although teratomas also frequently spread via lymphatics, blood-borne spread is common. It may occur in the setting of extensive lymph node involvement but is sometimes found in the absence of lymphatic metastases.

Choriocarcinoma is more likely to spread to the brain than the other types of teratoma. If choriocarcinoma is suspected (very high β-HCG or breast enlargement) biopsy of liver metastases is absolutely contraindicated since these tumours are highly vascular.

Investigations and Staging

When a patient presents with a testicular mass that may be cancer, the first investigation is to estimate the levels of potential tumour markers—β-HCG; alpha-fetoprotein (AFP); placental alkaline phosphatase (PLAP). This should be done prior to surgery since the levels will start to fall after operation. If the clinical diagnosis is not clear-cut a testicular ultrasound scan may help.

Once it seems likely that the mass may be cancer, an exploratory operation should be done. The testis is inspected through an inguinal incision and radically excised if a tumour is found. Trans-scrotal biopsy or excision are always contraindicated.

If cancer is confirmed the following tests are needed:

- bi-weekly tumour markers
- assessment of retroperitoneal lymph nodes (CT image or lymphangiography)
- chest X-ray and, if normal, CT scan of thorax

Other investigations are done if indicated by a likelihood of disease at other sites.

As with so many other tumours there is a plethora of different staging systems. Although they have much in common the details are different, making comparison of results very difficult. In general these classifications avoid the TNM notation. The

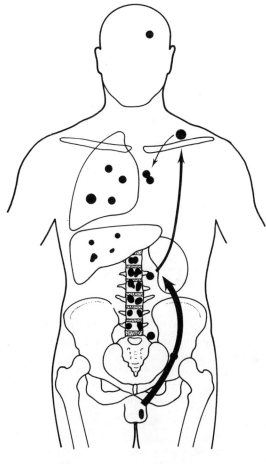

Spread
Along lymphatics of cord to the para-aortic
nodes and then to mediastinal and
supraclavicular nodes; and by blood to
lung and finally to liver, brain and other sites

Figure 20. Spread of testicular germ cell tumours and sites of metastasis

system developed by the Royal Marsden Hospital is widely used around the world, though not in the United States (Table 4).

Treatment

There is a variety of options and the key to optimal management is obtaining the very highest cure rate whilst limiting unnecessary treatment and reducing toxicity when therapy is needed. As well as estimating response by physical examination and imaging techniques, tumour markers are very helpful in gauging response and relapse and in

Table 4. The clinical staging classification system in use at the Royal Marsden Hospital describes extent of tumour, site(s) of involvement and tumour volume

Stage	Description
I	Lymphogram negative, no evidence of metastases
II	Lymphogram positive, metastases confined to abdominal nodes *Abdominal status*, three subgroups are recognized: A Maximum diameter of metastases <2 cm B Maximum diameter of metastases 2–5 cm C Maximum diameter of metastases >5 cm
III	Involvement of supra- and infradiaphragmatic lymph nodes, no extralymphatic metastases *Abdominal status*: A, B, C as for stage II
IV	Extralymphatic metastases *Suffixes as follows:* 0-lymphogram negative A, B, C as for stage II *Lung status:* L_1 <3 metastases L_2 multiple, none exceeding 2 cm diameter maximum L_3 multiple, one or more exceeding 2 cm diameter *Liver status*:* H_+ = liver involvement

*Criteria for liver involvement: of the 4 following parameters, 3 should be positive before liver involvement is diagnosed
1 Abnormal liver function tests
2 Positive CT scan
3 Positive ultrasonic or isotopic scan
4 Clinical enlargement

deciding on management (Figure 21). Treatment recommendations for various stages of seminoma and teratoma are given after a brief discussion of the available treatment modalities.

Surgery

There are three potential roles for surgery:

- radical orchidectomy
- retroperitoneal lymph node dissection for early stage teratoma
- resection of masses after chemotherapy for teratoma

Retroperitoneal surgery has become controversial since it is often done in patients without evidence of disease spread after proper staging. Even when there is microscopic, unrecognized, retroperitoneal tumour, one half of these patients have occult spread beyond the retroperitoneum which would not be treated by the surgery. These operations are discussed further below; such surgery requires a highly specialized and prolonged operation and often causes retrograde ejaculation.

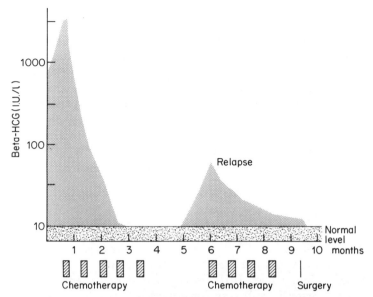

Figure 21. Beta-HCG as an indicator of response and relapse in germ cell tumours. The initial high level falls promptly with chemotherapy but has only returned to normal at the time of the fifth cycle of treatment. The level rises, indicating relapse, at 5 months and falls more slowly with further chemotherapy. Following surgical excision of a persistent mass, levels normalize again

Resection of persistent masses after treatment is done since the histological findings may be:

- malignant tumour
- mature teratoma
- necrosis and fibrosis

The finding of necrosis and fibrosis indicates that no futher chemotherapy is needed. Similarly, no more treatment is needed if mature teratoma is found, but an additional advantage of surgical resection is that such differentiated teratomas will often grow locally if left and may also become malignant. Clearly, more treatment may be indicated if malignant tissue is found in the resection specimen.

Radiotherapy

Seminoma is often regional in nature and is particularly radiosensitive, so that cure rates for low-volume disease are very high. Cure of bulky disease with radiotherapy is less common and chemotherapy is being increasingly used for the few patients with bulky seminoma.

Although radiotherapy has been used for teratomas, the introduction of effective chemotherapy has largely led to its abandonment.

Chemotherapy

The introduction, in the mid 1970s, of combinations of drugs including cisplatin has revolutionized the management of metastatic teratoma and bulky seminoma. The great majority of patients with low-volume teratoma are curable with a relatively short course of chemotherapy. Patients with bulky or very advanced teratoma still have a reasonable chance of cure, though increasingly intensive drug combinations are being used in an attempt to improve results. Bulky seminomas respond well to cisplatin alone or in combination with other drugs.

Currently, attempts are being made to reduce the toxicity of treatment, whilst maintaining effectiveness, in patients with highly curable disease.

Recommended Treatment by Stage

- Seminoma: Stage I or Stage II (non bulky)—radical orchidectomy and retroperitoneal radiotherapy.
- Seminoma: bulky stage II/III/IV—cisplatin-based chemotherapy.
- Teratoma: Stage I—still very controversial.
  Either—watch closely with sequential scans and tumour markers and treat relapsing patients (25%) with chemotherapy.
  Or—retroperitoneal lymph node dissection ± 2 cycles of chemotherapy.
    Although 25% of watched patients relapse all should have low-volume disease that is curable with chemotherapy, so that long-term cure rates of both policies should be virtually 100%.
- Teratoma: Stage II, low volume—again two options are available:
  Either—retroperitoneal dissection ± chemotherapy.
  Or—cisplatin-based combination (less intense treatment).
- Teratoma: Stage II bulky disease, Stage III/IV—chemotherapy with a cisplatin-based combination.

Outcome and Special Complications

The survival rates for testicular teratoma are continuing to improve and are amongst the highest of all solid tumours (Figure 18). Overall, well over 90% of these patients are cured. The figure approaches 100% for seminomas and less advanced teratomas. Even when chemotherapy is required for metastatic teratoma over 80% of patients are cured. Adverse prognostic factors include large tumour bulk, high marker levels and possibly CNS disease.

Chemotherapy remains toxic, though efforts are being made to reduce this further. Particular tumour-related problems include back pain, spinal cord involvement, renal failure from ureteric obstruction and metastatic disease to lung and brain.

Selected Papers and Reviews

Bagshawe, K. D., Newlands, E. S., Begent, R. H. (eds.) (1983) Germ cell tumours. *Clinics in Oncology*, 2(i): 3–279.

Einhorn, L. and Williams, S. D. (1980) Chemotherapy of disseminated testicular cancer. *Cancer*, **46**: 1339–1344.

Logothetis, C. L. and Samuels, M. L. (1984) Surgery in the management of Stage III germinal cell tumours. *Cancer Treatment Reviews*, **11**: 27–37.

Østerlind, A. (1986) Diverging trends in incidence and mortality of testicular cancer in Denmark 1943–1982. *British Journal of Cancer*, **53**: 501–505.

von der Masse, H., Rørth, M., Walbom-Jørgensen, S., Ørensen, B. L., Strøyer-Christophersen, I., Hald, T., Jacobsen, G., Berthelsen, J. G. and Skakkeboe, K. (1986) Carcinoma in situ of contralateral testis in patients with testicular germ cell cancer: study of 27 cases in 500 patients. *British Medical Journal*, **293**: 1398–1401.

Williams, C. J. (1977) Current dilemmas in the management of non-seminomatous germ cell tumours of the testis. *Cancer Treatment Reviews*, **4**: 275–297.

17 | Cancer of Unknown Primary Site

C. J. WILLIAMS

Although the primary site at which a cancer has developed is quickly obvious in most patients presenting with metastatic disease, the original site of the tumour is not found in up to 5% of cancer patients, and sometimes not even at post mortem examination.

Investigation

When a patient presents with metastatic disease, the sites to which the tumour has spread are a clue to the primary, as particular tumours have characteristic patterns of dissemination (Table 1 and Figure 1). Investigations designed to find the primary site will take into account this information, but should primarily be planned with a view to what treatment is available if tumour is found at those sites.

> Since the disease is already metastatic, intensive investigation is only warranted if there is a useful treatment for tumours at the sites being examined.

It is, for instance, questionable whether it is worthwhile looking hard for a pancreatic primary if there is a metastatic adenocarcinoma in the liver: treatment is probably not indicated, is never curative and is of little or no palliative value.

Because of this it is important to recognize the types of cancer that may benefit from treatment when they present as metastatic disease. These include:

- germ cell tumours of testis or ovary
- choriocarcinoma

Table 1. Sites of metastases from unknown primary (see Figure 1)

Site of metastasis	Likely primary site
High cervical nodes	Head and neck cancer Thyroid Lung
Lower cervical nodes	Head and neck Lung, breast Gut (especially L. supraclavicular node)
Axillary nodes	Lung Breast
Skin	Breast Lung Melanoma
Bone	Myeloma Breast Kidney Prostate Lung
Lung	Breast Kidney GI tract Bladder Germ cell Melanoma Lymphoma
Brain	Lung Breast Prostate Melanoma
Inguinal nodes	Vulva Anorectal Prostate Ovary
Disseminated intra-abdominal adenocarcinoma (including liver metastasis)	Ovary Stomach Pancreas Gut
Bowel	Malignant melanoma
Spleen	Malignant melanoma
Ovary	GI tract tumours Breast

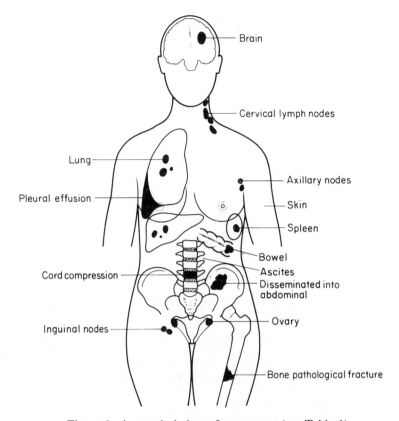

Figure 1. Anatomical sites of metastases (see Table 1)

- ovarian carcinoma
- breast cancer
- prostate cancer
- small cell lung cancer
- lymphoma and leukaemia
- thyroid cancer (well differentiated)
- bladder cancer

In some, cure is still possible despite tumour spread, whilst in others patients may have prolongation of life and relief of symptoms as a result of treatment.

The incidence of sites of primary disease (found at post mortem) in patients presenting with an unknown primary cancer do not correspond with the prevalence of various types of malignancies. This is presumably related to underlying tumour biology leading to spread and the difficulty of finding a small primary in certain parts of the body. Because of this, most tumours of unknown primary turn out, at post mortem, to have developed in the GI tract or lung (Figure 2).

It is not surprising that pancreas heads the list since it is notoriously difficult to investigate; the breast on the other hand is readily accessible so that primary cancer is rarely missed.

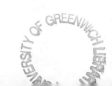

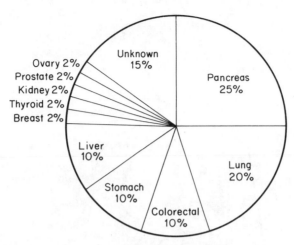

Figure 2. Proportion of tumours of unknown primary found, at post mortem examination, to have developed at various sites

Examination of Figure 2 will show that the majority of cancers of unknown primary have come from sites where treatment of metastatic disease is of little potential benefit for the patient. Investigation must be directed towards the less common but treatable tumours.

Factors in deciding an investigation include:
Patients' fitness, age and understanding of the situation.

Appropriate investigations will have to be planned according to the particular situation but are likely to include some of the following:

- Review of histology, special stains, immunocytology and EM as indicated. These may give further clues as to the primary site or reveal a potentially treatable cancer (e.g. germ cell or lymphoma). They may also show a metastatic cancer that is untreatable (e.g. malignant melanoma).
- Tumour markers—the finding of specific markers may reveal the tissue of origin (e.g. AFP/β-HCG).
- Routine blood tests (full blood count and biochemistry) are always indicated.
- Urine for microscopy may contain red blood cells, suggesting cancer in the urogenital tract.
- Chest X-ray—may reveal a primary cancer.
- Mammograms are rarely useful but are simple and occasionally reveal the source of the metastatic disease.
- Isotopic scan of the thyroid, if histology suggests this as a potential primary.

Other tests, such as computed tomography, radiological contrast studies and endoscopy are usually not indicated. They are time-consuming and uncomfortable for the patient and are expensive; if they do reveal the primary, treatment is probably not indicated.

Treatment

In general, treatment will be palliative in nature. Local radiotherapy may be used, such as for painful bone metastases, as well as analgesics and other drugs to improve symptoms.

Chemotherapy is only indicated, if no primary is found, in the following circumstances:

- Young men with a poorly differentiated carcinoma, with or without a raised AFP or β-HCG, may be treated as for a germ cell tumour (p. 339). Such an approach remains contentious.
- The histology suggests that the tumour may be chemosensitive, i.e. a small cell tumour.
- Young fit patients anxious to have therapy despite the uncertainty of benefit.

If such chemotherapy is given, response should be assessed early and treatment only continued in the event of good tumour regression.

The outcome is generally very poor; in one large series survival was 13% at 1 year and 3% at 5 years.

18 Cancers of the Central Nervous System

C. J. WILLIAMS

Primary tumors of the CNS are unusual in that they rarely spread beyond the nervous system itself; this is in spite of the fact that they comprise a remarkably diverse group of conditions. Since the brain and spinal cord are enclosed within the skull and spinal canal a mass lesion may cause symptoms early without destroying or invading adjacent tissue. Symptoms may be caused by displacement of structures, raised intracranial pressure or tissue destruction if invasion does occur.

Incidence and Epidemiology

Primary CNS tumours account for about 9% of all malignancies. Eighty-five percent arise within the cranial contents and 15% are spinal in origin. The incidence of CNS tumours in England and Wales is about 6 per 100,000, a figure which is similar to the United States. Incidence rates do not vary greatly around the world (Figure 1).

Most cases occur in two age peaks, one in childhood and the other in later life (50–70 years) as shown in Figure 2. As can be seen from this there is an excess of cases in adult males compared to females. Although the incidence in childhood is much lower than that in older adults, CNS tumours are the second leading cause of cancer death in childhood.

Aetiology and Pathogenesis

Little is known about the aetiology of the vast majority of primary CNS tumours. However, in a minority of cases genetic conditions may predispose to the development of malignancy. The conditions include:

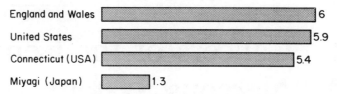

Figure 1. Incidence of primary CNS cancer around the world (per 100,000)

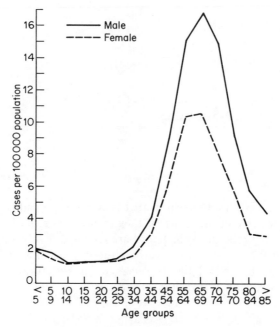

Figure 2. The incidence of all types of brain tumours in the United States by age. Data from U.S. Department of Health, Education and Welfare—Public Health Service (1968). *Vital Statistics Rates in the United States 1940-1960. Washington, D.C.*

- von Recklinghausen's disease (characteristic skin changes, autosomal dominant—develop tumours of brain and peripheral nervous system)
- tuberous sclerosis (skin lesions, epilepsy, mental retardation—intracranial or subependymal tumours)
- Lindau's disease (autosomal dominant—haemangioblastomas of cerebellum, spinal cord and retina)
- Turcot syndrome (familial polyposis of colon associated with gliomas)
- chromosome 22 is frequently abnormal in cases of meningioma.

There are no data to suggest that chemicals or viruses cause CNS cancer in man, though viruses can cause tumours after inoculation into the brain of experimental animals. Similarly, trauma does not seem to be a risk factor for subsequent CNS malignancy. A small excess of brain tumours was found in one study of children irradiated for scalp ringworm. An increased incidence of primary CNS lymphoma has also been shown in immunosuppressed patients (renal transplant, etc.).

Pathology and Natural History

The great majority of primary CNS tumours are gliomas though there is a wide spectrum of different tumours.

The peak age of incidence for these various tumours varies widely (Figure 3) and because of this a simplified classification is given for adults and children (see boxes).

ADULTS

Gliomas (50% of all CNS tumours)
   Astrocytoma—grades I–IV derived from astrocytes
   Ependymal—derived from cells lining CNS cavities
   Oligodendroglioma—derived from other supporting cells

Meningioma (10%)
   Parasagittal and sphenoid regions, benign and non-invasive but compress brain. Derived from meninges

Pituitary adenomas (15%)
   The majority are chromophobic and nearly always benign

Neurilemmoma (5%)

CHILDREN

Medulloblastoma (30%)
   Malignant tumour usually arising in posterior fossa, early dissemination within CSF

Astrocytoma (30%)

Ependymoma (12%)
   Usually fourth ventricle tumors

Optic glioma (5%)
   Usually well-differentiated gliomas

Craniopharyngioma (5%)
   Malformation, benign condition

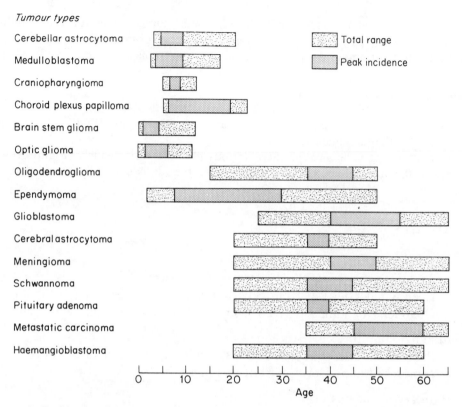

Figure 3. Incidence of brain tumours according to age. From Youmans, J.R. (ed.) (1982) *Neurological Surgery*. Vol. 5, W.B. Saunders Co., Philadelphia. Reproduced by permission

It should, however, be remembered that up to 40% of CNS malignant tumours in adults are metastatic in nature (lung, breast, kidney, melanoma and GI tract are the commonest primary sites).

Presenting Features

The symptoms and signs of CNS cancer are not surprisingly very diverse, reflecting the complex pathways of the brain and spinal cord. Table 1 outlines the sorts of symptoms and their frequency in glioma patients. Symptoms can be general or non-localizing, or the tumour may cause localizing symptoms by invasion or irritation of that part of the CNS.

Raised intracranial pressure may cause:

- early morning headache, worse on straining
- nausea and vomiting
- depressed level of consciousness
- papilloedema

These symptoms are largely dependent on the rate at which the tumour is growing. Slow-growing tumours of considerable size may cause no symptoms and signs. On the

Table 1. The frequency of symptoms at presentation in cerebral gliomas investigated at the National Hospitals, London (1955–1975)

Symptom	Relative frequency as initial symptom (%)
Epilepsy	38.3
Grand mal	15.9
Focal	14.7
Temporal lobe	7.2
Minor absence	0.5
No epilepsy	61.7
Headache	35.2
Mental change	16.5
Hemiparesis	10.3
Vomiting	7.5
Dysphagia	6.9
Impaired consciousness	4.6
Visual failure	4.3
Hemianaesthesia	3.4
Hemianopia	1.8
Cranial nerve palsy	1.8
Miscellaneous	2.3

Reprinted by permission from McKeran, R. O. and Thomas, D. G. T. (1980) The clinical study of gliomas. In: *Brain Tumours. Scientific Basis, Clinical Investigation and Current Therapy*, Thomas, D. G. T. and Graham, D. I. (eds.) Butterworth, Boston, p. 202.

other hand, rapid increase in tumour bulk or surrounding oedema frequently causes symptoms—as will tumours that block drainage of the ventricles, causing a sudden severe rise in intracranial pressure.

Localizing signs of intracranial lesions are complex and are summarized in Table 2.

Spread

As evidenced by the foregoing, CNS tumours are a mixed bunch; they vary from benign tumours which behave in a malignant fashion if they cannot be removed, to highly malignant tumours which may spread widely within the CNS. Spread is generally by direct invasion, though some tumours, such as medulloblastoma, may gain access to the CSF and seed extensively through the CNS. Spread outside the CNS is extremely uncommon.

Investigations and Staging

Investigation will depend on the exact clinical situation but will include some of the following:

- full physical and neurological examination
- ophthalmic and visual fields examination

Table 2. Localization of brain tumour by symptoms

	Frontal	Parietal	Temporal	Occipital
Symptoms	Often asymptomatic until late Symptoms of increased ICP Personality changes Libido changes Defective memory Urinary incontinence Seizures (generalized, becoming focal) Gait disorders Weakness Loss of smell Speech disorder Tonic spasms of fingers/toes	Symptomatic earlier than frontal lobe Symptoms of increased ICP Loss of vision Spatial disorientation Tingling sensation Dressing apraxia Loss of memory Seizures (focal sensory epilepsy) Weakness (anterior extension)	Speech disorders Loss of smell Disturbance in hearing, tinnitus, etc. Speech disturbance Uncinate fits Seizures with vocal phenomena in aura Hallucinations Dreams Déjà vu Space perception disturbances Dysarthria Dysnomia Disturbance of comprehension	Seizures, relatively less common, but with auras including flashing lights and unformed hallucinations Loss of vision Tingling (early) Weakness (late)
Specific cerebral functions	Behavioural problems Labile personality Mental lethargy Defective memory Motor aphasia	Anosognosia Autotopagnosia Visual agnosia Graphaesthesia (contralateral) Loss of memory Proprioceptive agnosia	Dysarthria Sensory asphasia Defective hearing Defective memory	Visual agnosia Visual impulses
Cranial nerve functions	Anosmia VI nerve palsy with increased ICP Papilloedema with increased ICP Foster Kennedy's syndrome Proptosis	Hemianopsia Papilloedema (with increased ICP)	Superior quadrantanopsia, could be homonymous hemianopsia with tumour extension Central weakness of the VIIIth cranial nerve Papilloedema with increased ICP	Macular sparing hemianopsia Horizontal nystagmus

Motor system	Contralateral weakness (late) Paresis (flaccid spastic) Disturbed gait (midline lesion) Automatism Persistence of induced movement (Kral's phenomenon) Diagonal rigidity (arm, contralateral; leg) Loss of skilled movement (X) (contralateral) Urinary incontinence (superior lesion)	Weakness Atrophy Clumsiness Dysdiadochokinesia Independent movements (unrecognized by patient)	Dysdiadochokinesia (early) Drift, secondary in later stages, involving arm more than leg	Motor signs appear late manifested by drift or dysdiadochokinesia
Sensory functions	Rarely involved initially	Dysaesthesias (tingling) (contralateral) Pallaesthesia (loss of vibratory sense) (contralateral) Loss of touch, press, and position sense (contralateral) but pain and temperature usually unaffected	Initially minimal	Somatosensory disturbances appear earlier than motor changes, as adjacent structures are involved Visual phenomena, such as persisting images, unformed hallucinations, auras, flashing of lights
Reflex changes	Tonic plantar reflex Hoffmann's sign Grasp reflex Babinski's sign	Babinski's sign Hoffmann's sign	May occur contralateral to tumour	Not affected in early stages

Adapted by permission from *Clinical Oncology*, 6th edition (1983) American Cancer Society.

- chest X-ray
- skull X-ray
- CT scan of brain
- EEG
- isotopic brain scan
- angiography (less common since CT introduced)
- lumbar puncture—contraindicated in the presence of raised intracranial pressure
- magnetic resonance imaging (MRI)—a new technique with particular promise in the CNS
- myelography if a spinal cord block is suspected

In view of the nature of spread and wide diversity of tumours there are no useful staging classifications.

Treatment

It is clearly not feasible to discuss the details of therapy in such a highly specialized field where there are so many different tumours arising in varying parts of the CNS. Discussion is, because of this, limited to the principles of treatment. Where intracranial tumours are suspected dexamethasone can provide useful, though temporary, relief of symptoms by reducing surrounding oedema—it is usually the first and simplest therapy. Childhood tumours are discussed in Chapter 21.

Surgery

Where possible, the initial treatment of all intracranial tumours is surgical excision. This makes the diagnosis and treats the tumour, but it may be limited by:

- location of the tumour
- invasiveness of the tumour

Meningiomas are nearly always benign and should, if possible, be completely removed. Partial removal may be beneficial since they are slow growing.

Malignant brain tumours are rarely cured surgically—by the time they are discovered they have often invaded deep-seated areas of the brain so that they cannot be completely excised. Partial removal may be of palliative use in selected patients. Where hydrocephalus is present surgical decompression by ventricular drainage can give dramatic relief. Surgical decompression of spinal cord compression can prevent paraplegia in selected patients. It is most useful when the onset of symptoms is slow and when paralysis is incomplete at the time of surgery.

Radiotherapy

Some *malignant* brain tumours respond to external beam radiotherapy. It is, however, generally palliative rather than curative, extending life and reducing symptoms.

Radiotherapy is used when:

- the tumour is centrally located when surgery would worsen the symptoms
- the tumour is adjacent to vital structures and when surgery would have an unacceptable mortality rate
- the tumour is metastatic—they are rarely single and are normally found in the setting of disease elsewhere

Radiation is also used as primary treatment for some chromophobe pituitary adenomas and for medulloblastomas when the area treated includes the whole cranio-spinal axis.

Postoperative radiotherapy is also recommended following incomplete removal of a number of tumours including:

- astrocytomas of higher grade
- ependymoma
- oligodendroglioma
- craniopharyngioma
- chordoma

Chemotherapy

Many anti-cancer drugs do not appear to cross the blood-brain barrier, though this may not be of paramount importance since abnormal tumour vasculature may already breach this. Lipid-soluble drugs which do cross this barrier are, however, among the most effective drugs in the management of CNS malignancy. Though a number of drugs can cause tumour regression, responses are generally brief (3–9 months) and long-term survival is rare. Chemotherapy has been extensively tested as an adjuvant after surgery and/or radiotherapy without much evidence of real benefit.

In general, chemotherapy is only indicated for selected patients with advanced disease. Its use as an adjuvant is not justified in routine practice.

Outcome and Special Complications

The outlook is gloomy for the majority of patients. Prognosis for the commonest tumour (astrocytoma) is closely related to grade (Table 3) but unfortunately most patients have high-grade tumours.

Complications of uncontrolled CNS tumours are legion. Dying patients with progressive symptoms from brain tumours (Table 1) or paraplegia from spinal cord involvement (Table 4) pose a major nursing problem—a team approach to care is needed (see Chapter 10).

Selected Papers and Reviews

Oldfield, E. H., Smith, B. H. and Kornblith, P. L. (1985) Tumours of the central nervous system. In: *Medical Oncology: Basic Principles and Clinical Management of Cancer*, Calabresi, P., Schein, P. S. and Rosenberg, S. A. (eds.), MacMillan, New York, pp. 1089–1192.

Sheline, G. E. (1975) Radiation therapy for primary tumours. *Seminars in Oncology* 2: 29–42.

Thomas, D. G. and Graham, D. I. (eds.) (1980) *Brain Tumours: Scientific Basis, Clinical Investigation and Current Therapy*. Butterworth, Boston.

Table 3. Estimated survival for the common brain tumours

	Percent survival	
	5-year	10-year
Astrocytoma		
Grade I (cerebellar)	95	90
Grade I (all sites)	55	35
Grade II	30	12
Grade III	20	5
Grade IV	5	1
Medulloblastoma	45	25
Ependymoma	42	40
Oligodendroglioma	65	25
Brain stem	25	5
Third ventricle and midbrain	30	7
Pinealoma	70	60
Pituitary adenoma	87	80
Craniopharyngioma	85	73
Optic	87	75
Meningiomas	90	55

Table 4. Spinal cord compression syndromes

Complete compression
Sensory level just below level of lesion
Loss of all modalities of sensation — variable in degree at first
Bilateral upper motor neurone weakness below lesion
Bladder and bowel dysfunction

Anterior compression
Partial loss of pain and temperature below lesion
Bilateral upper motor neurone weakness below lesion
Bladder and bowel dysfunction

Lateral compression (Brown-Séquard)
Contralateral loss of pain and temperature (touch much less affected)
Ipsilateral loss of proprioception and vibration
Ipsilateral upper motor neurone weakness

Posterior compression
Loss of vibration and position below lesion
Pain, temperature and touch relatively spared
Painful segmental paraesthesia at level of lesion

19 Sarcomas

C. J. WILLIAMS

Sarcomas are malignant tumours of mesenchymal tissue, affecting bone and soft tissues. Only an outline of the principles of their management can be given because, although they are uncommon, there are over 60 different tumours included under the term 'sarcoma'.

Incidence and Epidemiology

Although the incidence of bone sarcomas is highest in adolescence (3 per 100,000), bone tumours only account for 3–4% of childhood cancers. Incidence falls in early adulthood and then rises until at 60–70 years it equals the childhood rate (Figure 1).

Soft tissue sarcomas are rare, accounting for 0.8% of all cancers; the incidence rate is 2 per 100,000. They have a trimodal distribution pattern by age (Figure 1).

Variation in international incidence is small. Rates for soft tissue sarcomas range from 1 to 2.5 per 100,000, and bone tumours from 0.75 to 4 per 100,000. There is a small but consistent excess in males at all ages.

Aetiology and Pathogenesis

The finding of a high incidence of bone tumours in children suggests that bone sarcomas arise in areas of rapid and sustained growth. Tumours in adults may be associated with metabolic stimulation from Paget's disease, hyperparathyroidism, chronic osteomyelitis, fracture and bone infarcts. Tumours are more common in inherited conditions where there are exostoses and enchondromatoses. Radiation exposure has also been linked to the later development of bone sarcomas.

Soft tissue sarcomas are generally sporadic but are more common in von Recklinghausen's disease. They may also develop in irradiated areas, and one type of

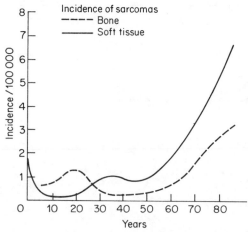

Figure 1. Age-specific incidence of soft tissue and bone sarcomas in England and Wales

sarcoma is common in oedematous limbs. Liver sarcomas are increased in frequency in workers exposed to polyvinylchloride. Kaposi's sarcoma is an uncommon tumour found in certain parts of the world (Africa, Jewish and Italian men), which has recently become common in patients with acquired immune deficiency syndrome (AIDS). A number of other genetically linked diseases (tuberous sclerosis, Werner's syndrome, intestinal polyposis, Gardener's syndrome and basal cell naevus syndrome) are all associated with soft tissue sarcomas.

Despite the wide variety of factors potentially associated with bone or soft tissue sarcomas, no clear-cut cause is found in the majority of cases.

Pathology and Natural History

Histogenetically, sarcomas arise from diverse connective tissue elements and are named after the dominant cell type within the tumour (Figure 2). However, there is often overlap between the various categories; for instance, 'bone tumours' can arise from soft tissues and soft tissue tumours may be quite unlike the tissue in which they develop. Grade is very important in sarcomas and should always be reported as it may influence the choice of therapy.

Table 1 (page 368) outlines a simple working classification of sarcomas. Table 2 (page 371) shows a classification of bone sarcomas and their distribution in a large series of patients treated at the Mayo Clinic.

Presenting Features

Because of the diversity of tumours the incidence of symptoms and signs cannot be given. Patients may present because of:

- Local signs and symptoms: mass, pain, fracture, paralysis or ischaemia, bowel or ureteric obstruction, depending on the site and characteristics of the tumour.

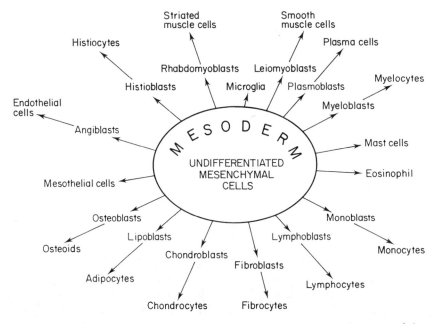

Figure 2. Primitive mesenchymal cells of soft tissue and bone may produce any of these forms, and mature cells may dedifferentiate to undifferentiated or poorly differentiated elements. From Hajdu, S.I. (1979) *Pathology of Soft Tissue Tumors*. Lea & Febiger, Philadelphia. Reproduced by permission

- Systemic effects: weight loss, fever and general malaise. Rarely, some sarcomas cause severe episodic hypoglycaemia, whilst others may cause thyroid and pituitary dysfunction. Such sarcomas are usually large retroperitoneal fibrosarcomas.

Spread

This will depend very much on the type of sarcoma since many have particular patterns of primary site and dissemination.

- local invasion and destruction is common and causes the symptoms leading to diagnosis in the majority of cases Tumours may spread long distances along tissue planes
- lymphatic spread is less common in many sarcomas
- blood-borne spread is a predominant feature in a number of sarcomas

Investigations and Staging

These will of course be guided by the site and type of sarcoma but may include:

- plain X-ray
- computed tomography } of primary lesion
- arteriography

Table 1. Simplified classification of the soft tissue sarcomas

Tissue of origin	Benign neoplasm	Sarcoma(s)
Fibrous tissue	Fibroma (single or multiple, as in fibromatosis)	Fibrosarcoma (including dermatofibrosarcoma protuberans)
Muscle *Striated*	Rhabdomyoma	Rhabdomyosarcoma Embryonal Alveolar Pleomorphic Botryoidal
Smooth	Leiomyoma (including uterine 'fibroids')	Leiomyosarcoma
'Histiocytic' tissue		Malignant fibrous histiocytoma of soft tissue or bone
Fat	Lipoma	Liposarcoma
Blood vessels	Angioma, haemangioma	Haemangiosarcoma, Kaposi's sarcoma, lymphangiosarcoma, haemangiopericytoma
Peripheral nerves	Neuroma, neurofibroma neurilemmoma (incl Schwannoma)	Neurofibrosarcoma, malignant neurilemmoma (including malignant Schwannoma and neuroepithelioma)
Pleura and peritoneum		Mesothelioma
Synovium		Synovial cell sarcoma
Others		Alveolar soft parts sarcoma (malignant non-chromaffin paraganglioma)

- biopsy
- serum biochemistry, including alkaline phosphatase
- radioisotopic imaging of bone
- chest X-ray
- thoracic computed tomography

The plain X-ray appearance of primary bone sarcomas is important and may be very helpful in deciding on the nature of the sarcoma.

There is no unified staging system.

Treatment

Bone Tumours

Malignant tumours of the bone are generally best treated with a combination of surgery, radiotherapy and chemotherapy (see boxes below).

SURGERY

Especially for osteosarcoma: there has been a move away from amputation and towards limb preservation, where appropriate. Local control is achieved in 90% of cases (skip lesions detected by isotopic bone imaging). May be used with pre-operative chemotherapy. Surgical removal of lung metastases may be curative in selected cases.

RADIOTHERAPY

Primary local therapy for Ewing's sarcoma: other common bone sarcomas are relatively radioresistant. High-dose irradiation to large fields of limbs requires special techniques if side-effects are to be minimized—a strip of skin is left unirradiated where possible.

CHEMOTHERAPY

Both osteosarcoma and Ewing's sarcoma respond to combinations of anti-cancer drugs. Extensive studies have suggested that pre- or perioperative chemotherapy improves survival, and recent randomized trials with osteosarcoma patients have confirmed these impressions. Chemotherapy is usually continued after primary local therapy.

The best chance of cure for patients with an osteosarcoma or Ewing's sarcoma lies with a multidisciplinary approach, chemotherapy being combined with optimal local control by surgery or irradiation.

Soft Tissue Sarcomas

Approaches similar to those for bone sarcomas are being tested: (see boxes below).

SURGERY

Because these tumours may spread extensively along tissue planes local excision needs to be radical. Despite this 30% or more of tumours recur locally. The extent of surgery will depend on the exact circumstances—sometimes amputation cannot be avoided if the tumour is to be completely removed. Occasionally, pulmonary metastases may be resected in selected cases.

RADIOTHERAPY

Poor results in these sarcomas are because of local and distant failure. Recently, radiotherapy (with or without chemotherapy) has been used to try to reduce local recurrence rates after radical surgery. CT imaging is useful for planning, and high radiation doses (5000–7000 cGy) are needed. Such irradiation has been used before or after surgery.

CHEMOTHERAPY

Combinations of anti-cancer drugs can produce objective responses in 50% or more of patients with metastatic disease, and because of this such treatment has been used in an adjuvant fashion. Although impressive results have been reported for combined modality therapy, randomized trials have so far failed to show that chemotherapy improves survival. Despite this many centres use a combined approach.

Sarcomas are rare tumours best managed in specialist centres. Special expertise is required in a variety of areas:

- pathology
- radiology
- surgery
- radiotherapy
- chemotherapy

In addition, concentration of patients in such centres is likely to offer the best chance that new, more successful treatments will be developed.

Outcome and Special Complications

Survival correlates with the histological type, grade and tumour extent at diagnosis. The introduction of combined modality approaches in specialist centres has resulted in much improved survival rates.

Table 2. Simplified classification of bone sarcomas: proportion (%) of 3634 patients treated at Mayo Clinic

Tissue of origin	%	Benign	%	Malignant	%
Chondrogenic	36	Osteochondroma	16	Primary chondrosarcoma	10
		Chondroma	4	Secondary chondrosarcoma	2
		Chondroblastoma	1	Dedifferentiated	1
		Chondromyxoid fibroma	1	chondrosarcoma	1
				Mesenchymal chondrosarcoma	
Osteogenic	33	Osteoid osteoma	4	Osteosarcoma	27
		Benign osteoblastoma	1	Parosteal osteogenic sarcoma	1
Unknown	17	Giant cell tumour	7	Ewing's sarcoma	8
		Fibrous histiocytoma	0.5	Malignant giant cell tumour	1
				Adamantinoma	0.5
Fibrogenic	6	Fibroma	1	Fibrosarcoma	4
		Desmoplastic fibroma	1		
Notochordal	5			Chordoma	5
Vascular	3	Haemangioma	2	Haemangioendothelioma	0.5
				Haemangiopericytoma	0.5

Complications will depend very much on the site of uncontrolled tumour.

Selected Papers and Reviews

Razek, A., Perez, C.A., Tefft, M., *et al.* (1980) Intergroup Ewing's sarcoma study: local control related to radiation dose, volume and site of primary Ewing's sarcoma. *Cancer,* **46**: 516–521.

Rosen, R., Marlowe, R. and Caparros, B. (1979) Primary osteogenic sarcoma: the rationale for pre-operative chemotherapy and delayed surgery. *Cancer,* **43**: 2163.

Shiu, M. H. and Hajdu, S. I. (1981) Management of soft tissue sarcoma of the extremity. *Seminars in Oncology,* **8**: 172.

Suit, H. D. and Proppe, K. H. (1982) *Multidisciplinary Decisions in Oncology: Soft Tissue Sarcoma.* Pergamon Press, New York.

20 | Lymphatic and Haematological Cancers

C. J. WILLIAMS

HODGKIN'S DISEASE

Hodgkin's disease has long been recognized as a disease entity (it was first reported by Thomas Hodgkin in 1832), and despite much improved therapy we are only just starting to understand the biology of this disease; current concepts are challenging long-held views.

Incidence and Epidemiology

There is a bimodal distribution by age in western countries, with a peak in the age range 20–30 and after 60 years of age (Figure 1). This pattern is absent in Japan and other Far Eastern countries. The disease is more common in men (sex ratio 1.5:1), especially before puberty (sex ratio 6:1). The variation in incidence around the world is relatively small (Figure 2).

Aetiology and Pathogenesis

Because fevers are among the symptoms of this condition, attempts to find an infective cause have been made for the past 100 years. A further reason for this search has been that the majority of cells in the tumour are inflammatory non-neoplastic cells. The putative cancer cells, Reed-Sternberg cells, are generally few in number. Despite all this effort no causative infectious agent has been found. In recent years most effort has concentrated on looking for a virus that might be implicated in the development of the disease; among suspect candidates have been the Epstein-Barr virus and the retroviruses.

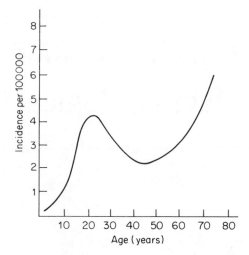

Figure 1. Incidence of Hodgkin's disease by age in England and Wales

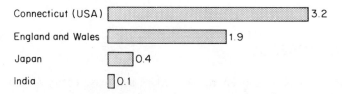

Figure 2. Variation in incidence around the world for Hodgkin's disease (per 100,000)

Reports of an increased incidence in the family of a patient with Hodgkin's disease have circulated for a long time. The risk of siblings is about six-fold that of a normal population; the risk is even higher (nine-fold) if the sibling is of the same sex. Occasional clusters of multiple cases of Hodgkin's disease have also been reported. Whether these arise because of chance or because of a transmissible agent remains an open question.

The increased incidence in families and finding of an excess of certain HLA types in Hodgkin's patients suggests the possible importance of genetic as well as environmental factors.

Pathology and Natural History

The requirements for the diagnosis of Hodgkin's disease are the finding of characteristic giant cells (Reed-Sternberg cells) in an appropriate setting. Classically, Hodgkin's disease has been divided into four major subdivisions (Rye classification) depending on the characteristics of the Reed-Sternberg and surrounding cells (Table 1). This has important prognostic implications (Figure 3). Figure 3 shows the effect of histological type on survival prior to 1970. Since the introduction of more effective treatment the survival differences are less marked.

Table 1. Rye classification of Hodgkin's disease

Subgroup	Major histological features	Approximate frequency (%)
Lymphocyte predominance (LPHD)	Abundant normal-appearing lymphocytes with or without benign histiocytes; occasionally nodular; rare Reed-Sternberg (R-S) cells	5
Nodular sclerosis (NSHD)	Nodules of lymphoid infiltrate of varying size, separated by bands of collagen and containing numerous 'lacunar cell' variants of R-S cells	70
Mixed cellularity (MCHD)	Pleomorphic infiltrate of eosinophils, plasma cells, histiocytes, and lymphocytes with numerous R-S cells	20
Lymphoctye depletion (LDHD)	Paucity of lymphocytes with numerous R-S cells, often bizarre in appearance; may have diffuse fibrosis or reticulum fibres	5

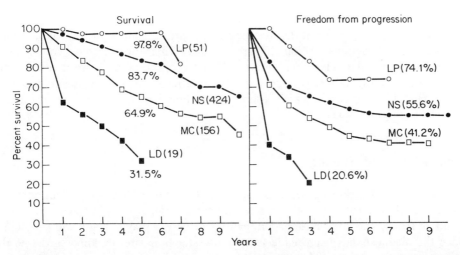

Figure 3. Survival and freedom from disease progression by histological type of Hodgkin's disease (LP = lymphocyte predominant; NS = nodular sclerosing; MC = mixed cellularity; LD = lymphocyte depleted; numbers of patients for each stage are shown in parentheses on the left-hand graph)

However, the very diversity of the appearance of the tissue in different subtypes of Hodgkin's disease has led recently to the suggestion that it is not one disease: indeed it has been suggested that some patients have a non-Hodgkin's lymphoma.

Reed-Sternberg cells are very difficult to study, partly because they are difficult to culture. They show aneuploidy and transplantability typical of malignant cells, but monoclonality has not been conclusively demonstrated. There is still much to learn about the biology of this disease before we can characterize it fully.

Presenting Features

Although patients may present with a wide variety of symptoms and signs most patients have:

- painless rubbery lymph node enlargement (cervical 70%, axillary 25%, inguinal 10%)

Patients may well give a history of fluctuating lymph nodes for months or years before diagnosis. Other features of Hodgkin's disease include:

- fever and night sweats (20% of patients)
- weight loss (>10% body weight in 15% of patients)
- generalized pruritus (5% of patients)
- respiratory symptoms from a large mediastinal mass (5% of patients)
- alcohol-associated pain (pain in a lymph node mass after drinking alcohol—2% of patients and highly suggestive of the diagnosis)

Spread

Many patients have a pattern of disease suggesting spread from one lymph node group to the next in a contiguous fashion (Figure 4). Mediastinal involvement is much more common in the nodular sclerosing subtype. When the disease has spread to the liver and bone marrow the spleen is almost invariably affected. CNS involvement is very rare and Hodgkin's disease is rarely found in the bowel or mesenteric nodes, unlike non-Hodgkin's lymphoma.

Investigations and Staging

The diagnosis of Hodgkin's disease is usually made simply by biopsy of an enlarged lymph node. Occasionally patients with severe constitutional symptoms (fever, weight loss and pruritus) and little lymphadenopathy can pose a major diagnostic problem.

Once the diagnosis has been made further investigations are designed to define the exact extent of the disease. These include:

- full blood count and ESR (high level suggests poor prognosis)
- routine biochemistry screen
- chest X-ray (mediastinal mass, pulmonary infiltrates)
- lymphangiogram (para-aortic lymph nodes are seen up to renal hilum)
- CT scan (thorax and abdominal lymph nodes)
- bone marrow biopsy and trephine

Staging laparotomy was introduced in the late 1960s as a technique to ensure that patients with apparently limited disease were suitable for radiotherapy. The most important aspect of the operation is splenectomy since involvement of this organ indicates increased risk of visceral spread. Simple enlargement of the spleen is

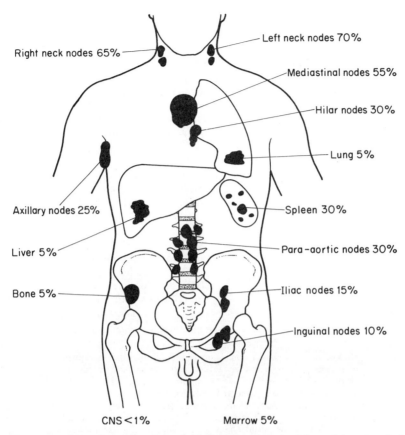

Right neck nodes 65%

Left neck nodes 70%

Mediastinal nodes 55%

Hilar nodes 30%

Lung 5%

Axillary nodes 25%

Spleen 30%

Liver 5%

Para-aortic nodes 30%

Bone 5%

Iliac nodes 15%

Inguinal nodes 10%

CNS <1%   Marrow 5%

Figure 4. Common sites of presentation of Hodgkin's disease. Adapted by permission from Souhami, R.L. and Tobias, J.S. (1986) *Cancer and Its Management*, Blackwell Scientific Publications, Oxford

insufficient evidence of involvement as only half of patients with an enlarged spleen have disease detected histologically. Recently, staging laparotomy has been used less frequently since chemotherapy and radiotherapy have been used together in selected groups of patients. Staging laparotomy should be done by an experienced surgeon; it includes biopsy of para-aortic nodes, splenectomy, splenic hilar node biopsy, biopsy of porta hepatis nodes and liver biopsy.

Hodgkin's disease is divided into four main stages according to the Ann Arbor classification (Table 2). Localized extension to an extra lymphatic organ (e.g. lung) is called an E lesion and does not upstage the patient to stage IV (visceral or diffuse involvement).

Treatment

Because the results of treating Hodgkin's disease have improved so much many physicians have the impression that management is simple. However, this is rarely

Table 2. Ann Arbor staging classification for Hodgkin's disease

Staging classification*	Features
Stage I	Involvement of a single lymph node region or of a single extralymphatic site (IE)
Stage II	Involvement of two or more node regions on the same side of the diaphragm, or of a localized extranodal involvement and one or more lymph node regions on the same side of the diaphragm (IIE)
Stage III†	Involvement of lymph nodes on both sides of the diaphragm, which may include the spleen (IIIS) or a localized extranodal site (IIIE) or both (IIISE)
Stage IV	Diffuse involvement of one or more extralymphatic organs

*Suffix A = no constitutional symptoms. Suffix B = constitutional symptoms present. These are fevers, night sweats and/or loss of 10% or more of body weight over 6 months. Pruritus is not included. Suffix E = localized extranodal involvement.
†Stage III disease can be subdivided according to the extent of intra-abdominal node involvement. Stage III_1 = involvement of spleen, splenic, coeliac or portal nodes or any combinations of these. Stage III_2 = involvement of para-aortic, iliac or mesenteric nodes with or without upper abdominal disease.

true and such curable patients are best looked after in specialist centres. Treatment is discussed under modality and then by stage.

Radiotherapy

When staging has shown disease localized and encompassible by radiotherapy this may be the primary treatment. Depending upon the pattern of disease, radiation may be given to lymph nodes above or below the diaphragm or both (Figure 5). Hodgkin's disease is very sensitive to radiation so that doses do not need to be very high, though outcome is clearly dose dependent (Figure 6). Doses are usually around 4000 cGy in 25 fractions.

There has been much debate regarding the extent of the radiation field to be used. In general large or extended fields are used because the recurrence rate is lower.

In the past 10 years chemotherapy has been used increasingly with radiotherapy.

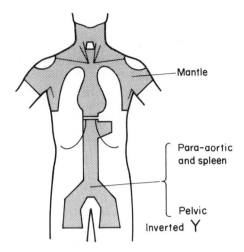

Figure 5. Radiotherapy fields for Hodgkin's disease. The upper field is called a mantle and the lower an inverted Y. When both are used together it is called total nodal irradiation

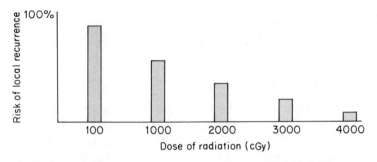

Figure 6. Radiation dose-response curve for Hodgkin's disease

Chemotherapy

The introduction of an effective combination of four drugs in the late 1960s revolutionized the care of Hodgkin's disease. Prior to this, the use of modern radio-therapy had started to cure an increasing number of patients with early stage disease. Only when effective chemotherapy became available was cure available to those with advanced disease or to patients relapsing after radiotherapy.

Since the introduction of the so-called 'MOPP' chemotherapy regime a number of other combinations of four or five drugs have been used with success. One of the reasons for developing new combinations was to reduce the acute and long-term toxicities of treatment as well as to find effective treatment for patients failing MOPP.

Treatment by Stage

Management of Hodgkin's disease is in a state of flux. This has been brought about by the decreasing use of staging laparotomy and a trend towards using combined modality therapy. Current practice includes:

- Stage IA or IIA   subtotal lymphoid irradiation (mantle or inverted Y [Figure 5] depending on whether disease is above or below diaphragm). If there is a large mediastinal mass (>one-third of transverse diameter of chest) chemotherapy should be given in addition to mantle irradiation used for stages I–III.
- Stage IB or IIB   total lymphoid irradiation (mantle + inverted Y) or chemotherapy.
- Stage III_1A total lymphoid irradiation.
- Stage III_2A chemotherapy or chemotherapy and irradiation. Combined modality may also be used when there is extensive splenic involvement.
- Stage IIIB, IVA and B   chemotherapy—may occasionally be in combination with irradiation for stage IIIB.

It is clear from the wide range of combinations of treatment that there is still much disagreement as to the optimal management. Choice may depend on:

- histology and grade
- stage, number of E lesions, extent of splenic involvement, size of mediastinal mass
- age
- B symptoms, level of ESR and LDH

Patients with asymptomatic limited disease should clearly be treated with radiotherapy whilst those with very extensive disease will receive chemotherapy. The problem patients are those with moderate amounts of disease potentially curable with radiotherapy, but at high risk of relapse. They may be treated with either radiotherapy or chemotherapy alone, or a combination of both (Table 3). The use of extensive irradiation (total nodal) and chemotherapy is more common in the United States, treatment being more conservative in Britain.

Recently, some patients with recurrent Hodgkin's disease refractory to conventional therapy have been treated successfully with high doses of drugs supported by autologous bone marrow transplantation.

Table 3. Hodgkin's disease: stages and clinical situations requiring combined modality therapy

Stage III_1A with extensive involvement of the spleen (>4 nodules) or Stage III_2A
Stage IIIB
Large mediastinal mass, >1/3 transverse diameter of the chest, of any stage
Multiple E lesions, i.e. lung, pleura, pericardium and bone, of any stage
Children, usually age 15 and younger

Outcome and Special Complications

The chances of long-term survival have improved greatly since the introduction of effective chemotherapy in 1970, so much so that the prognostic significance of staging has been reduced dramatically (Figure 7).

Uncontrolled Hodgkin's disease may cause many symptoms, depending on the sites of involvement, but characteristically patients waste away. They often have unusual infections since they are severely immunocompromised. Long-term complications of treatment include:

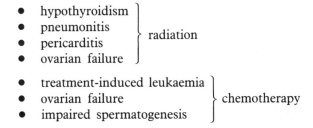

- hypothyroidism
- pneumonitis ⎱ radiation
- pericarditis
- ovarian failure

- treatment-induced leukaemia
- ovarian failure ⎱ chemotherapy
- impaired spermatogenesis

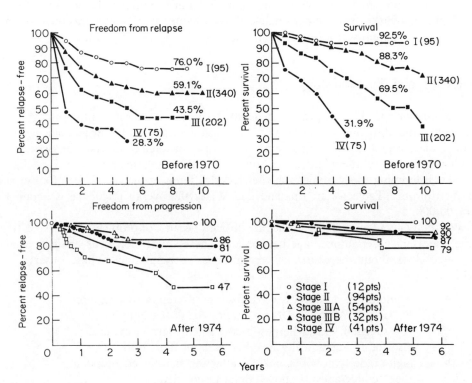

Figure 7. Survival and freedom from relapse by stage for patients with Hodgkin's disease treated at Stanford—prior to 1970 and after 1974

Selected Papers and Reviews

Coleman, C. N., Williams, C. J., *et al.* (1977) Hematologic malignancy in patients treated for Hodgkin's disease. *New England Journal of Medicine*, **297**: 1249–1252.

DeVita, V. T., *et al.* (1980) Curability of advanced Hodgkin's disease with chemotherapy: long term followings of MOPP treated patients at NCI. *Annals of Internal Medicine*, **92**: 587–595.

Gutensohn, N. and Cole, P. (1981) Epidemiology of Hodgkin's disease. *New England Journal of Medicine*, **304**: 135–140.

Kaplan, H. S. (1980) *Hodgkin's Disease* (2nd edition). Harvard University Press.

Rosenberg, S. A., *et al.* (1982) The Stanford randomized trials of the treatment of Hodgkin's disease 1967–1980. In: *Malignant Lymphomas. Etiology, Immunology, Pathology, Treatment*, Rosenberg, S. A. and Kaplan, H. S. (eds.), Bristol-Myers Cancer Symposia, Vol 3, Academic Press, New York, pp. 513–522.

NON-HODGKIN'S LYMPHOMA

Malignancy of lymphoid tissue has been divided into Hodgkin's disease and a ragbag of other neoplasms called the non-Hodgkin's lymphomas. These form a diverse group whose only common feature sometimes appears to be their derivation from lymphoid cells. They are distinguished from Hodgkin's disease by the absence of Reed-Sternberg cells, and from leukaemias on the arbitrary basis that the disease is primarily 'nodal' rather than bone marrow-based. The non-Hodgkin's lymphomas are monoclonal neoplasms thought to arise from a single cell (see Chapter 1), though occasional patients with disease apparently from more than one clone have been described.

Incidence and Epidemiology

Any discussion of these topics is bedevilled by the numerous different types of lymphoma and difficulty in separating them histologically and immunologically (see below). Because of this, comparisons of disease incidence around the world are unreliable. In general the incidence of non-Hodgkin's lymphoma rises with age (Figure 8), though lumping the subtypes together hides differences in typical age of onset and sex distribution (Table 4). In England and Wales the overall incidence is about 3.9 per 100,000.

Even though epidemiological studies are difficult because of problems of classification, some important observations have been made. These are of biological significance and may give clues about the causes of certain types of lymphoma. These observations include:

- The finding of an aggressive diffuse undifferentiated lymphoma in parts of Africa and New Guinea (Burkitt's lymphoma). It is associated with a herpesvirus (Epstein-Barr virus) and is also found sporadically in other parts of the world.
- A high-grade lymphoma, mainly affecting the bowel, found in the Mediterranean region. Alpha heavy chain immunoglobulin is secreted and the tumour appears to be

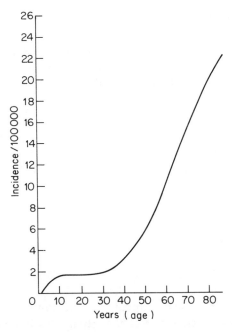

Figure 8. Incidence of non-Hodgkin's lymphoma by age in England and Wales

Table 4. Working Formulation of non-Hodgkin's lymphoma: age and sex ratio for 1175 cases

Subtype	Median age (years)	Sex ratio (M:F)
Small lymphocytic	60.5	1.2:1
Follicular, small cleaved cell	54.3	1.3:1
Follicular, mixed	56.1	0.8:1
Follicular, large cell	55.4	1.8:1
Diffuse, small cleaved cell	57.9	2.0:1
Diffuse, mixed	58.0	1.1:1
Diffuse, large cell	56.8	1.0:1
Immunoblastic	51.3	1.5:1
Lymphoblastic	16.9	1.9:1
Diffuse, small non-cleaved	29.8	2.6:1

related in some way to a non-neoplastic submucosal
infiltration of the bowel by mature plasma cells.
● A specific type of T-cell lymphoma is found in parts of Japan.
This appears to be associated with a retrovirus HTLV 1. A
similar lymphoma has been described in parts of the
Caribbean. Hypercalcaemia is a prominent feature of this
disease.

Aetiology and Pathogenesis

The cause of most lymphomas is unknown but the evidence presented above suggests that certain subtypes may be related to specific viruses. Some other lymphomas may be predisposed by a variety of inherited disorders (see box).

---

ataxia—telangiectasia
Bloom's syndrome
Chediak–Higashi syndrome
Klinefelter's syndrome
Swiss-type agammaglobulinaemia
X-linked lymphoproliferative disorder
Wiscott-Aldrich syndrome

Other acquired disorders, usually disturbing the immune system, also seem to predispose to subsequent development of non-Hodgkin's lymphoma. Some examples are given in the box below.

---

acquired immune deficiency syndrome (AIDS)
iatrogenic immunosuppression (organ transplant)
rheumatoid arthritis and Sjögren's syndrome
Hashimoto's thyroiditis (thyroid lymphoma)
systemic lupus erythematosus
coeliac disease

Characteristic chromosomal changes have also been described (usually chromosomes 8, 14 and 18) but their relationship to aetiology and function are unknown.

Although it seems likely that viruses play a role in the development of some lymphomas, Koch's postulates have not been fulfilled so that the exact role of viruses remains to be defined.

Pathology and Natural History

The pathology of the lymphomas is probably more confusing than any other area of histopathology. This has been caused by the plethora of different classifications and the rapid increase in biological and immunological understanding that has constantly shifted the ground upon which these classifications were developed.

Currently, there are at least seven major classifications, some used mainly in Europe and others in the United States. Recently the National Cancer Institute in Washington has tried to improve the situation by producing an internationally agreed unified classification—the Working Formulation (Tables 4 and 5). Although this is being increasingly used, it is still ignored by some groups who continue to use other classifications. The main alternative classification used in Europe is that of the Kiel group.

The introduction of immunological techniques has allowed pathologists to define the cell of origin of most lymphomas, and in the case of B-cell lymphomas to demonstrate monoclonality. This is not possible for T-cell lymphomas though gene rearrangement studies seem to confirm that these tumours are also monoclonal. The cell of origin of lymphomas is shown in Table 6.

This complicated scheme can be simplifed by assessing the overall pattern of the tumour (nodular or diffuse involvement) and the cytology of individual cells. In *general*:

- Lymphomas with a nodular pattern have a more favourable
    natural history than do diffuse lymphomas, excepting CLL-
    like lymphoma.
- Lymphomas with small mature or small cleaved cells have a
    better outlook than do those with predominantly large cells.

On this basis, the Working Formulation (Table 5) divides lymphomas into low, intermediate and high grade, which is useful in planning therapy.

A further complication in the assessment of pathological subtype is the finding of different histological patterns of lymphoma in the same node or in different nodes, and the tendency for low-grade lymphomas to transform into high-grade tumours with time.

Table 5. Working Formulation of non-Hodgkin's lymphoma

Low Grade
    A. Small lymphocytic*
    B. Follicular, predominantly small cleaved cell†
    C. Follicular, mixed small cleaved and large cells†

Intermediate Grade
    D. Follicular, predominantly large cell†
    E. Diffuse, small cleaved cell
    F. Diffuse, mixed small and large cells
    G. Diffuse, large cell
          cleaved or noncleaved cell

High Grade
    H. Large cell, immunoblastic*
    I.   Lymphoblastic
          convoluted or nonconvoluted
    J.   Small, noncleaved cell
          Burkitt's or non-Burkitt's

*May be plasmacytoid
†May have diffuse areas

Table 6. Cell of origin of various lymphomas

B-cell (85%)	T-cell (10%)
Follicular lymphomas—(small and large cleaved, non-cleaved cells)	Cutaneous T-cell lymphoma
Diffuse lymphomas—(small cleaved, small and large cells cleaved and non-cleaved)	Thymic T-cell lymphoma (diffuse large cell)
Lymphoplasmacytoid (Waldenström's)	Peripheral T-cell lymphoma
Chronic lymphatic leukaemia — (diffuse small lymphocytic)	
Burkitt's lymphoma— (small non-cleaved)	
Heavy chain disease	

Presenting Features

As might be anticipated presentation is very variable depending upon the site of involvement; spread to extranodal sites is common with some types of lymphoma. Disease frequently presents with a nodal mass in a similar fashion to Hodgkin's disease. Specific patterns of involvement include:

- lymphoid tissue in oropharynx (Waldeyer's ring)
- gastrointestinal tract and mesenteric nodes .
- salivary and lacrimal gland
- orbit and conjunctiva
- testis and ovary
- central nervous system
- bone marrow
- skin
- bone
- lung

As with Hodgkin's disease, patients may present with non-specific B symptoms (fevers and night sweats, pruritus and weight loss).

Spread

The likely sites of spread depend upon the subtype of lymphoma. For instance, follicular low-grade lymphomas frequently involve the bone marrow, whilst some diffuse high-grade lymphomas rarely do so at diagnosis (Figure 9). Involvement of more than one group of lymph nodes is common but spread to extranodal sites (see above) is also important.

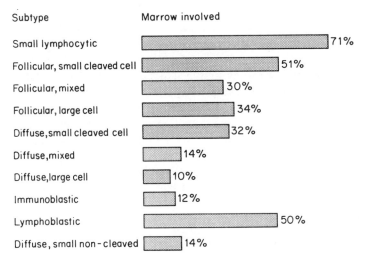

Figure 9. Non-Hodgkin's lymphoma bone marrow involvement

Investigations and Staging

Staging is similar to that used for Hodgkin's disease with the exception that staging laparotomy is not used. However, some patients will present with intra-abdominal pathology requiring a laparotomy to make the diagnosis. Common investigations include:

- biopsy of lymph node or other masses
- full physical examination
- full blood count, direct Coomb's test if haemolysis suspected
- blood chemistry
- blood and urine for immunoglobulins
- bone marrow aspirate and trephine
- chest X-ray
- lymphangiogram
- computed tomography
- ultrasonography
- lumbar puncture if CNS involvement is suspected and there is no mass effect
- myelogram if spinal cord compression is suspected

Staging uses the same system developed for Hodgkin's disease (page 378), though it is not always ideal as patterns of spread are often different from Hodgkin's disease.

Treatment

This will depend on the patient's general fitness, symptoms and sites and stage of disease, as well as histological subtype.

Radiotherapy

Non-Hodgkin's lymphoma is usually extremely sensitive to irradiation, but despite this radiotherapy has a smaller role than in the treatment of Hodgkin's disease. This is because, in spite of the apparent findings of clinical staging, nodal non-Hodgkin's lymphoma is nearly always generalized at presentation. Only the small proportion of patients (< 10%) who have stage I disease are suitable for irradiation as curative therapy. The dose employed is similar to that used for Hodgkin's disease but fields are generally smaller, there being no evidence that extended fields increase the chance of cure.

Radiation is sometimes used as a palliative therapy for patients with disease not controlled by chemotherapy, and it can also be used together with anti-neoplastic drugs as a curative treatment.

Cranial radiation may be used in patients with spread to the CNS or those rare patients who have primary brain lymphoma.

Chemotherapy

There are a number of drugs which are highly active when used alone, though responses are generally short lived. During the 1970s combinations of these were developed which can produce complete disappearance of all detectable disease in up to 80% of patients. Such responses do not seem permanent in patients with low-grade lymphomas but, so far, appear durable in many patients with high-grade lymphoma.

Because of this, chemotherapy is used to 'control' low-grade lymphomas (minimal treatment with the least side-effects), whilst intensive combinations of drugs are used in high-grade tumours with the intention of eradicating the disease. Overall, 50–60% of patients with certain subtypes of high-grade lymphoma appear to be cured by this approach.

Treatment Recommendations: 'Low-Grade' Lymphomas

- Stage I   Local radiotherapy—potentially curative.
- Stage II–IV Watch policy—only treat patient if they desire therapy, if masses become cosmetically unacceptable or if the tumour is causing untoward effects (i.e. ureteric obstruction). If therapy is necessary use minimal treatment to obtain response.

Using this policy, some patients will not require treatment for a number of years, and long-term survival (10 or more years) is seen in up to half of patients (Figure 10).

Treatment Recommendations: Intermediate- and High-Grade Lymphomas

- Stage I   Local radiotherapy; some centres will give adjuvant chemotherapy though benefit is not proved.
- Stage II–IV Combination chemotherapy (intensity depending on the favourability of stage and histology) is the mainstay of treatment. Intrathecal drugs may be used in patients at high risk of CNS

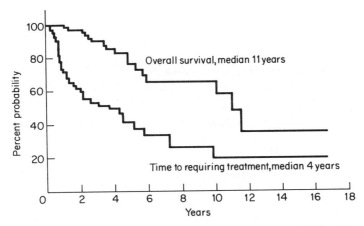

Figure 10. Survival and time to treatment of patients with low-grade lymphoma—treatment delayed until required (90% of patients had stage IV disease)

involvement. Recently high-dose chemotherapy and whole body irradiation with bone marrow transplantation has been used in patients failing conventional drug therapy. Results are encouraging so far and this approach is being extended.

Outcome and Special Complications

Low-grade or 'indolent' lymphomas are incurable even though they respond well to both irradiation and chemotherapy. However, because they are slowly progressive patients may live for 10 or more years (Figure 10). Spontaneous temporary regression of tumour is common (30% of patients) as is transformation to a high-grade histological type (20–30%).

High-grade tumours are rapidly fatal untreated, but intensive combination therapy will yield high complete remission rates; a good proportion of patients with certain histological subtypes will remain relapse-free.

The major complications of non-Hodgkin's lymphoma are related to involvement at extranodal sites. These include:

- CNS disease—brain and cord
- gastrointestinal tract—bleeding and perforation
- bone—pain, fracture, hypercalcaemia
- bone marrow—pancytopenia, immunosuppression; infections are a common problem

Amongst other problems arising from nodal involvement are:

- Mediastinal mass—SVC obstruction
- Retroperitoneal nodes—ureteric obstruction, pain, invasion of spine to cause cord compression and swelling of legs

Selected Papers and Reviews

Gatter, K. C., Heryet, A., *et al.* (1985) Clinical importance of analysing malignant tumours of uncertain origin with immunohistological techniques. *Lancet* i: 1305–1308.

Horning, S. J. and Rosenberg, S. A. (1984) Survival, spontaneous regression and histologic transformation in initially untreated non-Hodgkin's lymphoma of low grade. *New England Journal of Medicine*, **311**: 1471–1475.

Mackintosh, F. R., *et al.* (1982) Central nervous system involvement in non-Hodgkin's lymphoma: an analysis of 105 cases. *Cancer*, **49**: 586–595.

Mead, G. M. and Whitehouse, J. M. A. (1986) Modern management of non-Hodgkin's lymphoma. *British Medical Journal*, **293**: 577–580.

The Non-Hodgkin's Lymphoma Pathologic Classification Project (NLPCP) (1982) National Cancer Institute sponsored study of classifications of non-Hodgkin's lymphomas. *Cancer*, **49**: 2112–2135.

Ziegler, J. L. (1981) Burkitt's lymphoma. *New England Journal of Medicine*, **305**: 735–745.

LEUKAEMIAS

The group of illnesses known as leukaemia are a disparate collection of disease characterized by infiltration, with malignant cells, of the peripheral blood, bone marrow and other tissues. Their behaviour ranges from ones which are rapidly fatal if untreated to others which are very indolent and slow growing.

Incidence and Epidemiology

All types of leukaemia together represent just under 3% of cases of cancer in England and Wales. This figure is similar to that in the United States; incidence rates around the world do not vary greatly (Figure 11).

Acute and chronic leukaemias are roughly equal in incidence. However, most of the cases of acute leukaemia in adults (85%) are non-lymphocytic (myeloid). Nearly all chronic leukaemias are found in adults—two-thirds being lymphocytic in nature. Leukaemia in children is usually acute, and lymphocytic heavily outweighs non-lymphocytic in incidence. Leukaemia is rather commoner in males than females (3:2). The incidence of acute non-lymphocytic leukaemia rises with age, whilst that of lymphocytic leukaemia is bimodal (Figure 12) with peaks at ages 5–15 and 60+.

Aetiology and Pathogenesis

A wide variety of potential causative factors have been identified, though their importance is unclear.

Genetic

A number of inherited conditions appear to result in an increased risk of developing leukaemia; many of these are associated with somatic chromosome aneuploidy (see Chapter 1). They include:

- Down's syndrome (trisomy 21—caused by non-disjunction of the chromosome). The risk of leukaemias is increased 20-fold and is present at all ages, though the young develop acute lymphocytic leukaemia while older subjects develop acute non-lymphocytic leukaemia.
- Klinefelter's syndrome (XXY and variants)
- Patau's syndrome (trisomy D syndrome)
- Fanconi syndrome (autosomal recessive)
- Bloom's syndrome ⎫
- Ataxic telangiectasia ⎬ Spontaneous chromosomal breakages
- Kostman's syndrome ⎭

Radiation

There is a definite causal link between exposure to ionizing radiation and the development of acute leukaemia. This is based on study of those exposed to radiation in the atomic bombing of Hiroshima and Nagasaki in 1945 (Figure 13). There was an

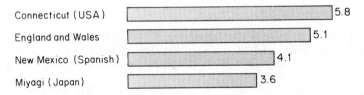

Figure 11. Incidence of acute and chronic leukaemias around the world (per 100,000)

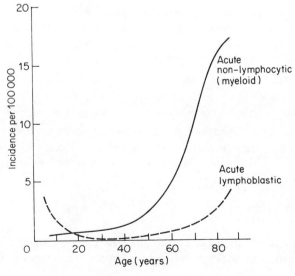

Figure 12. Incidence of acute lymphoblastic and acute non-lymphocytic leukaemias in England and Wales, by age

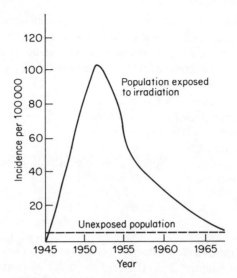

Figure 13. Incidence of leukaemia in those exposed to radiation at Hiroshima and Nagasaki compared to an unexposed Japanese population

enormous increase in incidence of leukaemia, which reached a peak 5–8 years after the event but which continued to show excess deaths for 20 years. The medical use of radiation confirms these data. Increased rates of leukaemia being found in:

- Early radiologists who did not perceive the need for adequate protection.
- Children exposed to radiation used as a treatment for ringworm.
- Those with ankylosing spondylitis treated with radiation.
- Cancer patients treated with therapeutic doses of radiation (Hodgkin's disease), though the risk, paradoxically, seems greater for patients receiving lower doses.

Viruses

Though viruses are established as having a causal role in a variety of leukaemias in animals (Chapter 2), such evidence is lacking in man. Recent evidence suggests that retroviruses (HTLV-1) may cause some types of adult T-cell leukaemia (especially that seen in Japan and the Caribbean).

Carcinogenic Chemicals

Chemicals and drugs which may lead to marrow aplasia can also cause acute non-lymphocytic leukaemia in affected individuals. Implicated compounds included:

- benzene
- chloramphenicol

- phenylbutazone
- anti-cancer drugs, especially alkylating agents.

In most cases the leukaemia occurs after a period of marrow failure. Chromosomal abnormalities are nearly always detectable.

Pathology and Natural History

In recent years there has been a marked improvement in understanding about the maturation of cells in the bone marrow and peripheral blood (Figure 14). The individual cells in acute leukaemia frequently retain the membrane, cytoplasmic and nuclear characteristics of normal cells. Because of this, it is possible to relate various types of acute leukaemia to various stages of myeloid and lymphoid maturation.

Diagnosis is based on examination of peripheral blood and bone marrow using:

- light microscopic appearance of stained sections
- staining pattern using Sudan black, peroxidase, PAS, acid
  phosphatase and naphthol ASD

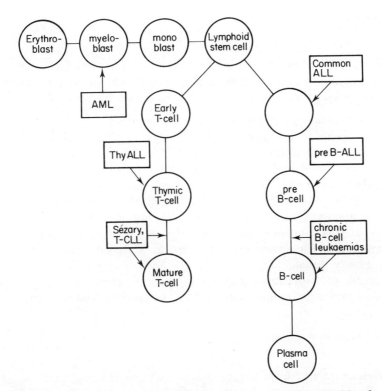

Figure 14. Haemopoiesis and leukaemia: the haemopoietic stem cell is capable of commitment to leukaemic erythroid, granulocytic and megakaryocytic precursors as well as lymphocytic cells of B, T or null cell type (ALL = acute lymphocytic leukaemia; AML = acute myelogenous leukaemia)

- membrane markers (common ALL antigen [CALLA],
  monoclonal antibodies to T-cell antigens, a DNA polymerase-
  TdT, antibodies to surface immunoglobulin-SIg, and a membrane glycoprotein Ia)

Using these criteria acute leukaemia is divided into lymphocytic and non-lymphocytic (myeloid) types. Non-lymphocytic leukaemia is further subdivided into six classes according to the French-American-British (FAB) classification (Table 7); this same classification divides lymphoblastic leukaemia into three classes.

Cytogenetics may give additional useful information for classifying the type of leukaemia. Abnormalities are found in 60–80% of patients, the chromosomal changes differing between lymphocytic and non-lymphocytic leukaemias (Table 8). Studies have shown that the Philadelphia chromosome (Ph[1]) is not specific for chronic myelogenous leukaemia (page 28), suggesting that a common stem cell may give rise to malignant cells with lymphoid or myeloid characteristics.

Presenting Features, Investigations and Staging

Acute Leukaemia

Most symptoms are non-specific, arising because of anaemia, leucopenia, thrombocytopenia and leucocytosis. Symptoms may seem to start abruptly but up to half of patients have symptoms present for 3 or more months. Common features are:

- Anaemia—fatigue, dyspnoea, pallor, palpitations.
- Neutropenia—local infections (abscesses, etc.) and systemic
  infections (pneumonia, etc.). In addition to low absolute
  levels of neutrophils, those present may function poorly.
- Thrombocytopenia—bleeding from gums, nose bleeds,
  gastrointestinal and urinary tract haemorrhage, intermenstrual
  or abnormal menstrual bleeding. Bleeding into skin
  (petechiae and purpura). Worse if sepsis is present.
- Symptoms of increased blood viscosity if white cell count is
  grossly raised.
- Fatigue and weakness is reported by half of patients.
- Bone pain is uncommon but may be very pronounced in some
  patients.

Physical findings may include:

- fever
- splenomegaly (usually lymphocytic) or chronic myelogenous
  leukaemia
- hepatomegaly
- lymphadenopathy (usually lymphocytic)
- evidence of bleeding (especially promyelocytic [M3] leukaemia)

Table 7. The French-American-British (FAB) classification of acute leukaemia

ACUTE LYMPHOBLASTIC LEUKAEMIA (ALL)

L1 A relatively homogeneous cell population with 75% or more small cells with scanty cytoplasm, finely dispersed chromatin and regular nuclear shape

L2 A heterogeneous cell population as regards size, chromatin pattern and nuclear shape. The cells are usually large with the cytoplasm occupying 20% or more of the surface area of the cell

L3 A large and relatively homogeneous cell population with regular nuclei and a fine chromatin pattern. Nucleoli are prominent. Lymphoblasts resemble those seen in Burkitt's lymphoma

ACUTE NON-LYMPHOCYTIC (MYELOID) LEUKAEMIA (ANLL)

M1 Myeloblastic leukaemia without maturation. Blasts show minimal evidence of myeloid differentiation with more than 3% of the blasts myeloperoxidase-positive and/or containing azurophilic granules, Auer rods, or both. No evidence of maturation is present

M2 Myeloblastic leukaemia with maturation. Some maturation of the granulocytic series is evident with more than 50% of the nucleated bone marrow cells consisting of myeloblasts and promyelocytes

M3 Hypergranular promyelocytic leukaemia. The predominant cells are abnormal promyelocytes packed with dense granulation and multiple Auer rods

M4 Myelomonocytic leukaemia. Evidence of both granulocytic and monocytic differentiation is present in varying proportions

M5 Monocytic leukaemia. Poorly or well differentiated monocytic leukaemia.

M6 Erythroleukaemia. Erythroblasts exceed 50% in the bone marrow, and bizarre morphological variants are found.

- evidence of infection
- skin rash, soft tissue and gum infiltration (especially monocytic [M5] and myelomonocytic [M4] leukaemia)

Initial tests include a full blood count: findings in the peripheral blood are given in the box below.

Anaemia.

Reduced reticulocyte count.

White cell count increased in most patients, but less than 5000 × 10^9/l in 30%.

Circulating leukaemia cells in peripheral blood in 95%.

Platelet count less than 100,000 × 10^9/l in 75%.

Once the diagnosis is suspected patients should be fully evaluated before therapy is begun. The aim of investigation (see box below) is to confirm the diagnosis, define

Table 8. Chromosome abnormalities in adult acute leukaemia: laboratory and clinical findings

Chromosome abnormality	FAB type (frequency)	Typical physical findings	Typical laboratory findings	Response rate and survival‡
Ph¹(22q−) t(9;22)	L2 (20% adult ALL)	Typical of ALL	Non-T, non-B, CALLA +* WBC>50,000/μl in 1/3 of cases	CR rate low; poor survival
t(4;11)	L2 (10% adult ALL)	Splenomegaly; 20 to 30% CNS and mediastinal involvement	Non-T, non-B, CALLA−* WBC very high	CR rate low; poor survival
t(8;14)	L3 (2% adult ALL)	CNS involvement common	B-cell; WBC low	CR rate low; very poor survival
t(8;21)	M2 (5% adult ANLL)	Young	Normal WBC	High CR rate and long survival
t(15;17)	M3 (5% adult ANLL)	Haemorrhage	DIC†	Long remissions and survival
del(16)(q22)	M2 or M4 (15% adult ANLL)	Typical ANLL	Marrow eosinophilia	Long remissions and survival

*CALLA = common ALL antigen.
†DIC = disseminated intravascular coagulation.
‡CR = complete remission.

the subtype, look for sepsis and bleeding, and to evaluate whether specific organ toxicity has developed.

Bone marrow aspirate: Morphology
(and trephine)   Cytochemistry
                         Cell markers
                         TdT
                         Cytogenetics

Blood chemistry: Liver function
                         Renal function
                         Calcium and phosphate
                         Glucose
                         Uric acid

Coagulation profile: Prothrombin time
                         Partial thromboplastin time
                         Thrombin time
                         Factor V
                         Fibrinogen
                         Fibrin split products

Chest X-ray

Lumbar puncture: Cytology   ⎫
                         Protein   ⎬ Acute lymphocytic
                         Glucose   ⎪ leukaemia
                         Microbiology   ⎭

Blood type and HLA typing if allogeneic bone marrow transplant a possibility.

Chronic Leukaemias

Chronic myelogenous leukaemia usually has an insidious onset. Symptoms are fatigue, malaise, fever, night sweats, weight loss and abdominal discomfort. Less commonly, bleeding or bruising may occur from platelet dysfunction. Symptoms of hyperleucocytosis are rarely the presenting features.

Physical findings include splenomegaly, which rarely may be massive, anaemia, lymphadenopathy and soft tissue tumour deposits.

The peripheral blood shows a very high leucocyte count (mean 200,000) with the whole spectrum of myeloid maturation present. There is usually an accompanying mild normochromic normocytic anaemia (9–10 g/dl). Thrombocytosis is common, with more than 50% of patients having a platelet count of greater than 450,000 $\times$ 10^9/l; however, platelet function and morphology may be abnormal. The level of leucocytes may appear to cycle, the period of oscillations varying from 1 to 3 months.

Bone marrow changes cause various features (see box).

Hypercellularity with granulocytic and megakaryocytic hyperplasia.
There is an elevated myeloid/erythroid (M:E) ratio.
Basophilia and eosinophilia are always present.
Myelofibrosis is present in some patients.

Investigations may result in other findings (see box).

Low level of leucocyte alkaline phosphatase
Increased levels of vitamin B$_{12}$
Philadelphia chromosome
Hyperuricaemia

Blasts crisis of chronic myelogenous leukaemia (see below) has similar features to acute leukaemia.

Chronic Lymphocytic Leukaemia

Chronic lymphocytic leukaemia is generally an indolent process, often detected as an incidental finding on routine blood count (25%). Typical findings are shown in the box.

Persistent lymphocytosis with small uniform cells
Demonstration that they are monoclonal B-cells (T-cell CLL is rare)
Lymphadenopathy
Hepatomegaly
Splenomegaly
Anaemia
Thrombocytopenia
Fevers, malaise and fatigue
Coomb's test positive in one-third of patients

Various attempts have been made to develop a classification in order to stage chronic lymphocytic leukaemia, though none is wholly successful. These classifications are generally based on the presence or absence of anaemia and thrombocytopenia, and the level of lymphocytosis, lymphadenopathy and organ failure.

Treatment

This is discussed according to the major subtype of leukaemia. In most situations chemotherapy is the only useful option—the aim of therapy will depend on the exact clinical situation. Where hyperuricaemia is likely patients *must* be started on allopurinol before treatment is started. Likewise, therapy for infections (especially abscesses) should be started urgently and metabolic complications corrected before treatment.

Acute Non-Lymphocytic Leukaemia (Myeloid)

Major improvements in treatment have yielded high response rates and a small proportion of long-term survivors. The main change in treatment philosophy in the past 20 years has been the development of drug regimes designed to cause profound pancytopenia—the initial goal is to obtain quickly a complete remission. Although intensive combinations of drugs are used to ablate the marrow, these give periods of profound neutropenia which are shorter than those produced when lower dose, less 'toxic', therapy is used since more courses are needed to obtain remission. Such intensive treatments are most successful in younger patients; response rates and survival are poorer the older the population being treated. Because of this treatments should be selected according to age and general fitness. The other reason for the better current results is improved patient support:

- transfusions of blood and platelets
- antibiotics
- antifungals
- antiviral agents
- mouth care
- use of long-term intravenous catheters
- management of electrolyte imbalances and renal failure.

Suitable patients (age and general fitness) are treated intensively with induction therapy (usually cytosine arabinoside, daunorubicin and thioguanine). Patients who are going to remit will usually do so with the first or second cycle. Such patients will receive similar therapy for several cycles (up to four) as a consolidation treatment—such treatment is usually better tolerated since the marrow has returned to normal. Maintenance therapy does not seem to improve survival. Young patients with a suitable donor may benefit from an allogeneic bone marrow transplant and high-dose chemotherapy. Recently, autologous bone marrow transplantation has been tested—patients in relapse receive their own remission bone marrow as a support during very high-dose chemotherapy.

Acute Lymphoblastic Leukaemia

Treatment of this disease in children is discussed in Chapter 21. This section refers to adults (more than 15 years). The results are not nearly as good as in children and worsen with increasing age. Combinations of drugs similar to those employed in aggressive lymphomas are used in an attempt to induce a complete remission. High response rates are achieved (75%), when further consolidation or maintenance therapy is given. These patients receive CNS prophylaxis (intrathecal drugs) since meningeal involvement is common. Despite good initial results most patients relapse within 18 months and the median survival is only about 2 years. Bone marrow transplantation is currently being tested.

Chronic Lymphocytic Leukaemia

The aim of therapy is to control the disease with as little treatment as possible. Asymptomatic patients will not benefit from treatment since despite marked responsiveness to chemotherapy cure is not an achievable goal. Such patients are best watched until disease progression results in symptoms that may be palliated. When treatment is required, alkylating agents with or without glucocorticosteroids are preferred. Resistant or rapidly progressive disease may be treated with drug combinations similar to those used in aggressive lymphomas, though results are not good.

Radiotherapy may be used palliatively, and in the past whole body irradiation has been used. Splenectomy may be helpful when hypersplenism is causing symptoms which are difficult to control.

Chronic Myelogenous Leukaemia

During the early chronic phase of this disease the aim of treatment is suppression of haemopoiesis. This results in reduced peripheral leucocyte count and spleen size, as well as an amelioration of the symptoms of the disease. Such control is usually achieved by the use of an oral alkylating agent, the dose being titrated so that the leucocyte count falls to about $20,000 \times 10^9/l$. Treatment is then stopped but may be reinstituted when the counts rise again or if the patient becomes symptomatic.

Other therapies include:

- leucopheresis if the count is very high and there are symptoms of hyperviscosity
- splenectomy ⎫ does not influence the course of the disease
- splenic radiotherapy ⎬ but may give symptomatic relief

After a period of time (2–3 years) the disease changes character, becoming more aggressive—this is known as 'blast phase' or 'accelerated phase' disease. The malignant cells may resemble lymphoblasts (20%) or myeloblasts, and chemotherapy appropriate to each type of acute leukaemia is used. Unfortunately, accelerated phase disease is generally unresponsive, though 'ALL-like' disease patients generally derive more benefit from treatment.

Allogeneic bone marrow transplantation has been used with some success in both the chronic and accelerated phases.

Selected Papers and Reviews

Burns, C. P. Armitage, J. D., Frey, A. L., Dick, F. R., Jordan, J. E. and Woolson, R. F. (1981) Analysis of the presenting features of adult acute leukaemia: the French-American-British classification. *Cancer*, **47**: 2460–2469.

Kreffler, H. P. and Golde, D. W. (1981) Chronic myelogenous leukaemia—new concepts. *New England Journal of Medicine*, **304**: 1201–1209, 1269–1274.

Kurzock, R., *et al.* (1988) The molecular genetics of Philadelphia chromosome-positive leukaemias. *New England Journal of Medicine*, **319**: 990–998.

Lister, T. A., Whitehouse, J. M. A., Beard, M. E. J., Brearley, R. L., Wrigley, P. F. M., Oliver, R. T. D., Freeman, J. E., Woodruff, R. K., Malpas, T. S., Paxton, A. M. and Crowther, D. (1978) Combination chemotherapy for acute lymphoblastic leukaemia in adults. *British Medical Journal*, **i**: 199–203.

Peterson, B. A. and Bloomfield, C. D. (1981) Long-term disease-free survival in acute non-lymphocytic leukaemia. *Blood*, **57**: 1144–1147.

The Third International Workshop on Chromosomes in Cancer (1981) *Cancer Genetics and Cytogenetics*, **4**: 95–142.

MYELOMA

Myeloma is a malignancy of B-cells which develops by proliferation of a single clone of plasma cells. This clone produces an excess of a single antibody molecule—this is referred to as a monoclonal or M protein.

Incidence and Epidemiology

This disease becomes more common as age increases (Figure 15) and is seen more often in men (1.8:1). The incidence in the United States is highest in blacks, in whom it is the commonest cancer of the lymphohaemopoietic system. There is a moderate variation in frequency around the world (Figure 16).

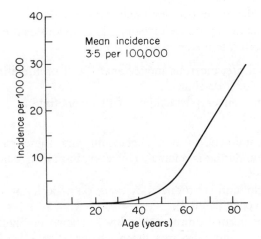

Figure 15. Incidence of myeloma by age in England and Wales

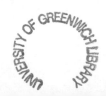

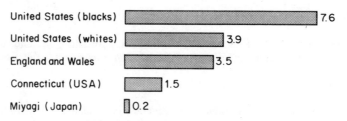

Figure 16. Incidence of myeloma around the world (per 100,000)

Aetiology and Pathogenesis

The finding of a monoclonal (M) protein suggests the malignant transformation of a single clone of cells derived from B-lymphocyte differentiation. It has been suggested, based on an animal model, that over-stimulation of the immune system as a result of chronic inflammation is a causal factor, though this is unsubstantiated.

There appears to be a modest excess of deaths from myeloma (4.7-fold) in atom-bomb survivors, and those occupationally exposed to chronic low doses of radiation have a small increased risk. Reports have also linked myeloma to a number of other occupations, including farming, smelting, plastics, woodworking and the food industry.

A number of reports of apparent familial myelomatosis have appeared, some cases appearing to have a recessive mode of inheritance.

Pathology and Natural History

Some otherwise healthy, often elderly, individuals have a monoclonal protein in their blood. This may remain stable or gradually increase over many years, the condition being known as 'monoclonal gammopathy of undetermined significance'. In one large study of such patients followed for 5 or more years, 60% showed no change in the M protein level and 10% developed myeloma.

Thus, it appears that the expanded clone may persist without additional expansion, or it may continue to expand to produce myeloma. Because of this it has been suggested that myeloma results from a two-step process:

- Emergence of a precancerous monoclonal B-cell proliferation partially under host control.
- A further event converts a member of this clone into a neoplastic cell.

Some myelomas are indolent in their behaviour and these patients have been described as having 'smouldering myeloma'. However, in most patients any preclinical phase appears to be brief.

Monoclonal immunoglobulin is produced by the great majority of myeloma cells and may be one of several types (Table 9).

The basic structure of normal immunoglobulins is shown in Figure 17. It consists of two polypeptide light chains and two heavy chains. These are held together by disulphide bonds. There is a variable region in the heavy chain, accounting for the

Table 9. Types of immunoglobulin produced by myeloma cells

Immunoglobulin	Proportion (%) of cases in which present
IgG	55
IgA	25
Bence Jones only	15
IgM	2
IgD	1
Biclonal	1
None	1

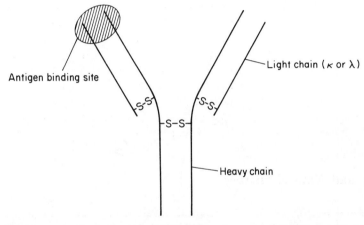

Figure 17. Schematic representation of the structure of immunoglobulin molecules. Two light chains are joined by disulphide bonds to two heavy chains. These are joined by further disulphide bonds. The heavy chain varies in each immunoglobulin class, but light chains do not. Figure 18 (page 404) gives a more detailed description of the molecule

five classes of immunoglobulin (IgG, IgA, IgM, IgD, IgE). There are two types of light chain (kappa and lambda).

The molecule can be cleaved by papain into two fractions (Figure 18). One is called the antigen-binding fraction (Fab) and the other, because it crystallizes, the crystallizable fraction (Fc). The complete molecule has two antigen-combining sites. The Fc portion is needed for complement activation, cell binding and placental transport.

Bence Jones protein consists of immunoglobulin light chains. The first case of myeloma was reported in 1847 when Bence Jones described a patient who excreted a protein (light chains) in the urine which precipitated when heated to 40–60°C and redissolved at about 100°C.

Cytological and histological preparations of myeloma tissue show infiltration with sheets of plasma cells. These may be atypical, the cytoplasm being ballooned with intracellular protein (Russell bodies). Bone marrow may show focal collections of plasma cells or may be diffusely involved.

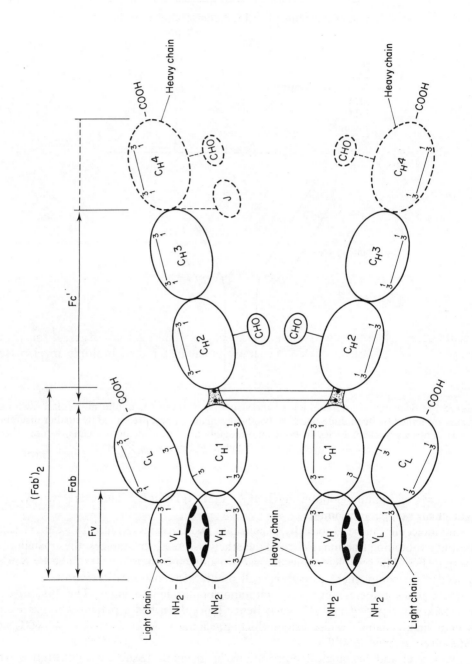

Presenting Features, Investigations and Staging

Symptoms and signs of myeloma are related to the effects on the bone marrow and skeleton as well as the distant consequences of the condition. They include:

- bone pain (70% of patients), usually ribs, spine and pelvis
- pathological fracture
- malaise and anorexia
- hypercalcaemia (nausea, altered level of consciousness, constipation, polydipsia and polyuria)
- anaemia
- infections (reduced normal immunoglobulins)
- spinal cord compression (fractures of vertebrae or paraspinal mass of tumour)
- abnormal bleeding
- renal failure
- hyperviscosity (especially IgM and IgA myeloma)

Spread

This is a disease of B-cells; the most commonly involved sites are:

- bone marrow
- bone

Extra-osseous plasmacytomas may occasionally be found in soft tissues; if this is the sole site of disease the outlook is generally much better than multiple myeloma or solitary plasmacytoma of bone.

Various staging classifications (based on haemoglobin, serum calcium, production rate of M protein, number of lytic lesions) have been proposed though none is especially useful.

Figure 18. Schematic diagram of the basic domain structure of the light and heavy polypeptide chains of immunoglobulins. The domains in the amino-terminal (NH_2) portion of each chain, the variant regions, are designated V_L and V_H for the light chain and heavy chain, respectively. The domains in the carboxyl-terminal (COOH) portion of each chain, the constant regions, are designated C_L and C_H for the light chain and heavy chain, respectively; the three C_H domains are designated C_H of immunoglobulins M and E and contain an additional domain designated C_H1, C_H2, and C_H3 (the C_H of immunoglobulins M and E contain an additional domain designated C_H4). An additional polypeptide chain, the J chain, is disulphide-linked to the C_H3 or C_H4 domains of polymeric immunoglobulins A and M, respectively. The carbohydrate moiety, usually exclusively on the heavy chain, is designated CHO. The polypeptide region between the C_H1 and C_H2 domains is termed the hinge region (indicated by the lightly stippled area); this region is particularly susceptible to proteolytic cleavage. Papain cleaves the heavy chain on the amino-terminal side of the interheavy chain disulphide bonds, resulting in the production of fragment Fc and the two monovalent antibody-combining fragments Fab; pepsin cleaves the heavy chain on the carboxyl-terminal side of the interheavy chain disulphide bonds, resulting in the production of the divalent antibody-combining fragment, $(Fab')_2$; and under special conditions of peptic cleavage the variant region (V_L and V_H) can be cleaved from the intact immunoglobulin molecule yielding the Fv fragment. (Adapted by permission of the *New England Journal of Medicine*, from Solomon, A.: Bence Jones proteins and light chains of immunoglobulins. *N. Engl. J. Med.*, 294:18, 1976.)

Investigations and Staging

Diagnostic procedures include the following:

- full blood count—mild anaemia
- ESR—invariably raised, usually greater than 100 mm/hr
- urea and electrolytes—renal insufficiency
- calcium—may be raised
- bone X-rays—fracture and/or multiple lytic lesions
- quantitative serum immunoglobulins—monoclonal band
- urine—Bence Jones protein (light chains)
- bone marrow—infiltration with abnormal plasma cells
- B2 microglobulin—good measure of disease activity

The diagnosis of myeloma is based on the findings shown in Figure 19. In most patients the diagnosis rests on marrow infiltration with plasma cells and the finding of lytic bone disease with or without abnormal plasma or urinary immunoglobulins. However, it should be remembered that immunoglobulins can be raised in other conditions (see box).

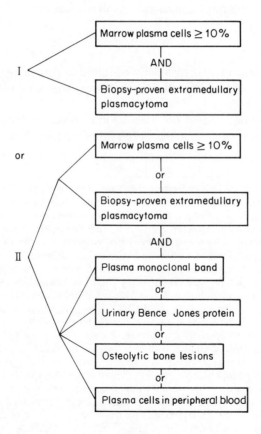

Figure 19. Criteria for the diagnosis of multiple myeloma

Benign monoclonal gammopathy of undetermined significance
Lymphoma, including Waldenström's macroglobulinaemia
Some solid tumours
Polyarteritis nodosa
Rheumatoid arthritis

Treatment

Myeloma is often a relatively indolent disease at presentation. This chronic phase may last a number of years, when the disease may be controlled by chemotherapy and radiotherapy. However, the terminal phase, when the disease becomes non-responsive, is usually short.

Supportive Care

A large part of the treatment of myeloma is managing the problems caused by the disease. Measures include:

Adequate analgesia ⎫   immobile patients are at risk of
Mobilization   ⎬   hypercalcaemia
Good fluid intake   ⎭
Treat infections
Transfusion
Pin fractures

Radiotherapy

Radiation is used primarily to treat painful areas of bone or lesions causing spinal cord compression. Only relatively low doses are required. Hemibody (upper or lower half body) irradiation has been used in some patients with diffuse bone pain unresponsive to cytotoxic treatment.

Chemotherapy

Alkylating agents together with prednisolone have been the standard therapy of this disease for the past 20 years. These are traditionally given intermittently and continued until the level of the M protein has fallen to a plateau. Treatment is then stopped until disease progression (and rising M band).

Recently, a number of combinations of cytotoxic drugs with high doses of steroids have shown a higher level of activity and apparently more prolonged survival. Despite this, control is incomplete and temporary.

High doses of alkylating agents with autologous bone marrow support have been tested in selected patients. The results show improved response rates, some patients having no detectable M band, and possibly better survival. This approach, however, remains experimental.

Outcome and Special Complications

The median survival for patients with multiple myeloma is about $2\frac{1}{2}$ years (Figure 20a); for patients with a solitary plasmacytoma the outlook is better (Figure 20b).

Complications of myeloma are legion. The more important ones are listed in the box below.

Hypercalcaemia
Fractures or generalized osteoporosis
Extramedullary plasmacytoma (especially nasopharynx)
Renal failure (up to 50% of patients)
Hyperviscosity
Cryoglobulinaemia
Clotting disorders
Anaemia
Susceptibility to infections
Amyloidosis (myeloma is relatively common cause of this condition)

Selected Papers and Reviews

Bergsagel, D. E. (1979) Treatment of plasma cell myeloma. *Ann. Rev. Med.*, **30**: 431–443.

Durrie, B. and Salmon, S. E. (1975) A clinical staging system for multiple myeloma. Correlation of measured myeloma cell mass with presenting clinical features, response to treatment and survival. *Cancer*, **36**: 842–854.

Kyle, R. A. (1978) Monoclonal gammopathy of undetermined significance. *American Journal of Medicine*, **64**: 814–826.

Pavlovsky, S., Saslavsky, J., Tezanos-Pinto, M., Palmer, L., Curachet, M., Lein, J. M., Garay, G., Dragosky, M., Quiroga-Micheo, E., Hubermann, A. B. and Pizzolatto, M. (1984) A randomized trial of melphalan and prednisolone versus melphalan, prednisolone, cyclophosphamide, MeCCNU and vincristine in untreated myeloma. *Journal of Clinical Oncology*, **2**: 831–840.

Soloman, A. (1978) Bence Jones proteins and light chains of immunoglobulins. *New England Journal of Medicine*, **294**: 17–23.

Solon, A. (1982) Bence Jones proteins: malignant or benign? *New England Journal of Medicine*, **306**: 605–607.

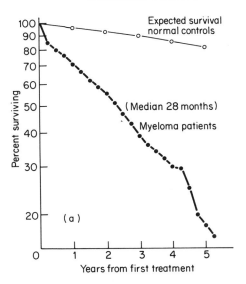

Figure 20a. Overall survival of 364 patients with myeloma treated with alkylating agents and prednisone. The expected survival of age- and sex-matched normals is shown in the upper curve. Adapted by permission of NEJM, from Bergsagel, R. *et al.* (1979), *New England Journal of Medicine*, **301**: 743–748.

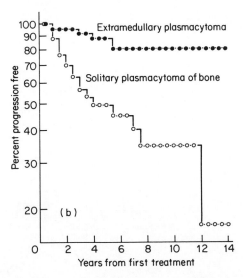

Figure 20b. Progression-free survival of patients with extramedullary plasmacytomas (49), or solitary plasmacytomas (36) of bone. (Note the scale of this graph is different from 20a). From De Vita *et al.* (1985). *Principles and Practice of Oncology*, Lippincott, Philadelphia. Reproduced by permission

21 | Paediatric Cancers

C. J. WILLIAMS

Incidence and Epidemiology

Although rare, childhood cancer is the leading cause of non-accidental death in children between the ages of 1 and 15 years.

The commonest tumours by site in western countries are shown in Table 1. The types and frequency of childhood cancers vary with age, sex, race, socio-economic status and geographical location. For instance, Ewing's sarcoma is a tumour of white children not black; acute lymphocytic leukaemia affects middle-class children more than lower-class children; neuroblastoma is commonest in the first 5 years whereas bone sarcomas are seen most often in adolescents.

Aetiology and Pathogenesis

The variations in incidence cited above suggest that genetic and environmental factors are important in the pathogenesis of childhood cancer.

Genetic Factors

Some childhood tumours have a clear genetic basis. These include:

- retinoblastoma—dominant inheritance in all bilateral tumours and 10% of unilateral (see Chapter 1)
- xeroderma pigmentosa ⎫
- neurofibromatosis ⎪
- Fanconi's aplastic anaemia ⎬ Increased incidence of various cancers
- Wiskott-Aldrich syndrome ⎪
- Bloom's syndrome ⎭

Table 1. Incidence of childhood tumours by site

Site	Incidence per 100,000	Proportion of childhood cancer (%)
Leukaemia	3.4	30
Central nervous system	2.1	19
Lymphomas	1.5	14
Sympathetic nervous system	0.9	8
Soft tissue	0.7	7
Kidney	0.6	7
Bone	0.5	5
Retinoblastoma	0.3	3
Liver	0.1	1
Others	0.6	6

Environmental Factors

Radiation has been demonstrated to cause cancers, data being derived from survivors of the atomic bombing of Nagasaki and Hiroshima: most childhood cancers were leukaemias. Thymic irradiation, used in the past for benign conditions, led to thyroid carcinoma and leukaemia.

Chemical exposure may lead to cancer. For instance, the use of diethylstilboestrol in pregnancy to prevent spontaneous abortion led to subsequent adenocarcinoma of the vagina in offspring.

Viruses

It has long been suspected that viruses may play a role in causing leukaemias and lymphomas. Despite demonstration of a causative role in animals, conclusive evidence in man is still awaited. The only virus which appears to be strongly related to childhood cancer is the Epstein-Barr virus which is associated with Burkitt's lymphoma.

Principles of Management of Children with Cancer

Childhood cancers differ from those in adults in a variety of ways:

- Leukaemias, sarcomas and 'blastic' tumours predominate in contrast to carcinomas in adults.
- Childhood cancers are more often related to genetic and developmental disorders whereas environmental exposure to carcinogens is of paramount importance in adults.
- Cancers in children appear to be more rapidly growing than the common adult cancers.
- Early blood-borne spread is commoner with childhood cancers.

- Cancers in children tend to be much more responsive to cytotoxic drugs.
- Cure rates for advanced childhood cancers are generally higher than for advanced adult tumours. Rapid improvements in therapy have been made (Figure 1).

When treating children with cancer it is important to remember that their body is growing and developing rapidly, so that cytotoxic treatment and irradiation may affect normal development (physically and socially). Particular points requiring emphasis in the care of paediatric tumours are shown in the box below.

Diagnosis and investigations should be prompt—these tumours grow quickly and may be rapidly life threatening.

Histopathological diagnosis may be difficult since the tumours are often undifferentiated. Immunohistochemistry and electron microscopy may be helpful.

Coordinated multi-disciplinary treatment is often required—this needs an experienced team of surgeons, radiotherapists and paediatric oncologists. These are supported by a team who can give optimum nursing and psychosocial support to the whole family.

Such expertise is, generally, only available in a specialist centre.

The long-term morbidity of treatment is of special importance since cure rates are high; this includes the psychosocial consequences of the illness. Paediatric oncology is a highly specialized field and in-depth discussion of the treatment of individual types of paediatric cancer cannot be given here. However, a brief description of management of the common cancers follows.

Acute Lymphocytic Leukaemia (ALL)

This is the commonest neoplasm in children, accounting for nearly a third of cases. Peak age of onset is 2–6 years (see Figure 12, Chapter 20, page 391). It is seen equally in girls and boys and is commonest in higher socio-economic groups.

The cells of 'common' ALL range from small lymphocytes to large lymphoblasts and primitive bizarre undifferentiated cells; cytochemical staining often shows:

- positive periodic-acid Schiff's (PAS) granules
- TdT activity
- common ALL antigen (CALLA) positive
- Ia positive

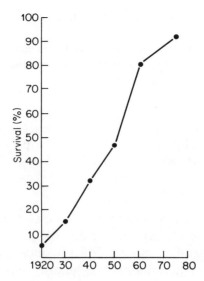

Figure 1. Two-year survival for Wilms' tumour patients treated at Children's Hospital Medical Center Boston: by decade showing rapidly improving results. Adapted from D'Angio, G.J. and Belasco, J.B. (1981) 'Wilms' Tumor', Table 1. In J.H. Burchenal and H.F. Oettgen (eds), *Cancer: Achievements, Challenges and Prospects for the 1980s*, volume 2. Grune & Stratton, Orlando. Reproduced by permission

Patients presenting with high leukaemia cell counts in the peripheral blood tend to have a worse prognosis although the initial response rates are the same as those with lower counts.

Treatment

The object of treatment is cure, and currently 50–60% of children with ALL are cured. The mainstay of treatment is chemotherapy. This is given in several phases:

- Remission induction. ALL is very responsive to chemotherapy and complete remission can be achieved with fairly simple drug combinations. During treatment care is needed to prevent the complications of rapid tumour lysis (page 146).
- Maintenance chemotherapy. Once a complete remission has been achieved a programme of maintenance treatment is begun. This most commonly includes weekly pulses of oral drugs with or without intermittent pulses of more intensive therapy. This may continue for as long as 2 to 3 years.
- Craniospinal therapy. There is a high risk of meningeal leukaemia if therapy is not directed to these sites. The commonest approach is cranial irradiation and a course of intrathecal chemotherapy.

- For boys testicular relapse may be troublesome and prophylactic testicular irradiation may be used, though some feel that relapse at this site is an indicator of inadequate remission induction chemotherapy.

Children may also present with thymic (T-cell) lymphoblastic lymphoma or thymic ALL as well as B-cell lymphoblastic lymphoma (Burkitt-like) and B-cell ALL. These tumours are particularly aggressive and require intensive chemotherapy. Relapse may occur early but those surviving disease-free for 2 years are generally cured. Some childhood ALLs have cells which lack features that enable them to be categorized—these are known as 'null cells'. They tend to have a high growth rate but are usually treated like common ALL.

Brain Tumours

Central nervous system tumours account for about one in five of childhood cancers. Mode of presentation is very variable (Chapter 7) but the commonest symptoms result from raised intracranial pressure (see box).

Enlarging head in infants
Headache
Vomiting
Neck stiffness and pain
Torticollis
Blurred vision

Other common symptoms include:

- ataxia
- nystagmus
- cranial nerve palsies

Treatment depends on histology, site and tumour extent. Radiotherapy is usually the most important available modality.

Astrocytoma

This is the commonest childhood brain tumour. It is usually low grade and *not* high grade as in adults. Cerebellar astrocytoma may often be curable with surgery. Where the tumour is cerebral, surgery is usually partial and postoperative radiation is given—survival rates may be as high as 50%. Thalamic and brain stem astrocytomas are treated with irradiation; long-term survival rates are about 30%.

Medulloblastoma

This is seen almost exclusively in children, usually in the roof of the fourth ventricle. Pathologically it is similar in appearance to neuroblastoma (see below). It has a tendency to spread via the CSF to distant meningeal sites. Surgery is undertaken to make the diagnosis and to insert a shunt to re-establish CSF flow. Radiation is the main treatment, the whole neuro-axis being treated owing to the tendency to CSF dissemination. Long-term survival rates are 30–40%; late relapses are not uncommon.

Ependymoma

In children ependymoma usually develops in the floor of the fourth ventricle. Prognosis is dependent upon grade and site. Radiotherapy is the primary modality; since subarachnoid seeding is relatively common the whole neuro-axis is often treated. Survival at 5 years is about 35%.

Craniopharyngiomas

These comprise the other relatively common group of childhood brain tumours. They may cause effects such as precocious puberty; treatment is surgery followed by irradiation.

Long-term Effects

There may be considerable morbidity from the tumour itself, from surgery and from irradiation of the immature brain. Complications include:

- neurological impairment
- mental impairment
- endocrine deficiencies
- bone growth impairment (due to neuro-axis irradiation)

Lymphoma

Most childhood lymphomas are high grade (page 302) in type. Some have been mentioned above in the context of acute lymphocytic lymphoma. Other high-grade lymphomas are treated with combination chemotherapy in a manner similar to lymphoma in adults.

Hodgkin's disease does occur in children; it is more common in underdeveloped countries. Because of the effects of high doses of radiation on bone growth and consequent skeletal deformity, low doses have tended to be combined with chemotherapy even for stage I and II disease. Results of treatment are similar to those in adults.

Neuroblastoma

This is the most common (7%) solid tumour of children after brain tumours. Half originate in the adrenal medulla and the rest can be anywhere along the sympathetic chain (Figure 2). Although the incidence of neuroblastomas is 1 per 100,000, *in situ* tumour is found in one in every 40 post mortems done in children dying without cancer. This implies spontaneous regressions. The peak age is 2 years (Figure 3) and the disease is rare beyond 6 years. The chances of cure also decrease with increasing age. Predisposing conditions include:

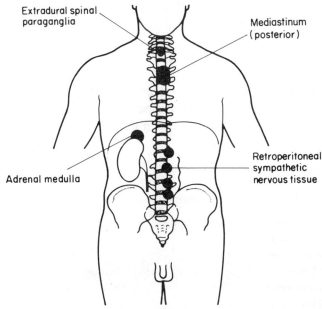

Figure 2. Primary sites for the development of neuroblastoma. Adapted by permission from Souhami, R.L. and Tobias, J.S. (1986) *Cancer and Its Management*, Blackwell Scientific Publications, Oxford

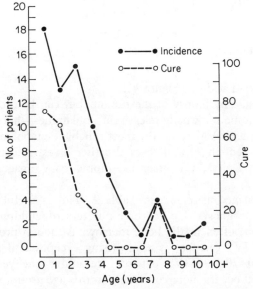

Figure 3. Incidence of neuroblastoma and the chances of cure by age. Reproduced by permission from Hassenbusch, S. (1977) *Journal of Paediatric Surgery*, **11**: 287–297, W.B. Saunders Co.

- von Recklinghausen's disease
- heterochromia aniscoria

The tumour is composed of small cells with a scanty cytoplasm which are often arranged in rosettes. Differentiation may be very variable. The main features differentiating neuroblastoma from other small and undifferentiated tumours of childhood are given in the box.

PAS positive, unlike Ewing's and other sarcomas.
Monoclonal antibody to neuroblastoma associated antigen positive.
Neurosecretory granules on electron microscopy.

Neuroblastomas may present in a number of ways:

- fever, malaise, weight loss and anaemia
- abdominal pain and mass ⎫
- mass in chest or neck ⎪
- cord compression ⎬ due to primary tumour
- Horner's syndrome ⎪
- loss of bladder control ⎭
- liver pain ⎫
- bone pain ⎬ due to secondary tumour
- proptosis of eye ⎪
- malignant meningitis ⎭
- hypertension ⎫
- diarrhoea ⎬ remote effects
- myoclonus/opsoclonus ⎭

These tumours spread widely (Figure 4).

The diagnosis is made by biopsy of the tumour but can be predicted biochemically in most cases. These tumours usually release catecholamines—homovanilic acid (HVA) and vanillyl mandelic acid (VMA) are the most reliable metabolites to measure. Raised 24-hour levels are present in 90% of cases. Further investigations include plain films (these tumours may calcify), CT images, isotopic bone images and bone marrow aspiration.

Neuroblastoma is staged as shown in Table 2. This is useful in selecting therapy and in deciding on prognosis. Up to three-quarters of children have disseminated disease at presentation, often in the bone marrow. Although prognosis worsens with increasing stage, the IVS category is a surprising exception to this rule (Figure 5). Despite the fact that 70% of IVS patients are under one year of age, and that spontaneous regression occurs more commonly in this age group, survival is good even in older children (Figure 5).

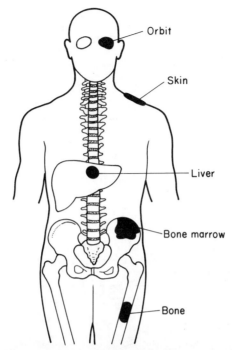

Figure 4. Common sites for metastatic neuroblastoma. Adapted by permission from Souhami, R.L. and Tobias, J.S. (1986) *Cancer and Its Management*, Blackwell Scientific Publications, Oxford

Treatment

The results have been rather disappointing in comparison with those achieved in many other paediatric tumours. Because chemotherapy is less effective, local management is of greater importance. In the minority of children with localized tumour, surgery and/or chemotherapy may be curative.

Chemotherapy is used for the majority of patients who have disseminated disease. Various intensive combinations have been tried and recently studies have tested the effectiveness of high-dose therapy with autologous bone marrow support (neuroblastoma cells in the marrow being 'purged' *in vitro*). Although results have improved they still leave much to be desired.

Wilms' Tumour

Most of these renal tumours occur before the age of 5 years. Results have improved dramatically (Figure 1): 80% of children with localized tumours are cured, as are 50% of those with advanced disease. There are well-recognized associations with a variety of genetic disorders; examples are given in the box.

Table 2. Staging system for neuroblastoma. Reproduced by permission from Evans, A. E. *et al.* (1971) *Cancer*, **27**:374–378

Stage	Anatomical description
I	Tumour confined to organ or structure of origin
II	Tumour extends in continuity beyond the organ or structure of origin, but does not cross the midline. Homolateral regional lymph nodes may be involved. Tumours arising in the midline structure (such as the organ of Zuckerkandl) penetrating beyond the capsule and involving the lymph nodes on the same side should be considered stage II. Bilateral extension should be considered stage III
III	Tumour extends in continuity beyond the midline. Bilateral regional lymph nodes may be involved
IV	Remote disease involving skeleton, parenchymatous organs, soft tissues or distant lymph node groups
IVS	A special category: stage I or II with remote disease confined to one or more of the following sites: liver, skin or bone marrow without radiological evidence of bone metastases on skeletal survey

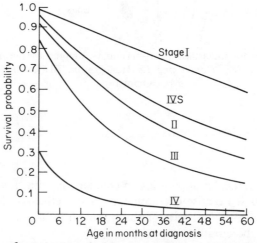

Figure 5. Probability of two-year survival by stage and age at diagnosis. Prognosis worsens with increasing stage, except for the surprisingly good survival rates in patients with stage IVS. Reproduced by permission from Breslow, N. and McCann, B. (1971) *Cancer Research*, **31**: 2098–2103

hemi-hypertrophy
Beckwith-Wiedemann syndrome
aniridia-Wilms' syndrome
hamartoma
genito-urinary malformations

Specific chromosomal defects are being identified and the aniridia-Wilms' syndrome has been associated with deletion of part of the short arm of chromosome 11 and children with other chromosome disorders have been shown to have trisomy 8 or 18 or XX/XY mosaicism. It is thought that a hereditary form of Wilms' tumour accounts for up to 40% of this type of cancer, transmission being autosomal dominant with penetrance of about 60%.

The tumour is thought to arise from the metanephric blastoma and is usually a single growing mass in the renal parenchyma. Up to 10% of patients have bilateral synchronous renal tumours (these are probably the hereditary form); these children are generally younger at presentation and have ten times the incidence of congenital anomalies compared to those with unilateral tumours.

The tumour contains a mixture of epithelial and mesenchymal elements, the neoplasm resembling developing embryonic renal tissue. Different patterns of differentiation of the tissue have been described; they correlate with prognosis and pattern of spread. A highly differentiated tumour, mesoblastic nephroma rarely spreads and is curable with surgery alone.

The commonest mode of presentation is the finding of a painless abdominal mass (80%). This may be large enough to be visible. Other presentations are:

- abdominal pain from the renal capsule (35%)
- fever (25%)
- haematuria (20%)
- symptoms from metastases (lung, liver, lymph nodes, bone or brain)

Assessment includes family history (looking for congenital anomalies), clinical assessment of the size and fixation of the mass, computed tomography or ultrasound, full blood count, biochemistry and urinalysis.

Isotopic bone imaging is useful as metastasis may be asymptomatic. Staging classification is usually that developed by the National Staging Wilms' Tumour Study and is based on the surgical findings (Table 3).

Treatment

As with many childhood cancers the approach is multi-disciplinary. Surgical excision is undertaken in all patients. Care to avoid tumour spillage has been stressed. The tumour bed should be marked with clips. Where there are bilateral tumours, surgery has to be individualized with as much viable normal tissue as possible being left. Radiotherapy is given to the tumour bed in stage II disease and wide field treatment is used for stage III disease and radiotherapy together with extensive surgery for stage IV disease. Postoperative chemotherapy is given to all stages—simple combinations for stage I and increasingly intensive chemotherapy for more extensive disease.

Outcome is closely related to stage and tumour differentiation. Patients with moderate amounts of disease spread (stage I–III) with favourable histology have a 2-year disease-free survival of greater than 90%; even patients with extensive disease of unfavourable histology have 2-year survival of more than 50%.

Table 3. National Wilms' Tumour Study Group Staging System. Reproduced by permission
from D'Angio, G. J., *et al.* (1980) *Cancer*, **45**: 1791–1798

Stage	Description
Stage I	Tumour limited to kidney and completely excised. The surface of the renal capsule is intact. Tumour was not ruptured before or during removal. There is no residual tumour apparent beyond the margins of resection
Stage II	Tumour extends beyond the kidney, but is completely excised. There is regional extension of the tumour, i.e., penetration through the outer surface of the renal capsule into perirenal soft tissues. Vessels outside the kidney substance are infiltrated or contain tumour thrombus. The tumour may have been biopsied or there has been local spillage of tumour confined to the flank. There is no residual tumour apparent at or beyond the margins of excision
Stage III	Residual non-haematogenous tumour confined to abdomen. Any one or more of the following may occur: a. Lymph nodes on biopsy are found to be involved in the hilus, the periaortic chains or beyond b. There has been diffuse peritoneal contamination by tumour such as by spillage of tumour beyond the flank before or during surgery, or by tumour growth that has penetrated through the peritoneal surface c. Implants are found on the peritoneal surfaces d. The tumour extends beyond the surgical margins either microscopically or grossly e. The tumour is not completely resectable because of local infiltration into vital structures
Stage IV	Haematogenous metastases. Deposits beyond stage III, i.e. lung, liver, bone and brain
Stage V	Bilateral renal involvement at diagnosis. An attempt should be made to stage each side according to the above criteria on the basis of extent of disease prior to biopsy

Soft Tissue Sarcomas

Although these tumours only account for about 1% of all malignancies they are more common in children, accounting for 7% of paediatric cancers. The sarcomas found in children (in descending order of frequency) are:

- rhabdomyosarcoma
- liposarcoma
- angiosarcoma
- fibrosarcoma

Because rhabdomyosarcoma is seen so very much more frequently than the others the rest of this section refers specifically to this tumour. The other sarcomas are generally less responsive to chemotherapy and radiotherapy and they are treated in much the same way as adult sarcomas.

The aetiology of this tumour is unknown; there are no known environmental factors associated with it. Congenital malformations are more common in patients with rhabdomyosarcoma than in unaffected children. The incidence by primary sites is shown in Figure 6. The age distribution shows an early peak in the first 5 years of life because of the frequency of head and neck and genito-urinary tumours and a larger peak in the teens due to extremity and male genito-urinary tumours.

The tumour arises from embryonic mesenchyme and shows histological and ultrastructural evidence of varying stages of embryonic muscle differentiation. Electron microscopy and immunocytochemistry are very useful in making the diagnosis. Rhabdomyosarcoma is divided histologically into several subtypes, as shown in the box.

Embryonal—primitive spindle-shaped small cells with elliptical nuclei (63% of childhood rhabdomyosarcoma, of which 6% are botryoides subtype of embryonal)

Alveolar—alveolar architecture with occasional giant cells; usually in older children with extremity lesions (19% of childhood rhabdomyosarcomas)

Pleomorphic—an uncommon subtype, much commoner in adults (1% of childhood rhabdomyosarcomas)

Undifferentiated mesenchymal tumours account for the remainder: most are in extremity or head and neck sites (17% of childhood rhabdomyosarcomas)

These tumours commonly present as a diffuse asymptomatic swelling. Specific presentations by site include:

- Orbit: swelling proptosis, discoloration, reduced eye movement.
- Other head and neck sites: polyps, dysphasia, epistaxis, reduced hearing, persistent 'otitis', 'sinusitis' and 'parotitis', cranial nerve palsies.
- Retroperitoneum: abdominal pain and signs of a mass lesion.
- Genito-urinary: urethral, vaginal, perineal masses, haematuria, urinary frequency/retention.

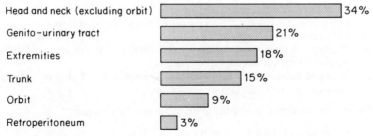

Head and neck (excluding orbit)	34%
Genito-urinary tract	21%
Extremities	18%
Trunk	15%
Orbit	9%
Retroperitoneum	3%

Figure 6. Incidence of rhabdomyosarcoma according to primary site

Diagnostic and staging investigations will of course depend very much on the primary site but will include a full blood count and biochemistry. X-rays of the primary site (computed tomography and/or contrast studies), plus other imaging techniques are used to look for metastatic disease.

Staging uses a simple classification based on resectability, regional spread and the presence of metastases (Table 4).

Treatment

Surgical excision is only possible in one in six cases. With the introduction of more effective chemotherapy, often integrated with radiotherapy, radical surgery has started to play a lesser role. The exact plan of treatment will depend very much on the site of the tumour as well as the extent of spread. Many patients will be treated with surgery (biopsy or resection where possible), followed by radical radiotherapy to the tumour or the site of the resected mass. Combinations of cytotoxic drugs are given after primary treatment to control the local tumour. As can be seen from Figure 7 good survival rates are found for patients with localized disease, but results are much poorer when there is metastatic disease.

Ewing's Sarcoma

This is a highly malignant non-osseous tumour that usually arises in bone, though it is also seen in soft tissues. It is the commonest bone tumour in the first decade of life and is second to osteogenic sarcoma in the teens. Distribution of Ewing's sarcoma according to site and age is shown in Figure 8. Although primarily a childhood sarcoma

Table 4. Intergroup rhabdomyosarcoma study staging system. Reproduced by permission from Mauer, H. M. *et al.* (1981) *Journal of the National Cancer Institute Monograph* **56**: 61–68

Stage grouping	Description
Group I	Localized disease, completely resected. Regional nodes not involved a. Confined to muscle or organ of origin b. Contiguous involvement — infiltration outside the muscle or organ of origin, as through fascial planes; totally resected
Group II	Regional disease a. Grossly resected tumour with microscopic residual disease. No evidence of gross residual tumour. No clinical or microscopic evidence of regional node involvement b. Regional disease, completely resected (regional nodes involved completely resected with no microscopic residual) c. Regional disease with involved nodes, grossly resected, but with evidence of microscopic residual
Group III	Incomplete resection or biopsy with gross residual disease
Group IV	Metastatic disease present at onset

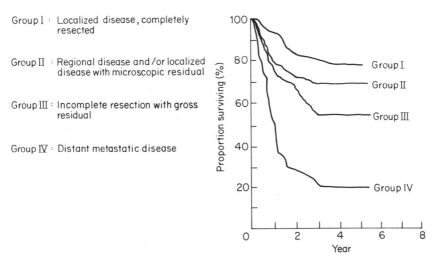

Group I : Localized disease, completely resected

Group II : Regional disease and/or localized disease with microscopic residual

Group III : Incomplete resection with gross residual

Group IV : Distant metastatic disease

Figure 7. Survival of patients with childhood rhabdomyosarcoma by stage grouping. Reproduced by permission from Gehan, I. *et al.* (1980) *Journal of the National Cancer Institute Monograph* **56**: 193–199

it is seen relatively often in the third and fourth decades. The common sites are the femur and pelvis. The diaphyseal region is most commonly affected. It is thought to arise from reticulum cells in the marrow cavity. Histologically the tumour is composed of solidly packed cells of a dimorphic pattern with undifferentiated small and large cells.

The typical presentation (80%) is with localized pain and swelling of the involved bone. Symptoms are often present for some months (mean 9) before diagnosis. A palpable mass is present in 60% of patients. Systemic symptoms (fatigue, weight loss, fever) are common and may lead to an erroneous diagnosis of osteomyelitis.

Investigation consists of radiography of the affected area. The classical appearance is described as 'onion-skin like'—periosteal reaction in the form of periosteal elevation and subperiosteal new bone formation as the tumour extends through the cortex. Biopsy is necessary to establish the diagnosis, but surgical excision is *not* recommended. Other investigations looking for metastatic disease include:

- Isotopic bone imaging.
- Chest X-ray and, if negative, thoracic CT.
- Bone marrow aspiration.
- Full blood count and biochemistry.

There is no staging classification, patients simply being classified as localized or disseminated.

Treatment

Surgery is generally used to establish the diagnosis and radical operations are generally not undertaken. Radiotherapy is used to gain local control since this sarcoma is unusually radiosensitive and the tumour is frequently locally extensive. Large fields of

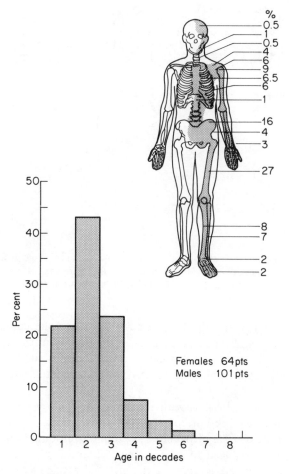

Figure 8. Distribution of Ewing's sarcoma by site of primary disease and by age at onset: 165 patients seen at Mayo Clinic. From Dahlin, D.C. *et al.* (1961) *Journal of Bone and Joint Surgery*, **43A**: 185–192; reproduced by permission

high-dose irradiation are used for primary treatment, in conjunction with combination chemotherapy. Good localized tumour control (Table 5) is gained from this approach though disease-free survival rates are less good—results vary according to the primary site involved.

Osteogenic Sarcoma

This is the commonest of the bone tumours, being derived from bone-forming mesenchyme. The peak age range is 10–25 years, there being a small male excess (1.7:1). The aetiology of this tumour is unknown. Its high incidence in adolescents undergoing rapid bone growth and in adults with Paget's disease of bone suggests that

Table 5. Disease-free survival and local control rates for Ewing's sarcoma. Reproduced by permission from Perez, C. A., *et al.* (1981) *National Cancer Institute Monograph* **56**: 262–271

Site	Local control (%)	Disease-free survival (%)
Pelvis	85	47
Humerus	79	50
Femur	91	56
Tibia	89	59
Fibula	97	62
Ribs	94	56
Skull and spine	100	100
Sacrum	100	29
Ulna, radius, hand	80	80
Feet	75	75

factors associated with increased bone production are important. Its relationship to trauma is unclear.

Most of these tumours start in the diaphysis of bones, lower limbs being more commonly involved. About half are found in the femur, 80% involving the distal end. Other primary sites (in decreasing frequency) are proximal femur, proximal humerus, tibia, pelvis and jaw.

The common presenting features are pain and a palpable mass. Systemic symptoms are uncommon. Diagnostic tests include X-ray of the primary site which characteristically shows bone destruction and periosteal new bone formation. When the tumour spreads through the cortex the formation of new bone spicules produces a so-called 'sun burst' appearance on X-ray. Other staging investigations include chest X-ray and, if normal, thoracic CT imaging. CT may also be useful in delineating the primary. Isotopic bone imaging may reveal metastatic disease elsewhere in the skeleton.

Histologically, osteosarcoma is divided into several subtypes. The diagnosis requires the presence of osteoid tumour cells.

- Classically, the osteoblasts show pleomorphism, hyperchromaticity and bizarre mitosis.
- Juxtacortical or parosteal osteosarcoma is an uncommon variant in which new bone formation is particularly dense. These tumours are generally less malignant in their behaviour.
- Periosteal osteosarcoma is a variety of intermediate malignancy.

There is no formal staging classification.

Treatment

Amputation used to be the standard and only curative therapy. However, many patients (80%) died of metastatic disease. Since the introduction of more effective chemotherapy and radiotherapy the role of surgery is being rethought. Currently, there is, where possible, a trend towards conservative surgery. Following excision of affected bone a prosthesis is placed (usually at the knee joint). Such operations are now done after initial chemotherapy has been given to 'shrink' the primary. Complicated combinations of cytotoxic drugs are used before and after surgery. Radiotherapy is less often used primarily, being reserved for local relapse.

Early uncontrolled studies of the approach of chemotherapy/surgery/chemotherapy showed apparent improvement in survival, a finding which has recently been borne out in two randomized trials.

Selected Papers and Reviews

D'Angio, G. J. and Evans, A. E. (1985) *Bone and Soft Tissue Sarcomas*. Edward Arnold, London.

D'Angio, G. J. *et al.* (1981) The treatment of Wilms' tumour. Results of the second National Wilms' Tumour Study Group. *Cancer*, **47**: 2302–2311.

Knudson, A. G. and Meadows, A. T. (1980) Regression of neuroblastoma IV-S: a genetic hypothesis. *New England Journal of Medicine*, **302**: 1254–1256.

Pinkel, D. (1979) The Ninth Annual David Karnofsky lecture: treatment of acute lymphocytic leukaemia. *Cancer*, **43**: 1128–1137.

Gjerris, F. (1976) Clinical aspects and long term prognosis of intracranial tumours in infancy and childhood. *Dev. Med. Child. Neurol.* **18**: 145–159.

NIH (1985) Consensus developmental panel on limb sparing treatment. *Cancer Treatment Symposia Vol. 3*. National Institutes of Health, Bethesda.

Sutow, W. W., Fernach, D. J. and Wietti, J. J. (eds.) (1984) *Clinical Pediatric Oncology, 3rd Edition*. Mosby, St Louis.

Index

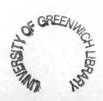